The Bridge between Neurology and Psychiatry

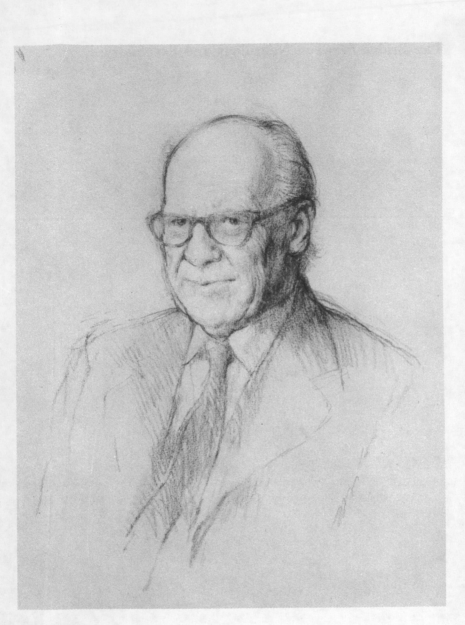

Sir Denis Hill

The Bridge between Neurology and Psychiatry

EDITED BY

E. H. Reynolds MD FRCP FRCPsych
Consultant Neurologist, Bethlem Royal
and Maudsley Hospitals, and King's College Hospital,
London

M. R. Trimble FRCP FRCPsych
Consultant Physician in Psychological Medicine,
National Hospital for Nervous Diseases;
Raymond Way Senior Lecturer in Behavioural Neurology,
Institute of Neurology, London

WITH A FOREWORD BY

Denis Williams CBE MD DSc FRCP
Honorary Consulting Physician, National Hospital for
Nervous Diseases, London, and Royal Air Force

CHURCHILL LIVINGSTONE
EDINBURGH LONDON MELBOURNE AND NEW YORK 1989

CHURCHILL LIVINGSTONE
Medical Division of Longman Group UK Limited

Distributed in the United States of America by
Churchill Livingstone Inc., 1560 Broadway, New
York, N.Y. 10036, and by associated companies,
branches and representatives throughout the world.

© Longman Group UK Limited 1989

First published 1989
  Reprinted 1990
ISBN 0-443-03344-7

British Library Cataloguing in Publication Data
The Bridge between neurology and psychiatry.
  1. Neuropsychiatry
  I. Reynolds, E. H. (Edward Henry)
  II. Trimble, Michael R.
  616.8

Library of Congress Cataloging in Publication Data
The Bridge between neurology and psychiatry/edited
  by E. H. Reynolds, Michael R. Trimble; with a
  foreword by Denis Williams.
        p.   cm.
  Includes index.
    1. Mental illness.   2. Nervous system —
Diseases.
3. Neuropsychiatry.   I. Reynolds, E. H. (Edward
Henry)
II. Trimble, Michael R.
  [DNLM: 1. Mental Disorders.   2. Nervous
System Diseases.
3. Neuropsychology.   WL 103 B8508]
RC455.B738 1989
616.8 — dc 19
DNLM/DLC
for Library of Congress   88-16209
                                           CIP

Produced by Longman Singapore Publishers (Pte) Ltd.
Printed in Singapore

Foreword

If Sir Denis Hill had lived to draft a foreword to this volume of essays upon
'The Bridge between Neurology and Psychiatry', which he had envisaged,
he would have been concise, as I intend to be, but his pen would have been
that of a professed psychiatrist; mine of a professional neurologist. Yet he
might well have written what I now write.

Denis and I first met at the war's end in the National Hospital, Queen
Square, in strangely obverse circumstances. For my war I joined the Royal
Air Force from, and also because of, our infant department of electrophysiology there. Denis, working in London, joined the Emergency Medical
Service which was responsible not only for the whole civilian population
of the United Kingdom, but for most of the Service personnel in it, too.
He was appointed to that unit in the National Hospital. On my demobi-
lisation I came, as the statute ruled, to resume my deserted post. Although
we had been separated by the years of war, we had actually been sailing
parallel courses on the newly charted seas, with the slow and fast waves,
of the EEG in the brain damage of war. Whilst he was working in a
militantly neurological hospital, I was paradoxically engaged with the
psychological disorders of air crew, which indeed became the subject of an
Air Ministry publication.

So 'for the duration', as the phrase was, the psychiatrist turned his hand
to neurology, the neurologist to psychiatry. This was the bridge which
linked me closely to Denis Hill, his work and his interests; and unlike
Arnhem it was not at all a bridge too far.

That rudimentary device, the electroencephalograph, gave each of us not
merely a novel tool to use at the time (and I write of over 40 years ago),
but also a signpost for the future. It encouraged Denis Hill's interest,
through epilepsy and brain damage, along the wide road of British
psychiatry, based as it was upon the pathology of the brain as well as of
the psyche; and Denis Williams away from the straight but narrow pathway
of British neurology, firmly based as it then had to be on morbid anatomy,
but with little evident room for its related psychopathology. The EEG took
Denis Hill with his patient into the laboratory and so into academic work

and thence into administration at increasingly high levels — in which he was so successful, but for which I was not equipped.

I cannot leave this blunt appraisal without reference to our seniors; notably, for each of us, Sir Charles Symonds, who spent his long life striding back and forth over the bridge between neurology and psychiatry. Others have written about Sir Aubrey Lewis and the School at the Maudsley, which Denis Hill inherited. It is interesting historically that whilst Symonds fittingly was the civil consultant in neuropsychiatry to the Royal Air Force, Lewis, on R. D. Gillespie's death, became consultant in psychiatry only. Symonds learnt his psychopathology from the great Adolph Meyer, whilst a generation later Lewis his neuropathology from that equally great neuropathologist Alfred Meyer.

So the pages turn from Hill to the present generation of medical scientists who have made their contribution here. This intellectually handsome volume of dedication says more, and leaves much more unsaid, about Denis Hill's place on the bridge between neurology and psychiatry than the notices could have at the time of his death. For me to write more would be presumptuous tautology. The quality of the essays speaks for us all. It is happy symbolism that one of the two physicians who initiated and edited the volume is a psychiatrist in the Institute of Neurology, the other a neurologist in the Institute of Psychiatry, of London University.

The two disciplines divided very recently as part of the fragmentation of medicine, itself inevitable when the growth of medicine transcended the understanding of one physician and the skills of any one group. Let us keep perspective though and remind ourselves that the bridge between neurology and psychiatry is the oldest bridge in medicine. The name of the bridge *is* medicine, the care of body and mind, or more properly of body *with* mind, traced backwards through all history in writings and practice; its practitioners have had many names — doctors, priests, medicine men. Call us what you will, the divisive words mislead; none more so than 'bridge' and none more evident than here; but there are, in truth, as many of those bridges as there are skills in medicine, and every one of those bridges spans the whole length of medicine — and its breadth too.

This, our chosen path — or is it a high road? — of medicine is what this volume, dedicated to the work of the late Professor Sir Denis Hill really forces us to see — that our work on this ancient bridge is just a very short step on the long devious road of medicine. Whether we are employed as neurologists or psychiatrists, we are all physicians. The bridge we are engaged upon here, with the memories of Denis Hill, may seem to the short-sighted to create a barrier. He sees on one side the body and on the other, the mind, for it strides the hyphen in brain-mind. Let us get on with our work on the bridge, leaving that unprofitable dispute to others.

London, 1989   Denis Williams

Preface

This book arose from our mutual conviction that the divergence of
neurology and psychiatry has gone too far. It is undeniable that there is a
large common ground, interface, or in Sir Denis Hill's term, 'bridge',
between neurology and psychiatry. Both neurologists and psychiatrists are
interested in cerebral function and disease. Both bring to these problems
similar techniques of observation and measurement but different perspectives based on traditional differences in interest and approach, the former
more often concerned with mechanism, the latter with motivation and
meaning. In the UK, the gulf between neurology and psychiatry has been
greater than in most other countries. There has been little communication
between the two disciplines despite the recent obvious growth in their
common ground. This book is an attempt to reverse this trend.

We have, therefore, brought together British neurologists and psychiatrists,
and an American neurologist closely associated with British neurology
and psychiatry, to explore the bridge between neurology and psychiatry.
We must emphasise that this is not a textbook of neurology and psychiatry;
nor is it a treatise on mind-brain relationships. It is a series of essays
exploring the common ground of neurologists and psychiatrists as viewed
from one or other end of the bridge.

Although neuropsychiatry has always been to some extent a bridge
between the two disciplines, in the first half of this century the domination
of dynamic psychiatry, together with the steady progress of scientific
neurology, contributed to the progressive separation and isolation of
neurology and psychiatry from each other (Chapter 5), encouraged also
perhaps by differences in the personalities of neurologists and psychiatrists
(Chapter 4). The latter half of this century has seen a remarkable growth
in the application of the neurosciences to psychiatric disorders (Chapters
12–15) and to functions of the nervous systems of common interest to
neurologists and psychiatrists, such as consciousness (Chapter 6), sleep
(Chapter 7), speech (Chapter 8), body image (Chapter 9), memory (Chapter
10), and movement (Chapter 11). At the same time, the study of epilepsy
(Chapters 16–20) has continued, as in the past, to illuminate both neurology

and psychiatry. Scientific fields of common interest to both disciplines that that are represented here include neuropsychopharmacology (Chapter 21), genetics (Chapter 22), and neurotransmitter function (Chapter 23). As Denis Hill saw in 1964 (Chapter 3), this bridge or common ground is expanding, as evidenced by the growth of such fields as organic psychiatry, biological psychiatry, behavioural neurology and neuropsychology, of interest to practitioners of both neurology and psychiatry. Psychiatrists have rediscovered the wisdom of the great nineteenth century neurologists and, assisted by modern imaging techniques, have renewed their interest in brain pathology and localisation of function in the nervous system, just at the same time as neurologists are beginning to perceive the enormous complexity of nervous system function and the influence of psychological and social factors on brain function and, therefore, on neurological disease (Chapter 5).

The title of this book is taken from Sir Denis Hill's 1964 address, reproduced in Chapter 3. Shortly before his untimely death, we discussed with Sir Denis our plans for this book. He gave it his enthusiastic support and offered very useful and constructive advice, as well as his essay on states of consciousness (Chapter 6). Others in this volume have described Sir Denis's great contribution to British psychiatry (Chapters 1 & 2). However, this book celebrates his wider view of the bridge between neurology and psychiatry, as illustrated by his two contributions reproduced here and by the establishment of an academic department of neurology at the Institute of Psychiatry during his stewardship. We hope and believe this book is a fitting memorial to him and that it will bring the two disciplines of neurology and psychiatry into closer communion in a common cause, as he would have wished.

London, 1989

E. H. R.
M. R. T.

Contributors

D. Frank Benson MD
Augustus S. Rose Professor of Neurology, UCLA School of Medicine, Los Angeles, California

R. H. Cawley PhD FRCP FRCPsych
Joint Professor of Psychological Medicine, King's College School of Medicine and Dentistry, and Institute of Psychiatry, London

A. H. Crisp MD DSc FRCP FRCP(E) FRCPsych
Professor of Psychiatry, University of London at St George's Hospital Medical School, London

John Cutting MD MPhil MRCP MRCPsych
Consultant Psychiatrist, Bethlem Royal Hospital, Beckenham, Kent

George W. Fenton MB FRCPsych FRCP(E)
Professor of Psychiatry, University of Dundee, Ninewells Hospital and Medical School, Dundee

Peter Fenwick DPM FRCPsych
Consultant Neuropsychiatrist, The Maudsley Hospital; Consultant Clinical Neurophysiologist, St Thomas's Hospital; Senior Lecturer, Institute of Psychiatry, London

Denis Hill MB BS FRCP FRCPsych
Late Emeritus Professor of Psychiatry, Institute of Psychiatry, London

W. A. Lishman MD DSc FRCP FRCPsych
Professor of Neuropsychiatry, Institute of Psychiatry; Honorary Consultant Psychiatrist, The Maudsley Hospital, London

C. David Marsden DSc FRCP FRS
Head, University Department of Clinical Neurology, Institute of Neurology, National Hospital, London

Robin M. Murray MD MPhil FRCP FRCPsych
Dean, Institute of Psychiatry, London; Honorary Consultant Psychiatrist, Bethlem Royal Hospital, Beckenham, Kent

M. J. Owen PhD MRCPsych
MRC Research Fellow, Department of Biochemistry and Molecular Genetics, St Mary's Hospital Medical School; Honorary Lecturer, Institute of Psychiatry; Honorary Senior Registrar, Maudsley Hospital, London

John Oxbury PhD FRCP
Consultant Neurologist to Oxfordshire and Oxford Regional Health Authorities; Clinical Lecturer in Neurology, University of Oxford

S. Oxbury MA
Principal Clinical Psychologist, Department of Neurology, Radcliffe Infirmary, Oxford

Michael A. Reveley PhD MD MRCPsych
Senior Lecturer and Consultant in Psychiatry, London Hospital Medical College; Honorary
Senior Lecturer in Psychiatry, Institute of Psychiatry, London

E. H. Reynolds MD FRCP FRCPsych
Consultant Neurologist, Bethlem Royal and Maudsley Hospitals, and King's College
Hospital, London

M. Rossor MA MD MRCP
Consultant Neurologist, National Hospital and St Mary's Hospital, London

Martin Roth MD ScD FRCP FRCPsych FRCP&S(Glas)
Fellow, Trinity (Cantab & Lond) College Cambridge, Professor Emeritus of Psychiatry,
University of Cambridge

Brian Kenneth Toone MPhil MRCPsych MRCP
Consultant Psychiatrist, King's College Hospital; Honorary Consultant Psychiatrist,
Maudsley Hospital; Honorary Senior Lecturer, Institute of Psychiatry, London

Michael R. Trimble FRCP FRCPsych
Consultant Physician in Psychological Medicine, National Hospital; Raymond Way Senior
Lecturer in Behavioural Neurology, Institute of Neurology, London

Stephen A. Whatley PhD
Lecturer in Molecular Neurobiology, Institute of Psychiatry, London

Contents

Sir Denis Hill

Denis Hill was born in Herefordshire, and his boyhood years were shared between Shrewsbury School and the still remoteness of the countryside, where he had few companions of his own age. His early interests in natural history soon matured into curiosity about biological processes and theories, and became balanced by a fascination with radio, valves, electronics and associated gadgetry. Dependent upon his own resources, as he grew up he became increasingly aware of the uniqueness of the individual and the rich complexity and pre-eminence of personal inner experience. He was much influenced by reading Freud's *Collected Works*, given to him on his 21st birthday, Jung's lectures, and other literature of psychoanalysis. And so, long before he qualified in medicine, the foundations were laid for his parallel interests in biological processes and in the adaptations and subjective experiences of the individual — the dual approaches of mechanism and meaning — which provided impetus to so much of his work and his thinking and stayed with him throughout his life.

At Maida Vale Hospital in 1937–38 he came under the influence of Grey Walter, then occupied with the electroencephalogram as an exciting new device for measuring the electrical activity of the brain, capable even of locating cerebral tumours. Denis Hill was intrigued by this technology, both for its own sake and for what he saw as its potential for psychiatry. Meantime he continued his psychiatric training, having started at the Bethlem Royal Hospital and later moving on to St Thomas's. When the war came, he was appointed to develop an EEG department at Belmont Hospital, where some members of the Maudsley staff were exiled. At first he worked with a home-made two-channel EEG with a smoked drum kymograph, but after some months a new, purpose-built, machine arrived from America. During his years at Belmont, he saw a great many patients with epilepsy and a great many with personality disorders. From the latter group he was able to put forward his hypothesis linking psychopathic behaviour with immature slow-wave patterns in the EEG.

After the war, his reputation in the EEG field well established, Denis Hill spent two years in charge of the EEG department at the National Hospital Queen Square, and in 1947 was appointed Senior Lecturer in charge of the

Department of Clinical Neurophysiology at the Institute of Psychiatry. There he stayed for 14 years and during this time achieved world renown for his work in electroencephalography, its bearing on the elucidation of the pathological mechanisms of epilepsy, and its applications to psychiatry. Particularly notable during those years was his work with Alfred Meyer and Murray Falconer on temporal lobe epilepsy and its pathology and treatment, and his report with Desmond Pond on a series of 100 murderers, reviewing studies in relation to alleged abnormal states of consciousness in which the crime was committed. This investigation had much impact on criminological debate and practice at the time and laid the basis for Denis Hill's growing reputation in the field of forensic psychiatry.

At the Maudsley during those years his teaching conveyed his endless fascination with the antinomies between mind and brain. His unit recognised this concern in its targets, which were the management of epilepsy associated with behaviour disorders and emotional problems, and in its methods, which emphasised the importance of intrapersonal processes and interpersonal communication between patients and staff. Ward 2 at the Maudsley was, in advance of its time, a therapeutic community taking patients of all ages and both sexes. Not surprisingly, Denis was an admired figure among Maudsley registrars. Moreover, he had been a founding trustee of the Institute of Psychiatry and was active on the academic board and committee of management. Despite this involvement, the mainstream activities of those who shaped the policies of the Maudsley at the time seemed to pass him by. He was not conspicuous among the leaders of the tribe; his role was that of a clinician and clinical scientist practising his own special interests with distinction.

The pattern of his career at this time was balanced by strong interests in the world outside the Maudsley, where his influence was growing. He was the physician in charge of psychological medicine at King's College Hospital, in which he was vigorous in providing a clinical service in all aspects of psychiatry, especially those appropriate to a general hospital, and it was there that his inspiration and success as a teacher of medical students became so well known, and is remembered to this day. And in the wider world he was becoming recognised as a determined fighter for his subject. His strengths as a committee man, so notable in the second half of his life, were coming to the fore. As a member of the Medical Research Council he carried out enquiries into the status of psychiatric teaching and research in Britain and came out with some disquieting results. In the London undergraduate teaching hospitals, there was no research in the subject, the teaching to medical students was inadequate by the most modest standards, and there was no reference to psychiatry in the final examinations. As a result of these findings, the University Grants Committee sought rapidly to establish the principle that each school of medicine should have its own academic department of psychiatry. Soon after this, in 1961, he was appointed to the newly established Chair of Psychiatry at the Middlesex

Hospital Medical School. This move brought an end to his first Maudsley period and his association with King's College Hospital.

Arthur Crisp (Ch. 2) has written compellingly about Denis Hill's achievement during his five years at the Middlesex. It was a hugely successful department. Psychiatry had entered a period of unprecedented growth and change. Hitherto, its main focus had been on the big mental hospitals, whose medical superintendents had exercised total power over their colleagues and the profession in general. In this country, certainly in London, only the Maudsley had adopted a disciplined approach to psychiatry's conceptual problems and sought for the scientific foundations of the subject. The rigorous study of aetiology, natural history and psychopathology, and a command of the clinical methods apt for the subject, were the Maudsley's raison d'être. It was a centre of excellence for exceptional standards of clinical practice and for postgraduate teaching and research. It was as a result of what had been happening at the Maudsley that the tides were beginning to turn against those who misguidedly believed that a sceptical outlook was of necessity clinically void, leading only to a pessimistic, indeed nihilistic, approach.

But now, as far as academic psychiatry was concerned, the hegemony of the Maudsley was over. Psychiatry was becoming more widely recognised as a medical discipline with its own body of knowledge and rigorous procedures for clinical practice and advancement. And Denis Hill was one of those whose destiny had been to make it so.

But even if the Maudsley was no longer supreme, its power and influence on both a national and international scale were advancing apace. Over years of distinguished leadership of the Institute of Psychiatry, Sir Aubrey Lewis had increased and diversified the scientific approaches to the teaching and practice of the subject and, in keeping with his achievements and further plans, the Institute was growing rapidly. By 1966, the year of Lewis's retirement, the Institute contained four academic departments in addition to psychiatry. The Department of Psychiatry itself had an academic staff numbering over 40, 11 of them occupying senior posts. Every year it contributed massively to the psychiatric literature. Over 150 postgraduate students, from all corners of the world, were in regular attendance. It was a magnificent department.

Among students of people and events in the medical academic world, few can have doubted that Denis Hill would be sought after as Aubrey Lewis's successor. He was an energetic and ambitious man with a sense of destiny. His impact in teaching and in advancing the cause of psychiatry as a uniquely placed medical discipline had already been great. He was by nature an enthusiast, but he had never lost sight of the fact that enthusiasm is potent only if tempered by scepticism and a regard for consistency and truth. He had the confidence, seemingly, of everybody in the world. The Chair at the Institute was the premier chair. The man and the opportunity seemed well matched.

Over the ensuing 13 years, Denis Hill built steadily and with imagination on the foundations laid by Aubrey Lewis. He was responsible for a great many new developments. On his appointment the Institute moved into a brand new home — another part of his predecessor's legacy. Soon, thanks to Denis Hill's efforts, funds were available for extending this, providing the East Wing and the Neurology building. The Department of Psychiatry grew in its size and in its contribution to research. The programme of education and training for Maudsley registrars was revised and extended, with new developments in forensic psychiatry, neuropsychiatry, psychotherapy and social psychiatry. Links with undergraduate teaching hospitals were forged by the establishment of rotational senior registrar posts. Hill's policy of encouraging the growth of a range of specialist interests in his department and, at the right stage, allowing a budding off of new departments or sections, had led to the establishment of independent departments of child and adolescent psychiatry, neurology and pharmacology. Returning to his old affinities with King's College Hospital and Medical School, Hill worked hard to promote the establishment of a joint Chair in Psychological Medicine and thus opened the way for Maudsley trainees to gain experience of general hospital psychiatry and medical student teaching.

It was a difficult post and it demanded very hard work, huge commitment and great resources of energy, wisdom and diplomacy. The large numbers of ambitious men and women over whom he presided were as copious in their demands as in the promise of their achievements. Their inevitable searching for personal research opportunities, facilities and funds laid heavy responsibility on the department's head. There was no-one whose specific and acknowledged job it was to provide him with continuing help in his task of viewing the balance of interests within the department, between this and other departments in the Institute, and between the Institute and other organisations competing for recognition and money. Moreover the Institute and Bethlem/Maudsley were under threat, for the idea of 'centres of excellence' was becoming distinctly unpopular in some official circles. Denis was a vigorous defender of the continuing need for a postgraduate university hospital and multidepartmental institute for the teaching and advancement of psychiatry. He contributed in large measure to the survival and indeed expansion of the place.

In these years at the Institute it was understandable that the head of the Department of Psychiatry should feel some sense of isolation. In his earlier roles — both as a clinical research worker and as a head of a medical school department — Hill had been the leader of united and coherent teams working on well-defined enterprises in which the pioneer spirit was ever-present, success was undisputed, and the rewards plain for all to see. Now, in a post unsustained by close professional companionship, he was exposed to the perils faced by all who fight in isolation — the inevitability of self doubt, and the lack of the contentment which comes from the certainty of achievement. Sometimes his position offered little in the way of assurance that particular tasks were either complete or well accomplished. He was not insensitive to matters in which he considered he had not been wholly successful: and as a man who could be hurt he was sensitive to the hurts of others. Peace of mind came less easily, perhaps, than in earlier days. But his leadership and commitment were confident and he supplied them with perceptiveness, imagination, good humour and a shrewd appraisal of what was right for his department and Institute. On all necessary criteria the man was indeed suited to the post. The extent of the innovation in the department was really remarkable. The diversification of the department's territory and interests — in clinical work, teaching and research — was plain for all to see. It had started as a large department and by the time of Denis Hill's retirement it had become very much larger. There were now professors of addiction behaviour, epidemiological psychiatry, experimental psychopathology, forensic psychiatry, neuropsychiatry, neuropsychology, psychological medicine and social psychiatry, together with 22 senior lecturers, a number of lecturers and a band of powerful and articulate research workers — a total staff approaching 200. The enhanced survival, and indeed expansion, of psychiatry and related disciplines in the Institute as a whole was evident to all. There is every reason to conclude that in this stage of his career he reached his ultimate success.

Two things saddened him. At an early stage he had to recognise that the demands of his job, together with his outside commitments, were not consistent with continuing personal clinical responsibility. This restriction was made bearable because he never lost his role as a teacher, in which his zest, his expository skills and his gifts for empathy ensured, to his great satisfaction, that he remained closely in touch with day-to-day clinical problems. In this part of his teaching he was able to deliver elegantly reasoned and balanced clinical assessments, as a result of which he was consistently in demand as a second opinion. Another cause for regret was that he had insufficient time to devote to the personal creative work which, in view of his fascination with ways of advancing our grasp of mind-body relationships, he valued so greatly. His life-long interests in the contrasts and parallels between biological processes and personal inner experience continued to tax him. His Ernest Jones lecture (1970) on *The contributions of psychoanalysis to psychiatry: mechanism and meaning* provided a definitive statement of his professional and intellectual standpoint. It was masterly in its informed, thoughtful and imaginative treatment of a topic which, though so plainly central to psychiatry, has eluded clear definition and caused the expenditure of so much heat with the production of so little light. On this topic Denis Hill said in his lecture at least the beginnings of the important things he had to say. Many who knew him suspect that, when he died, he was working on further salient contributions to this debate.

In the wider world outside the Institute, the list of Denis Hill's achievements is imposing. Conspicuous were his contributions to forensic psychiatry — its theory, its empirical base, the framework within which it operates, and its opportunities and interests in providing a bridge between psychiatry and the law. Building on the interest generated by his earlier clinical experience and research, he was a member of official working parties on special hospitals (1959–61) and on the organisation of the prison medical service (1964). In the second of these he and others strongly favoured the Prison Medical Service becoming part of the National Health Service, an objective which remains at the forefront of discussion in forensic psychiatry. In 1972 he was a member of the Aarvold Committee whose brief was to consider criteria for release from special hospitals of dangerous persons. He was also influential on the Butler Committee on Mentally Abnormal Offenders, which did so much to remedy the isolation of the special hospitals and lay the foundations for an integrated and comprehensive service for treatment and rehabilitation of mentally disordered people who clash with the law. His contributions to forensic psychiatry have been fittingly commemorated since 1985, when the new Regional Secure Unit at the Bethlem Royal Hospital was named after him.

Notable too was Denis Hill's long service to the General Medical Council (1961–82). Over the years he served on all its major committees: for a time he was acting president of the council. As chairman of the special committee on mental health he set the scene for the present arrangements whereby the Health Committee deals with the problems of the sick doctor. This work provided yet another opportunity for him to combine his talents and knowledge in diverse fields with his imagination, perceptiveness, fair-mindedness and unfailing compassion.

Denis's professional achievements at so many different levels — as clinical psychiatrist, clinical researcher, teacher, educator, administrator and leader of medical opinion — were staggering. No less impressive were his personal qualities of warmth. humour and generosity of spirit. He carried with him a sense of occasion which made him a most agreeable companion and a much loved man.

Sir Denis Hill at the Middlesex

I first came into contact with Denis Hill in 1960 when, with two and a half years training in psychiatry and a DPM recently acquired, I was uncertain as to whether I wished to stay in the field. I had left neurology and neurosurgery for the seemingly more interesting arena of psychiatry and had received a sound classical clinical training from exceptionally able teachers, who were also excellent diagnostic clinicians and who cared deeply and genuinely for their patients, and yet I was slightly dissatisfied. I had not been able to discern many of the links between human nature and the constitutional aspects of many of the illnesses now confronting me and for which I sought. Nor had I developed substantial psychotherapy skills. Then I applied for a senior registrar job with Denis Hill at King's College Hospital, the post having been drawn to my attention at the last moment by someone who closely understood my interests. I had had the inestimable luck to refer a patient to him just a few weeks before at the request of my consultant. The patient had complicated complaints suggestive of either primary psychological illness or possible brain stem and diencephalic organic brain disease. I had laboured to produce a balanced referral letter and, drawing on my neurosurgical experience, postulated the existence of a rather amazing and meandering angiomatous malformation as the only possible basis for an organic contribution. Fortunately, I had also done justice to the potential primacy of the patient's psychopathology, not least because this ultimately proved to be the basis of the disorder!

To begin this article in honour of the memory of Denis Hill by referring to the above episode is intended only to help to make sense of my subsequent relationship to this exceptional man. His knowledge of the brain and mind was profound and it was of a kind that enabled him to develop his own thinking and stimulate that of others throughout his life. I learned much from him week by week (and continued to learn from him until the time of his death). At King's College Hospital at that time he walked the corridors as a respected senior physician. He was a world authority on epilepsy and especially on temporal lobe epilepsy. His book on electroencephalography was pre-eminent in the United Kingdom and well known throughout the world. Although he had earlier done a significant amount of systematic research, his interest lay in synthesis and communication of ideas. His notion that induced epilepsy for the treatment of depression worked through the mechanism of restoring the individual's capacity for denial was elegantly argued along both psychodynamic and psychophysiological lines. He always pondered on the nature of epilepsy. A 19th century man, in the sense of being a shrewd observer and reader and a teleologist, he believed that its widespread existence within the developed central nervous system reflected an inherent subclinical homeostatic role. He collected and carefully documented a series of patients with temporal lobe epilepsy whom others were subsequently to write up, and in this patient group he noted the alternation between periods of depression and bouts of epilepsy, regarding the two as dynamically related to each other, again whether construed in psychodynamic or neurophysiological terms. As the new senior registrar I slotted immediately into the clinical liaison service that he had established throughout the hospital. Deeply interested in human aggression and its role in human destiny and human nature he taught me how to recognise its existence lurking beneath the surface in so much human psychopathology and underlying both 'somatic' and 'psychiatric' disorders. His Saturday morning clinical demonstrations to medical students at this time were formidable, even for a senior registrar, in terms of the standards he set, and a great source of pleasure because they were so enthusiastically received by the students. He had already attracted excellent medical psychotherapists to his department and all junior doctors and other staff were well supervised in their psychotherapy training.

Then, within a year, he accepted the offer of the Chair in Psychiatry at the Middlesex Hospital Medical School. He had been for some years the active leader of a group committed to establishing psychiatry in the medical undergraduate curriculum and had persuaded the University Grants Committee of the importance of such a development. It was no coincidence, therefore, when he took the Chair on the basis of the strong support offered by the Dean of the day, Sir Brian Wyndeyer. My own dismay at his imminent departure from King's turned to relief when he indicated that he hoped I would apply for the lecturer post in the new department. Within a few months the department was established with John Hinton as senior lecturer and myself as lecturer in psychiatry, Victor Meyer as senior lecturer and Miller Mair as lecturer in clinical psychology. Under his direction, the development of undergraduate training within the Department of Psychiatry was revolutionary. From the outset he was quite emphatic that our task was to enable undergraduates to become doctors with a sound understanding of social and psychological aspects of medical practice. The students came to psychiatry itself for a full three months and during this period they had a great deal of general teaching concerned with human psychopathology and the further development of interview skills, as well as learning their mainstream psychiatry. The clinical and research interests of the members of the department inevitably centred on psychosomatic processes. For instance, John Hinton had just completed his definitive study on psychological aspects of dying people and had also developed a motility bed for the study of sleep, whilst Denis Hill continued to write about his idea of 'the depressive position', which proved to be the forerunner of much of the best psychobiological thinking about depressive disorders. In clinical psychology at that time there were great developments in behaviour therapy and personal construct theory and both these flowered within the new department. His other contribution was to develop psychotherapy and to this end he secured, over the course of time, university sessions at senior lecturer level and spread these over several part-time appointments. Over the years that he remained at the Middlesex these appointees included John Klauber, Eugene Wolf, Heinz Wolff, Joseph Sandler and Walter Joffe. His hope that this level of inspiration might bear fruit in terms of research was not to be fulfilled. Even the most able psychotherapists resolutely refused to submit their skills to such base scrutiny! But the increased breadth of clinical wisdom which they brought was outstanding and, both directly and indirectly, inspirational to the education of undergraduates and the practice and research of postgraduates. Margaret Bailey came as senior social worker and later Oscar Hill and Raymond Levy were to come as senior lecturers. I know that Denis Hill regarded these years as the happiest period of his career.

He always regarded psychotherapy as an important clinical skill. Pilloried by many on this account, he simply insisted that it was logical to believe that one individual could sometimes bring about important change in another through the medium of their relationship. The world worked on this basis. The task for psychiatry and medicine was to identify the mechanisms at work and optimise and harness them for the purposes of symptom relief and, occasionally, personal growth. Furthermore, to people practising psychotherapy with relatively high levels of skill, such as was by now the case at the Middlesex, its effectiveness was self-evident. He realised what an invasive process it could be, infinitely more so than the usually reversible effects of medication, and he understood and tolerated the anger and resistance of others to his views.

The holistic approach that he achieved through structuring the department in this way influenced the medical students in particular. For him and hence for them, psychiatric illness became one more illustration of the psychosomatic process become pathological. The potential dissonance that always existed for the medical student between his acceptance of the psychiatric and the medical orientation, wherein the former then usually loses out, did not exist. This process was facilitated by the students' regular contact with the psychiatrists within the liaison service, which was now modelled on the Rochester system of specific attachments to medical, surgical, obstetric firms, etc. Two of my own working days each week (including a Saturday morning) were taken up with such work since psychiatrists were expected to undertake joint ward rounds with physicians and others and explain themselves within the testing circumstances of busy medical and surgical wards with medical students present.

Within a year or so psychiatry had an important stake in the new introductory course in clinical method, teaching elementary interview skills but already requiring the student to recognise the need to understand himself and his impact on the transaction. A few months after this a major behavioural sciences course had become established within the preclinical curriculum organised by the department and with teaching from all its members, much of it designed to demonstrate the clinical relevance of the subject matter.

The first two senior house officers appointed to the new department had been Peter Mellett and Sidney Crown, both Middlesex graduates and the forerunners of many junior doctors appointed to the department, often Middlesex graduates, who have gone on to distinguished careers. Many other Middlesex graduates at that time also paradoxically opted for careers in psychiatry.

By this time Denis Hill was heavily involved in national medical affairs. His advice was much sought after by government and his knighthood was imminent. He became a respected senior member of the General Medical Council. Subsequently he was to play a crucial role in rewriting its constitution in respect of the handling of sick doctors. He shunned several high offices within the profession that were his for the taking despite much encouragement. Modest and shy, he usually preferred to work behind the scenes. He was remarkably shrewd and generous with friendship, ideas and support. He fought for recognition of psychiatry within the Royal College of Physicians rather than that it should develop a separate Royal College but, sadly, and for many well-known reasons, that ultimately was not to be. In 1966 the Middlesex Hospital Medical School lost him to the Institute of Psychiatry, but his impact on those who came into contact with him during the six years he spent at the Middlesex was such that it may not fade.

3

The bridge between neurology and psychiatry*

Neurology and psychiatry are specialties within the main corpus of medicine, and it may be asked what makes a specialty. Specialisation comes about as a result of four processes which proceed together but at unequal rates, so that one may appear to develop before another.

There is first the intense and prolonged observation by a few outstanding individuals of the part-functions of individual patients. For neurology and psychiatry this occurred in the early and middle 19th century. This stage can be called the stage of syndrome recognition.

The next process is the utilisation of knowledge, derived perhaps from branches of science quite alien to medicine, to develop techniques, either for more accurate observation, e.g. the stethoscope, or for bringing measurement of the altered function which observation has revealed. The early neurologists were outstanding observers and the instruments they used were, at the start, simple. For psychiatry the problem of measurement has always been very difficult and still is. Psychiatrists have always had to rely upon their eyes and ears. The recognition of inherent biological differences between men, which so preoccupied Francis Galton, led to the application later of statistical methods to study those differences and led ultimately to the appearance of a new subject, clinical psychology. But order out of the chaos of syndrome-medicine in psychiatry was achieved by intense and prolonged observation alone, and notably by Kraepelin, who separated the two large groups of functional mental disorders, the manic-depressive disorders from dementia praecox.

The third process in the development of a specialty is the appearance of new knowledge specifically concerned with normal and abnormal functions of the system concerned. At this point a high degree of sophistication begins to appear and the sources of knowledge become diverse. The function of the specialist is to put them together: to collate facts from different sources in a meaningful way, so that abnormal function can be understood,

---

* Address at Birmingham on October 25, 1963, on the occasion of the 50th anniversary of the foundation of the Birmingham Nerve Hospital. Reprinted from *The Lancet*, March 7 1964.

aetiology of disease explained, and logical treatment sought for. This is the fourth process.

PSYCHIATRY WITHOUT DOCTORS

It is often pointed out that psychiatry is a far older subject than neurology. For centuries men had been concerned about, thought about, and wrote about madness, and the insane had been recognised for what they were and treated one way or another ever since the time of Ancient Greece. Neurology as a specialty developing out of general medicine began to appear at the beginning of the 19th century, and by this is meant that it did so as a scientific discipline. The application of scientific knowledge and principles to psychiatry came nearly a century later. Those who thought and wrote about the mind and its disorders during the three preceding centuries had not usually been doctors at all. In fact medical men, with a few notable exceptions, had little interest in what we now call psychiatry. This activity was carried on by scholars and philosophers.

During the medieval period, and even into the 18th century, the pathology of humours based on the Hippocratic dogma dominated medicine. With the development of science medicine began to escape from this intellectual imprisonment after the Renaissance. There was no great difficulty in replacing a pathology based upon imaginative ideas about the functions of the heart, liver, and spleen with one based upon the observed facts of morbid anatomy and pathology and supported by the great new discoveries about the circulation of the blood. Once it became clear that the sensorium lay not in the heart but in the brain, from which muscular activity originated and in which the senses were perceived, the development of neurology as a science became inevitable. But for psychiatry the matter was different. Side by side with the Hippocratic humoral theory which saw melancholy, for example, as a liver disturbance of black bile, there existed another ideology which ascribed mental illness to demon possession. The insane were regarded with loathing and fear. The origins of mental disorder were considered to be due to witchcraft, evil, and the loss of the patients' souls to the devil. In this the Church took a leading role, and it was held by most that the identification and treatment of the insane were not matters for the laity or for the medical profession, but were the sacred duty of the Church itself to carry out. Hundreds of thousands of insane persons were burnt to death in the towns of Europe over several centuries. Theological experts and professors gave their attention to these matters.

At the end of the 15th century the textbook of the Inquisition, the *Malleus Mallificarum*, or Hammer of the Witches, was published by Papal Decree. It went through 10 editions before 1669 and through 9 more before a century had passed. It was translated into a modern language in the 20th century, and an English translation appeared in 1928. The last witch executed in Germany was a woman decapitated in Bavaria in 1775, in Switzerland another woman in 1782. Torture, beating, and ducking continued, of course, for longer. Ducking was still used both in this country and in America hardly more than a century ago. Indeed the idea that the neurotic and mentally ill are in some way evil, bad, or weak persists even today, and the age-old conception of punishment for them is one from which we have only escaped with the greatest difficulty. Pierre Janet, the great French psychopathologist, looked upon hysteria as a result of 'degeneracy' and an essential psychic weakness. Sigmund Freud, more than anyone else, freed the 'witch' from the odium which surrounded her (Zilboorg 1941).

In the climate of opinion regarding the mentally ill it is therefore not surprising that medical men and the scientists who were helping them had little interest in their problems. Indeed, in the 16th and 17th centuries it was dangerous for them to involve themselves. On the other hand, scholars and philosophers could argue about the mind and reflect upon the nature of mental disorder with relative impunity, and things were easier in England after the Reformation.

PHYSICIANS AND PHILOSOPHERS

Occasionally an outstanding physician made a contribution, but he did so in a manner which we would now call 'double-think'. Thomas Willis (1621–75), the neuroanatomist, styled 'the first inventor of the nervous system' and who is remembered for the circle of arterial anastomoses at the base of the brain, tried to localise nervous diseases by correlating clinical signs with postmortem examination of the brain. He was the first to use the term 'Neurologie', but he also turned his attention to what he called 'Psychology', which was the study of the 'nature and essence, the parts, powers and affections of the corporeal soul or mind'. He became convinced that the uterus did not cause hysteria, nor that the humoral pathology was responsible for mental illness. He placed his pathology squarely upon the 'Brain and the Nervous Stock' (Hunter & Macalpine 1963). Yet we learn that his treatment of a young mentally disturbed girl was to order that 'in the middle of the night she should be carried by women forth of doors and put into a boat, and her clothes being pulled off, and she tied fast with a cord, should be drenched into the depth of the river' — but with the caution that 'she might not be stifled in the water'.

Whatever they might do in practice if confronted with the mentally sick, the scientist and the physician had become aware that only careful observation and the painstaking collection of facts would unravel the problem of the nature of man. If, for social and ethical reasons, medical men were prevented from looking at psychiatric cases in this way, there were no obstacles to the thinkers and scholars who did not have to dirty their hands. Almost to the end of the last century, a chapter of history concluded by William James, the development of ideas about psychological functions was in the hands of philosophers. Nevertheless one such man, possibly a genius, suggested where the studies which would unravel psychiatric problems should go, and in the main history has proved him right.

Francis Bacon (1561–1626) was a philosopher, and happened to become Lord Chancellor of England. He was not a physician. Hunter and Macalpine (1963) say of him that he 'refuted the contention which had long impeded study of the sick mind that mental illness was the result either of bodily disease, i.e. the humoral theory, or of divine punishment'. Instead he suggested four lines of research along which psychiatry has, in fact, mainly advanced since his time.

The first should be the investigation of mental faculties, their sites of action, and the disturbances which can occur in them. In the study of what he called 'Physiognomie', 'which discovereth the disposition of the mind', he drew attention to the bodily configuration. Neurology and psychiatry have followed this idea, but in different ways. We no longer believe, with Gall, in phrenology — that by examining the cranial configuration we can determine the psychological characteristics of a man — but there can be no doubt that the scientific study of cerebral localisation of function, which started 140 years ago with the work of Bell and Magendie, owed its origin to these ideas. Both physiognomy and cerebral localisation have had a long history for both our specialties, but neurology has come off the better. Gall, an example of a fanatical localiser, asserted that the site of hysteria was in the cerebellum because the latter was the seat of carnal love. Naive as this may sound to modern ears, we still attribute the highest intellectual functions to the frontal lobes, think of the limbic system as the site of organisation of the emotions, and regard the mid-brain reticular system as the activator for instinctual drives. Physiognomy too, first in the hands of Francis Galton, later in those of Kretschmer, and now in the scientific studies of Sheldon on somatotyping, has had a respectable career. It can be said of this first of Bacon's recommendations that its realisation in different ways, using different techniques and approaches, has provided all that hitherto has been common ground for neurology and psychiatry. It has been the basis of what some call 'neuropsychiatry'.

Bacon's second recommendation was to study individual cases; but, as far as neurology was concerned, this had to wait until the beginning of the 19th century and for psychiatry until the end of it. His third advice was to study by 'Anatomy', by which he meant necropsy findings correlated with clinical findings. The first neuropsychiatric clinicopathological entity, general paralysis of the insane, was identified by Calmeil in 1826, exactly 200 years after Bacon's death. The fourth and most remarkable recommendation, to study the interaction between society and the individual — what today we call social psychiatry — was realised only in our own period, 300 years after Bacon lived. Anticipating the roles of individual psychology on the one hand and of social psychology on the other, Bacon wrote, 'Human philosophy, or humanity, hath two parts: the one considereth man segregate or distributively: the other, congregate or in society'.

PERSISTING SEPARATION OF PSYCHIATRY FROM MEDICINE

These few references to the ideas and events of the 16th and 17th centuries illustrate the divergence of approach which inevitably separated the body of developing medicine from the study of the mentally ill. In the 19th century, which saw the start of nearly all the present major specialties in medicine, including neurology, this division remained, and in fact had been increased.

The situation of psychiatry at the beginning of the last century when neurology had its birth, was grim. The appalling prison-like conditions in which the mentally ill were confined, and the brutality and cruelty with which they were treated, began to affect the conscience of mankind. Perhaps the French Revolution, with its upsurge of humanism and the stimulus it gave to liberal ideas, was partly responsible. The story of Philippe Pinel, who induced the revolutionary tribunal to give him permission to free his wretched patients from the Bicêtre, is well known. He did this in peril of his life and nearly lost it. The example and the teaching of Pinel in France were taken up and extended by humanitarian reformers in many countries. Just as in the 16th and 17th centuries such objectivity towards the mentally ill as was achieved came not from physicians and scientists but from scholars and philosophers, so in the 18th and 19th centuries aid came from non-medical social reformers with a keen conscience and humanistic ideas. A school teacher, Dorothea Dix, in America did more than anyone else in that country to bring decent treatment to the insane, and in England the movement for reform was led by a Quaker family, the Tukes, who founded the Retreat at York in 1792. There were four generations of Tukes, but only the founder William's great-grandson, who died in 1895, studied medicine and became a psychiatrist. There followed a period of social reform carried out by people who were not doctors and who had no pretensions to scientific knowledge or skill, and the care of the mentally sick passed into their hands. It seemed to many of them that kindness and fair treatment were enough. During the middle period of the last century the great mental hospital building programme began, with results that are still with us. Doctors were, of course, involved — but in small numbers — and the physician interested in the mentally ill devoted himself almost exclusively to hospital administration and to the training and organisation of appropriate staffs of attendants.

Although psychiatry owes a debt to many of these first psychiatrists, the superintendents of large mental institutions, their standing in the medical profession as a whole was not high. Few of them had any contacts with medical schools, and they were wholly ignorant of the contemporary scientific advances of their times. When psychiatry reached our medical schools it did not come from the psychiatrists working in the mental hospitals in the main, but from practitioners of a new subject, 'psychological medicine'.

The topographical, social, and intellectual isolation of those who worked in the old mental hospitals throughout the last hundred years was made all the more absolute by the fact that the hospitals themselves were built for economic reasons in the country at some distance from the main centres of population. Only now in the last five years is this process being reversed. It has become a positive policy of the Ministry of Health never to build a psychiatric hospital again in the old style or the same size, and where new psychiatric hospitals are required, to put them in direct physical contiguity with and as part of general hospitals.

Neurology in the end was responsible for reclaiming psychiatry as a subject which could be studied by scientific methods, but at the beginning of the 19th century this was still a long way ahead. Neurology itself had to develop, and 50 years were to elapse before Wernicke and Freud, both neurologists and both pupils of Meynert in Vienna, were to start the streams of thought which have done so much to invigorate both subjects. Nevertheless, throughout the century there were a few prominent men in all countries who reaffirmed the principles which Bacon understood and which had been repeatedly stated only to be forgotten. Hunter and Macalpine (1963) have quoted from the writings of such men, both from the side of general medicine and from the side of mental hospital psychiatry, against this unhappy state of affairs, even a hundred years ago. One such, a descendant of the first William Tuke, deserves quotation; for what T. H. Tuke wrote in the *Journal of Mental Science* in 1859 might have been written in the last decade with reference to other psychiatric conditions. Tuke was describing the prevalence of general paralysis of the insane, then so common a condition that in some hospitals a sixth of the admissions were of patients suffering from it. He went on to deplore the regrettable exclusion of psychiatry from medicine, the consequence of the fact 'that so few of even our most accomplished professors have any knowledge of the various types of mental derangement', and this in turn was because:

> the study of mental disorders is studiously excluded from the medical curriculum. Alienist physicians, as they are well called, work in a department of science the first principles of which are not even recognised by their medical brethren, and seem often to speak a language not understood by those around them; and thus indisputable facts and conclusions in psychological medicine become liable to be ignored or passed over.

He goes on:

> 'That this should be the fate of deductions from speculative or metaphysical theories is not surprising; but it does seem most marvellous that General Paralysis, a disease so frequent in its attack and so serious in its result, the form of insanity that is, perhaps, of all the most clearly marked out by physical and mental symptoms, should still remain unknown to the great mass of the profession.

THE NEUROLOGIST'S CONTRIBUTION

When finally psychiatry emerged as a scientific subject at the end of the last century, the men who were responsible were in fact neurologists. They were entirely convinced that the brain is the organ of mind and that all mental derangement is the result of derangement of the brain. Meynert, who had taught both Wernicke and Freud, objected to the term 'psychiatry'. In his theories the psychoses were due to a variety of changes in the circulatory system. Delusions and hallucinations, he thought, were due to subcortical irritation of the brain; melancholia and mania, to changes in the cortical blood vessels or cortical cells. This school of thought has been called that of 'brain mythology' by those who take an entirely different view of the nature of mental events, but of course in one form or another it has persisted to the present day — and the experimental evidence to support it, which was so conspiciously lacking in 1880, has here and there been provided.

By the beginning of the 20th century two pathways for psychiatric theory, two quite different methods of approach to the patient and his problems, had emerged. Both came from Meynert's school in Vienna and they were started by two of his pupils, Wernicke and Freud. Both had done original work on aphasia, but Wernicke will always be remembered as a great neurologist, Freud as the originator of the psychodynamic theories of mental illness.

NEUROPSYCHIATRIC OR PSYCHODYNAMIC?

Wernicke's success in discovering sensory aphasia and of relating a specific type of memory failure to lesions in a local area of the brainstem provided a pattern for all subsequent attempts to relate psychological phenomena to discrete brain areas. The pure 'brain mythology' of Gall's phrenology was translated into a scientific occupation. This was the beginning of neuropsychiatry. It had close links with neurology, using the same concepts, the same methods of observation and the same techniques. It has inspired much useful work. It differed fundamentally from the science which Freud carved out. The neuropsychiatrists studied the phenomena of mental illness from the outside. The patient's behaviour, reflected in the clinical symptoms and the signs he presented, were the hard data of observation. When they looked within the patient it was not at his feelings, wishes, frustrations, or character, but at his brain as an organic structure. They had to wait to look within until after the death of the patient.

Freud, of course, soon gave up his interest in these things. His vision of what went on within was determined not so much by the manner in which the patient spoke, but what he said. Psychoanalysis, for reasons that are wholly false, has been accused of dualism. In fact, the theory of psychoanalysis as developed by its founder is essentially a biological theory.

An important difference between the two approaches is that, while the neurologist and the neuropsychiatrist observe the patient as an object and are prepared to use a variety of techniques, psychological and physical, to demonstrate the behaviour which the object produces, the psychodynamic observer regards the patient only as part of the field of observation. He is more concerned with the interaction between the patient and those around him, and in particular the interaction between the patient and the observer himself. This means that the raw data are social and psychological, not physical or physiological, and the techniques of physical science cannot be used. There has been much time wasting and unnecessary polemic between the extremist adherents of these two approaches. The 'either-or' disputation is no longer relevant. Few believe that *either* a study of the nervous system alone *or* a study of interpersonal relations alone will provide all the answers for psychiatry, but it is certain that we cannot do without either.

The early neuropsychiatrists did not understand this. Wernicke, like Hughlings Jackson, based his theories on the reflex arc as a functional unit within the nervous system, and believed that the principles it involved could be extended to the highest mental activities (Mayer-Gross et al 1960). Like Pavlov after him, he viewed the operations of the nervous system as a series of ongoing processes from sensory input through interneuronal association to motor output. Wernicke believed that the whole field of psychiatry could be explained by disturbances at one level or another in these processes. Kraepelin, whose classification of the mental disorders was the first major breakthrough in knowledge of prognosis, believed that all mental illnesses were due to organic disease in the brain. He did not recognise the role of emotional disorder and psychogenesis in his system. The study of personality was unknown to him and would have appeared irrelevant. Kraepelin's immense influence on European and British psychiatry led to great efforts to find the 'lesions' responsible for all the mental disorders, and so for many decades these efforts were directed to the brain. When the microscope, using every refinement known, failed to reveal lesions of structure in any part of the brain in any groups of psychiatric patients except those with the organic psychoses, attention was directed to the endocrine glands, particularly the testes, and for several decades abnormalities of structures in them were claimed.

This has had a long history. Henry Maudsley, who left money to found the Maudsley Hospital, was essentially a neuropsychiatrist, and developed his own version of a 'brain mythology'. A chair of mental pathology of London University, which preceded the chair of psychiatry, was created at his hospital, and most of Sir Frederick Mott's work was concerned with studies of the testes in mental illness. This was the neuropathologist's answer to the Freudian idea that somehow or other sex was involved in mental disease. But with the development of many means of studying functional changes, both biochemical and electrophysiological, a new era began, and the search for lesions of structure appears to be over. The last word as far as the brain is concerned may well have been that of Professor Alfred

Meyer, who declared that his studies of schizophrenic brains had revealed that the more typical the case, the more nuclear the syndrome had been during the life of the patient, the more certain it would be that from the histological point of view the brain would reveal no lesions.

THE GULF AND THE BRIDGE

The great schism which has rent the theory and practice of psychiatry in the present century began to appear in the first decade of it. It has had profound effects upon psychiatry itself and has done much to separate psychiatry from neurology. It is surprising perhaps that Freud, the main architect of this, was himself a distinguished neurologist. Stengel (1954), who is responsible for the authorised translation of Freud's book *On Aphasia*, sees in this phase of Freud's work the origins of psychoanalytic theory. There can be no doubt that Freud was much influenced by Hughlings Jackson, just as Hughlings Jackson was influenced by the philosopher, Herbert Spencer. At the time this book was written, physiologists and neurologists were greatly preoccupied with the exact localisation of cerebral functions. The early neuropsychiatrists imitated them. The cerebral cortex appeared to them as a mosaic of areas, each with a separate function, and the localisation of mental activity seemed almost within grasp. Stengel (1954) points out that Freud was the first in the German-speaking world to subject these ideas to critical analysis and to show that unbiased clinical observation in the case of the aphasias failed to confirm the theory. The speech apparatus, conceived by the physiologists and neurologists of the day as an organic organisation, was conceived by Freud as a borderline concept with phenomena which can only be described in psychological terms.

It is of great interest that Freud, while still thinking in neurological and physiological terms, used the words 'projection', 'representation', 'cathexis' and 'overdetermination' to describe physiological phenomena of the cerebral cortex in his account of aphasia. The ideas implicit in them were, of course, taken over and have become the household words of psychoanalysis. It is of even greater interest that some of these terms and the ideas implicit in them have been taken over by neurophysiologists using electrical methods to study cerebral function. The phenomena of aphasia induced by cerebral lesions were explained by Freud in evolutionary terms, and here he was greatly influenced by Jackson and Spencer. As a result of pathological lesions (to quote Freud),

> the modes of reaction represent instances of functional retrogression (disinvolution) of a highly organised apparatus and therefore correspond to previous states of its functional development. This means that in all circumstances an arrangement of associations which, having been acquired later, will be lost, while an earlier and simpler one will be preserved.

From this it was but a short step to the concept of regression, a fundamental concept of psychoanalytic theory.

Freud, however, gave up thinking about the organic apparatus and turned totally to the psychic apparatus which he found at work in his study of the aphasias, with results that are well known. In doing so, he turned away from the observation of matters which are common to all people and became preoccupied with matters that are peculiar to the individual person. In a sense, this is the difference of approach which distinguishes those who are concerned with the organic apparatus from those who are concerned with the so-called psychic apparatus.

There are important consequences. While it is true that the adherents of both have as ultimate goals the identification of a sufficient body of facts that general laws about human behaviour and mental activity can be derived, there are significant differences. The distinction is that between the sciences using deductive generalisation mainly of a physical nature and the sciences using the processes of history. The first are concerned with 'testing universal hypotheses having the character of natural laws' and in prediction, the second are concerned in explaining past events by interpretations about causes (Popper, quoted by Lewis 1958). The raw material of the generalising sciences is for biology the species in aggregate; for the historical sciences it is the individual in isolation. From this point of view, the generalising sciences are not so much concerned with the characters of individuals which make them unique, but with the characters of individuals which make them similar, or at least which place them in classes or categories. By contrast, the historical sciences are concerned primarily with the past of a given individual in so far as it is unique to hm. In so far as it may be possible thus to categorise or classify members of the species into groups, this is derived as a secondary result. It is not the main issue.

Neurology, clinical and academic psychology, and some sociology have followed one path, psychoanalysis and all the derivative schools of dynamic psychiatry have followed the other. The techniques, the language used, the hypotheses themselves are different. Psychiatry, which is so dependent on both, is rent by the division. Lewis (1958) in his Bradshaw lecture deplores this situation and believes that in recent years there has been a move away from the search for general laws towards preoccupation with the individual. He quotes Manfred Bleuler (1957), who said that, 'the most essential feature in the recent development of psychiatry has been that the diagnosis of disease has given place to absorption in the personal tragedy of individuals'. The good psychiatrist, like every other good clinician, is inevitably swayed by his powerful motivation to help the suffering of his patients. He must inevitably be a psychotherapist. To the extent, however, that psychiatry becomes a historical science dependent for its ideas and progress upon the 'personal tragedy of individuals', it moves away from neurology and the sciences of brain from which it took origin. Yet, to the extent that psychiatry continues to take cognisance of those characters of individuals, whether well or sick, which they have in common, it retains a bridge with neurology, irrespective of the techniques which it may employ. These may be physical or psychological, but they are all concerned with making observations on behaviour, whether of the isolated neurone, the neuronal net, the reflex arc, the whole individual, or individuals in aggregate. But the methods we use for study of such behaviour depends upon what we have to observe. Psychological methods will never throw light on the functions of the isolated neuron, nor will physiological techniques illuminate the behaviour of social groups.

SHARED GROUND

This is so obvious that perhaps it is not worth saying, but out of the argument a conclusion is easily reached. If psychiatry is the study of abnormal behaviour and abnormal experience, it is only in the first part, abnormal behaviour, that we can see over the bridge which leads to the brain sciences. It would be unfair to neurology to assert that it is concerned with the organic apparatus alone. If preoccupation with sensory and motor functions, with equilibrium and co-ordination and the mechanisms by which local and general disease affect these functions, is the neurologist's first task, there is a large area of common ground which he shares with the psychiatrist. This is just that borderland area which Freud encountered in his studies of aphasia, which he saw was shared by the organic and the psychic apparatus. These words, coined so long ago, are now out of date, for the psychic apparatus is also part of the organic apparatus, and few will dispute this. If this is so, one should speak of functions in terms of whether they are physiological in expression or psychological in expression, both being aspects of brain activity. Failure in fact to do this led to the mistaken idea that psychoanalytical theory was based on metaphysical dualism and was an unbiological theory.

What, then, is the common ground which neurologists and psychiatrists share? When we study the disorders of consciousness, sleep, memory, speech, perception, and motility we must have common knowledge and use the same techniques of observation and measurement. Clinical psychologists, being reared on a diet from the generalising sciences and avoiding all phenomena they cannot measure, are not interested in consciousness and sleep; but neurologists and psychiatrists, being scientifically hybrid, are. Consciousness is both an experience and an observable phenomenon. The great light which has been thrown on the basic cerebral mechanisms upon which consciousness depends came as the result of neurophysiologists and neuropathologists interpreting the data of clinical experience. Electrophysiology, a science common to both psychiatry and neurology, has played a major role in this. Functional neuronography has complemented, and even bids to replace, the histological methods upon which neuronanatomy depended.

Whenever we are concerned with understanding disorders of mechanism, which in the case of consciousness may give rise to coma, stupor, epilepsy, akinetic mutism, narcolepsy, parasomnia, and many others, we are dependent upon the derivative neurological techniques. But as soon as these disorders demonstrate the workings of motivation, which is specific to the individual patient, we are concerned with the historical methods which dynamic psychiatry has developed. Thus in twilight states, hysterical fugues and fits, and states of amnesia, for example, we are concerned with functions of the nervous system which reflect the activity of the individual as a whole person — the old psychic apparatus. But the borderland is not clearly marked; for stupor (another example of disordered consciousness) may be the consequence of disordered mechanism or may be an expression of motivational behaviour. This was Freud's observation in the case of aphasia, when he noted that many of the repetitive utterances and the paraphasias could not be understood in terms of the disordered mechanism alone. Thus he moved from a study of functions commonly called conscious to those which are commonly called unconscious, and from the study of what could be described as a result of direct observation to phenomena whose existence had to be inferred to explain those observations.

The story is similar for the other examples mentioned, such as sleep, memory, perception, and motility. The borderland is broad, and with every advance of technique and extension of knowledge becomes broader; and the bridge — so narrow when Freud started his work 70 years ago — has become a main traffic way. The territory on either side is distinguished by one difference at least, which has already been outlined. On the side of neurology and the brain sciences, the field of study, the methods, and the techniques evolved are directed to understanding mechanism and the disorder of mechanism, and are therefore applicable to all brains of human or of subhuman species. On the side of psychiatry, on the other hand, the field of study and methods are directed to understanding not mechanism in the organic sense, but motivation, and the object of study is the whole person rather than a part of him, and is concerned with man alone rather than subhuman species.

In this country, for historical and social reasons already outlined and because of the very success of clinical neurology as a branch of medicine, the division between neurology and psychiatry has become more profound that in other countries. In America, with its shorter history and its liberal tradition, this division is less apparent. Psychiatry and neurology have both had easy and ready access to medical schools and research establishments. As a consequence, so-called interdisciplinary research has flourished and it is now commonplace to find psychiatrists and neurologists, psychologists and neurophysiologists, histologists and the students of animal behaviour, working together.

FROM BRIDGE TO BRIDGE

The bridge, therefore, which is observed to be a firm structure joining these two subjects has hitherto been a bridge of necessity; and many famous men have spent useful and creative lives working on the borderland area between neurology and psychiatry. The bridge itself has been constructed from the materials of common techniques, shared ideas, and an endeavour to solve the same problems. But essentially it has been created from a common intellectual curiosity, not from a need to provide the patient with the best that science can do.

This academic orientation of medicine, which centred what was done around the doctor's curiosity, is now changing and will give way to an orientation of medicine in which the patient's needs are paramount. To a certain extent this will inevitably lead to a blurring of the edges which separate one subject from another. In the new reticulum of medical sciences devised and developed to serve first the needs of the community, there will be a need within the network to preserve the academic function and the research function. Many new bridges will be built.

REFERENCES

Bleuler M 1957 Schweizerische Medizinische Wochenschrift p 113. Quoted by Lewis 1958
Hunter R, Macalpine I 1963 Three hundred years of psychiatry. Oxford, London
Lewis A 1958 Between guesswork and certainty in psychiatry. Lancet i: 227–230
Mayer-Gross E, Slater R, Roth M 1960 Clinical psychiatry. Bailliere, Tindall and Cassell, London
Stengel E 1954 Re-evaluation of Freud's book 'On aphasia'. International Journal of Psycho-Analysis (London) 35: 85–89
Zilboorg G 1941 A history of medical psychology. George Allen and Unwin, London

Neurologists and psychiatrists

The masterly review by Sir Denis Hill, reprinted here as Chapter 3, was more than an academic exercise alone. It reflected his clinical wisdom and his orientation to practical problems. He saw that neurology and psychiatry must collaborate with one another if progress were to be made, and he saw that 'the patient's needs are paramount' in considering joint endeavours between the two. Indeed his own life's work was built around the cardinal requirements of clinical practice, which remained always his chief motivating force.

That Denis Hill surveyed the gulfs and bridges between the major disciplines of neurology and psychiatry, and pondered so deeply upon them, reflected his breadth and open-mindedness in relation to psychiatric problems. He was neither overly 'organic' nor overly 'psychodynamic' in orientation to clinical matters, while being deeply skilled in both avenues to understanding. He combined, in fact, the essential virtues of both the neurologist and the psychiatrist.

We may ask what are these virtues, and how it comes about that medicine has grown to embrace two distinct and demarcated specialities. Neurologists and psychiatrists, after all, are united in their fascination with the brain and mind — with movement, thinking, feeling, perception and communication — yet they differ very considerably in their approaches and their definitive fields of study. In essence, when doctors are drawn to deal with malfunctions of the brain and mind they have to make a choice — should they become neurologists and concentrate on the problems of the physical apparatus, or become psychiatrists and deal with disorders of the mind directly? Few seem to experience substantial conflict over the decision; the die becomes cast quite early in their careers. What can shape such a choice, and what are the qualities in the persons concerned that lead them into one field or the other?

A further set of questions follows on. Why, for example, have the two specialities increasingly split apart in one country after another? And having split, why do they tend to follow divergent paths, leaving a borderland between which stands at risk of suffering neglect? In 1980 Dr Gerhardt

Table 4.1 Specialisation in neurology and psychiatry — 1980

Two separate specialities		Dual specialisation possible	One single speciality
Australia	Nigeria	Argentina	Austria
Bulgaria	Norway		
Canada	Peru	Egypt	East Germany
Columbia	Poland		
Czechoslovakia	Romania	Hungary	Greece
Denmark	Singapore		
Finland	Spain	Iran	Korea
Ghana	Sweden		
Hongkong	Switzerland	Kenya	Saudi Arabia
India	Thailand		
Israel	Turkey	Lebanon	Zaire
Japan	UK		
Malta	USA	Netherlands	
Morocco	USSR		
		West Germany	

Lenz made available his survey of the then situation worldwide as shown in Table 4.1. A small minority of countries retained neurology and psychiatry as fused and indivisible, and these in terms of population were mostly small. Since 1980 the number has fallen further — in Greece the specialities split apart in 1981 and in Korea in 1983.

In all such matters complex determinants must be at work. Neurology and psychiatry may each have become too complicated for one person to encompass both together. Problems of training, of the delivery of services, or of the organisation of research may play a considerable part. But beyond such factors there may be something still more fundamental which has served to perpetuate the division. It seems possible that there may be something that is distinctive about the practitioners of neurology and psychiatry which has tended to draw them apart.

In what follows we will explore the idea that the answers to these questions may lie, at least in large degree, with the *sorts of people* who become neurologists and psychiatrists. We may be dealing with personal attributes, matters of 'personal style', definable attitudes in relation to science and clinical practice. It may be an aspect of *human diversity* rather than any external constraint that has conspired towards the present situation.

First we will review what these two groups of clinicians do in their everyday work and how they set about accomplishing it. We will then look at the processes involved in more abstract terms and try to identify essential differences in approach, in guiding principles and in sources of satisfaction. A brief glance at the historical background to neurology and psychiatry will help us to appreciate the present situation to the full. Finally we shall join with Sir Denis Hill in examination of the bridges, as they appear now some 25 years further forward.

ACTIVITIES AND EXPERTISE

Table 4.2 attempts to summarise the clinical arenas of neurologists and psychiatrists. The neurologist starts out with physical disorders of the brain, cord and nerve. It just so happens, in a sense, that the brain is also the apparatus of the mind. The psychiatrist, by contrast, takes affections of the mind as his immediate point of departure. It just so happens, for him, that mind is subserved by the physical apparatus of the brain.

Table 4.2 Clinical arenas of neurologists and psychiatrists

	Neurologist	Psychiatrist
Field	Affections of the brain and nervous system	Affections of the mind
Observational data	Motor and sensory abnormalities. Disorders of language, recognition, etc	Change of affect, thought disorder, abnormal subjective experiences & beliefs
Clinical history	Detailed exploration of physical symptoms and their evolution	Life history, personality development, interpersonal interactions

So the neurologist is expert at evaluating motor abnormalities, reflex changes, subtle sensory disturbances. He also understands disorders of language, recognition, and other complex functions in the sense that they may be disturbed by a lesion of the brain. His skills in examining the patient are finely focused, more so perhaps than in any other area of medicine. MacDonald Critchley (1979) said of Sir Gordon Holmes that he 'could coax physical signs out of a patient like a Paganini on the violin . . . It was a sheer delight to watch him evoking one physical sign after another . . .'. In approaching the clinical history the neurologist excels at a detailed exploration of symptoms, paying scrupulous attention to their nature and evolution.

The psychiatrist deals with much blunter instruments. His expertise lies in assessing abnormalities of mood, qualities of thought disorder, false beliefs and abnormal subjective experiences such as compulsions and hallucinations. Human behaviour and experiencing are his primary concern. This leads him into diverse territories — minds can interact with other minds and can be profoundly influenced by circumstance and social processes. In taking a history he explores biographical data and processes of personal development. He must consider the patient's environment, and the nature of his interactions with people and things. Henry Maudsley wrote at the age of 25: (see Lewis 1951):

> In an account of insanity in any form there are thus two elements to be taken into consideration, one almost as important as the other; these are the subject and the environment, the man and his circumstances, subjective force and objective forces, both passive and active . . . .

SYNTHESIS

Further interesting differences come when, armed with this information, the clinician has to decide what is afoot (Table 4.3). Both sets of specialists have a daunting task. The neurologist is confronted with the intricacy of the nervous system, the psychiatrist with the complexity of human behaviour.

Table 4.3 Synthesis of clinical information

	Neurologist	Psychiatrist
Relates clinical information to:	Knowledge of well-defined disease entities	Knowledge of 'mental diseases'
	Knowledge of anatomy and physiology of nervous system	Conversance with range of variation in human personality, situations, reactions
Uses knowledge of:	Matters common to all	Matters unique to individuals

The neurologist relates the data he has gathered to a knowledge of certain well-defined disease entities. He must be well-informed on matters of clinical nosology. Of Sir William Gowers we are told (Critchley 1949):

> To him [Gowers] the neurological sick were like the flora of a tropical jungle, and his keen eye and collector's flair enabled him to identify, arrange and classify . . . . Furthermore, he was able to pick out a species which had not previously been described or labelled.

The neurologist must also rely on detailed acquaintance with the anatomy and physiology of the nervous system. He has to know how this complex machinery works in order to decide where the trouble lies and what may be its nature.

The psychiatrist tends to do something very different. He tries to relate his clinical information to a corpus of knowledge concerning 'mental diseases' where this may be applicable. But in many parts this corpus is shaky indeed. The vagaries of mental disorder and of personal distress cannot be encompassed by a neat classificatory system. He must always be ready, furthermore, to think in terms of a 'range of variation' which has nothing to do with disease — aberrations of personality, changes of mood, responses to conflict, threat or disaster. The psychiatrist relies very little on a detailed knowledge of the nervous system, but rather on an appreciation of human situations and crises and the way predispositions can shape human behaviour.

Thus we see the force of the differences set out by Sir Denis Hill (Ch. 3). The neurologist's decisions and inferences hinge on matters that are common to all men and women — their neural physiology and anatomy. The raw material for his science is the 'species in aggregate'. The psychiatrist's conclusions, by contrast, hinge very often on matters peculiar to individuals — knowledge of persons in particular settings, of the 'characters which make them unique'.

REWARDS AND SATISFACTIONS

When we consider the intellectual rewards deriving from either discipline still further contrasts appear. Perhaps it is here that we find the nub of the differences that attract persons to one specialty or the other. The neurologist may be said to achieve satisfaction from near-complete understandings. The psychiatrist must rest content with much less.

The neurologist aims for precision, certainty, feed-backs from his hunches. He can investigate with biochemical tests and radiological procedures. In neurology the clinico-pathological conference has always flourished. The psychiatrist must largely forego such rewards, and indeed must learn to live with uncertainty. Instead he enjoys room for 'imaginative endeavour', processes of empathy, creative attempts at explanation. He is drawn to abstract concepts, and he must often involve himself in discussion of sharply contending opinions. In essence the neurologist's inferences are finely drawn from carefully marshalled evidence; the psychiatrist must often infer on a wide, far-reaching scale from rather slender clues.

When it comes to therapy, similarly, the neurologist will usually understand a good deal about the nature of the pathogenic process, but he may have little scope to alter things with treatment. The psychiatrist understands much less at a fundamental level, but this does not impede his room to manoeuvre — he can often obtain a striking response to simple interventions, such as ventilation of distress, assurance of concern, or discussions with the patient and his family.

These, of course, are broadly drawn abstractions from a very complex whole, gross generalisations extracted to make a point. In practice a good deal of overlap occurs. Nevertheless, they enable us to see how different the practitioners of neurology and psychiatry are liable to be from one another. Core differences emerge in a multitude of respects — in their activities, expertise and styles of thinking, and in the nature of their rewards from clinical practice. These may be powerful influences in drawing doctors to one or other specialty and, very importantly, in sometimes turning them away from the other.

Some evidence for this can be found from surveys conducted on medical students. Walton (1969), for example, investigated personality attributes, as measured by standardised questionnaires, among students declaring positive or negative attitudes to psychiatry as a possible career choice. A 'complexity trait' was high among those drawn to psychiatry — high scoring here indicates a liking for diversity and shows that the person is not discomforted by ambiguity; low scorers seek a definite structure, dislike uncertainty, and tend to react against unfamiliar ideas. Another trait was even more influential — high scorers (drawn to psychiatry) have a liking for abstract ideas, are more idealistic than realistic, and have a penchant for analysing their motives; the low scorer is a person of action and less prone to reflect.

HISTORICAL DEVELOPMENT

Turning from the present situation we may review some aspects of history to see how the distinctions have come about. Neurology and psychiatry have had very different origins, likewise different impulses to their development. Psychiatry, starting earlier, has had a complex evolution; neurology has grown throughout with more straightforward ties to mainstream scientific progress. Yet an important intertwining of ideas has shaped each discipline from the earliest stages of their joint existence.

17th–18th centuries

Psychiatry's development did not begin with discoveries in the field of science, but with the pressing need to care for a class of persons — the insane. From the late 17th century onwards medicine began to take an interest in what had traditionally been the provenance of others, notably the Church. Denis Leigh (1961) has traced the early attempts made in Britain to explain insanity, employing the physiology of the day, first in terms of bodily malfunction (Purcell 1702) then with attention gradually focusing on the brain and nervous system (Whytt 1765). With Thomes Arnold (1786) we find early mention of the role of disturbed emotions in leading to mental disorder — a radically different conception of aetiological forces.

What strikes us during this early history is the enormity of the task confronting early thinkers about mental disorder. Imaginative endeavour was certainly required. Where they turned for physiological explanations they found little to guide them. Attempts at neuropathology yielded negligible results. The roles of 'passions' and emotions were championed, but there was no systematic psychology, no hint of a descriptive psychopathology to provide a framework for such ideas. The range of disorders was daunting — from 'vapours' and 'hypochondrias' to flagrant states of insanity. These last brought additional perplexities and responsibilities that had nothing to do with the unravelling of causes, namely how to manage and care humanely for the mentally deranged. This in itself was to become a major area of concern and endeavour.

Early 19th century

Through the early 19th century such turmoils continued. John Haslam (1764–1844) at Bethlem thought almost exclusively in terms of neuropathology as the basis for mental disorder, Benjamin Rush (1745–1813) in the

USA in terms of the cerebral vasculature. Esquirol (1772–1840) in Paris meanwhile tabulated the psychological causes of insanity in great detail. The French, as Zilboorg (1941) points out, had already 'a keen sense of psychological discernment of individual trends'. Meanwhile Anton Mesmer was at work on the European scene, with his remarkable theories of cause and cure which are considered further below.

It was during the early 19th century that neurology began to take shape. In 1817 James Parkinson wrote his essay on the shaking palsy, in 1837 multiple sclerosis was described, in 1847 locomotor ataxia. And here we note that such studies were immediately quite different in their promise. The signs and symptoms of neurological dysfunction were more definite, more constant from one patient to another, thus enabling disease entities to be spotted. More importantly, fundamental discoveries about the structure of the nervous system began to provide the background against which to view the effects of coarse brain lesions. Abercrombie's work in 1828 rested on clinicopathological correlations on a large series of carefully studied cases. Here was the start of a much richer and more rewarding set of enterprises than confronted the psychiatrists who looked to brain pathology in attempts to clarify mental illness.

Later 19th century

Later in the century decisive events took place. In England the National Hospital for the Relief of Paralysis, Epilepsy and Allied Disorders was opened at Queen Square in 1859 as the first neurological centre in the world. Hughlings Jackson and Ferrier were making their now classical observations. In Paris, Charcot at the Salpêtrière was the first professor of neurology ever to be appointed. Such men were the beneficiaries of an expanding knowledge of brain anatomy and physiology, to which they in turn contributed. Dax, Broca and Wernicke clarified the seat of language in the brain. Fritsch & Hitzig (1870) showed that discrete motor movements followed discrete stimulation of the cortex. Neurology was well set on its course and had clearly found its way forward. Soon Sherrington, Gowers, Holmes and Kinnear Wilson were deeply involved in the process.

Psychiatry in the later 19th century remained prey to schisms and uncertainties. The main centre of interest in the mid-1800s lay in Germany, where the psychiatrists of that period were strongly oriented to neurology and neuropathology. Griesinger, before his death in 1868, had written: 'Psychiatry and neuropathology are not merely two closely related fields; they are but one field in which only one language is spoken and the same laws rule'. Such determined attempts to follow neurology's path were reinforced by the success achieved in relation to general paresis. Bayle and Calmeil had delineated the clinical picture in 1826 and its pathological basis was now becoming clearer. Here was a conspicuous mental disorder with a conspicuous pathological basis.

Henry Maudsley in England (1867) shared the belief that mental diseases were brain diseases. Meynert in Vienna taught that psychoses were due to circulatory changes in the brain, delusions and hallucinations derived from subcortical irritations, melancholia and mania from the cortex. Psychiatry was vying with medicine, jealous of the successes achieved in relation to clinical medicine and pathology.

The Germans set about psychiatric nosology too in a systematic and vigorous manner. Hecker described hebephrenia in 1871, Kahlbaum catatonia (1874) and later cyclothymia (1882). The great nosological triumphs of Kraepelin were achieved at the turn of the century.

Meanwhile, however, attention had centred on hysteria and on the curious phenomenon of hypnosis. Such a turn of events had profound repercussions for psychiatry. Moreover, the leader in this remarkable historical development was a neurologist, Charcot himself.

Charcot took up the study of hypnosis in 1878 at the Salpêtrière. As is well known, he applied it to large numbers of patients under his care to whom a distinct neurological label could not be given. They suffered from all manner of crises, seizures and other peculiar symptoms. Many were impressionable young women. He found that they were unusually susceptible to hypnosis and that, when hypnotised, their crises could be provoked at will.

Charcot believed that he was witnessing a phenomenon produced by purely physical means. With the keen observation of a neurologist he described the successive stages of lethargy, catalepsy and somnambulism, each being initiated and terminated, he thought, by definite physical procedures. To Charcot these were the outward signs reflecting changes occurring in the nervous system. He believed, furthermore, that the capacity to be hypnotised was a definite manifestation of abnormality, of the organic morbid state that was hysteria itself. He was applying the principle of disease delineation that had served him so well in his neurological studies.

Charcot's conclusions were, however, denied by parallel workers in Nancy. There Liébeault, a country doctor, and Bernheim, a professor of medicine, had themselves been studying hypnosis. Bernheim published his observations in 1886. In opposition to Charcot the workers in Nancy claimed that hypnosis was by no means a pathological condition found only in hysterics. The effects, moreover, were produced by suggestion — 'the aptitude to transform an idea into an act' — a propensity that everyone possessed to different degree. Psychological factors alone were responsible for the induction of hypnosis; the operator worked by means of mental influences over the patient.

The clash of opinion between Charcot and Bernheim achieved resounding intensity. Sigmund Freud visited both, and it was soon clear to him where the most fruitful hypotheses lay. He later wrote (Freud 1925):

Before leaving Paris I discussed with the great man (Charcot) a plan for a comparative study of hysterical and organic paralyses. I wished to establish the thesis that in hysteria paralyses and anaesthesias of the various parts of the body are demarcated according to the popular idea of their limits and not according to anatomical facts. He agreed with this view, but it was easy to see that in reality he took no special interest in penetrating more deeply into the psychology of the neuroses. When all is said and done, it was from pathological anatomy that his work had started.

Bernheim's views in the end prevailed. A psychological conception had won over a physiological model of a complex mental state. Human motivations, wishes and expectations had found a respectable place in medical thinking. Psychiatry had in effect started out on the road to an explanatory psychopathology.

What happened thereafter has had continuing influence on psychiatry. Pierre Janet succeeded Charcot at the Salpêtrière and developed psychopathological conceptions further. With his theory of 'dissociation' he opened the field of unconscious mental processes to careful enquiry. Freud commenced his own studies of hysteria with Joseph Breuer, and developed his own remarkable edifice of psychodynamic theory.

A process had unwittingly been set in motion which drove home a core difference between the disciplines of neurology and psychiatry — the process whereby psychological systems of explanation came to supplement, in some cases to supplant, explanations based on purely physiological knowledge. In embarking on this road, moreover, psychiatry was no longer seeking direct evidence by way of tissue pathology, but was relying on the intuitive deductions of observers of human behaviour.

Psychiatry has, of course, proceeded along other roads as well during the past 100 years. Study of environmental, social and cultural factors, attention to interpersonal relationships and group interactions, have all served to enrich the subject. In continuing attempts to understand and ameliorate mental disorder, psychiatrists were to continue to draw heavily on disciplines remote from physiology.

Gall and Mesmer

Before leaving history it is intriguing to consider two men, Gall and Mesmer, whose theories can be seen with hindsight to have had a cardinal influence on the development of neurology and psychiatry. Both, moreover, share certain remarkable parallels. Each propounded a 'system', on shaky foundations to say the least, and acquired ardent disciples who spread their teaching throughout Europe. Both started in Vienna, left under a cloud, and came to establish their teaching in Paris. Neither the one nor the other could have foreseen where their ultimate impacts would lie.

Franz Joseph Gall (1757–1828) was a neuroanatomist of very considerable achievements. But along with his anatomy he developed corresponding psychological doctrines — that the mind could be analysed into independent faculties, each with their seat in the cortex, that the size of each cerebral organ indicated its functional capacity, and that this could be determined by inspection of the contours of the skull. He and his pupil Spurzheim promoted these 'phrenological' ideas widely. In the absence of all evidence, the system evolved out of reasonable control, with claims for centres reflecting 'hope', 'benevolence', even 'philoprogenitiveness'. Certain prominent medical men lent credence to the system, one such being John Elliotson, holder of the Chair of Physic in London.

Ultimately, of course, such ideas were firmly exploded. But the lasting outcome for science was indubitable. The prevailing conception of holistic brain functioning had been thoroughly challenged and shaken, and a powerful impetus given to studies of brain localisation. *The Phrenological Journal*, which ran through the early 19th century, was replete with reports in which symptoms and signs were correlated with the site of cerebral lesions. Gall's work, when stripped of its claims for divining personality and intelligence, can be seen as a spur to the process by which neurology was to advance and prosper.

Anton Mesmer (1734–1815), a charismatic and bizarre figure, founded his own school of thought. He taught that a subtle physical fluid with magnetic properties filled the universe, forming a connecting medium between man, the earth and the heavenly bodies. Disease originated from imperfect distribution of the fluid in the human body — but with appropriate techniques it could be channelled, stored or conveyed to other persons. He attracted a huge following, undoubtedly among the neurotically sick, and held séances and sittings in which remarkable cures were obtained. The magnetic principles were carried to fantastic lengths: his disciple, the Marquis de Puységur, seated patients beneath a 'magnetic' oak tree from which long ropes descended to be wrapped around affected body parts.

The spread of mesmerism to England brought it to the attention of James Braid (1795–1860), a Scottish surgeon working in Manchester. Braid investigated the mesmeric influence in detail, coined the new term 'hypnotism', and gradually substituted a psychological for a physical explanation of the process. He intuitively perceived that the suggestive effect of ideas aroused in the patient's mind were the real and potent forces. Braid was a forerunner in this regard to the fierce debates which later occupied Charcot and Bernheim.

In effect, therefore, Mesmer can be seen to have set in train the whole sequence of events which came ultimately to catalyse the growth of psychological systems of explanation. In this he benefitted psychiatry. Moreover, mesmerism had left its mark in another significant respect: it had drawn attention to the great mass of neurotically ill patients who, till then, had attracted scant attention from psychiatry.

Finally it is useful to consider, as a cautionary tale, how the derivatives of each of these movements — phrenology and mesmerism — bore fruit for one particular discipline, but ran into error when interpreted for the other. Phrenology, in encouraging clinicopathological correlations, enriched neurology, but as a system for character delineation, for determining individual differences, it was a sham. Mesmerism, in leading to an appreciation of the power of unconscious processes in mental functioning in effect revolutionised psychiatry, but when Charcot attempted to apply neurological reasoning to the phenomena of hypnosis he blemished an otherwise splendid record in history.

Conclusions from history

The broad conclusions we can draw from this history support in many respects the contention made at the beginning — namely, that neurologists and psychiatrists are very different types of people. They complement each others' major functions in a most important way. They trespass on one anothers' domains with a certain degree of risk. And we see more clearly some of the trends that have come to shape their thinking and practice.

Both neurologists and psychiatrists have at some point in their course descended from physicians. But the neurologist has had a straight-forward ontogeny — through the classical process of the evolution of medical knowledge generally. He has relied on clinical observation, the study of identifiable pathological processes, and the discernment of the links between the two. This has led to clear definition of syndromes and disease entities. The success of neurology in such enterprises has been great, and this very success is attractive to doctors who like tidiness and certainty, the challenge of putting clinical skills and clinical memory to the test.

Psychiatry by contrast has had a chequered evolution, more chequered than in any other branch of medicine. It had first to secure its territory from the theologians and philosophers. It had to contend with severe disappointment in seeking clinicopathological correlations. It had to subsume variations from the norm, when dealing with such matters as the neuroses and personality disorders. And it had to deal all through with controversy, debate and a plethora of explanatory systems. Such a course has been necessary for psychiatry to reach even partial, tentative explanations for the phenomena with which it must deal.

In essence we see that the neurologist is a committed physiologist, drawn to the challenge inherent in the most complex organ and system in the body. He is the specialist par excellence. The psychiatrist, by contrast, has had to be remarkably versatile; he has required something of physiology, but something of psychology and sociology as well. He needs an additional large investment in something as vague and ill-defined as 'human understanding'. The neurologist has had to intensify to unravel mechanisms; the psychiatrist to diversify to find his explanations. It is perhaps small wonder that their strivings have tended to draw them apart.

Thus the neurologist has found his richest rewards in matters over which he could feel on firm ground — matters he could measure, quantify and dissect, mechanisms he could clearly understand. Disorders of higher mental function have come well within his purview, but few have made this their special area of concern. Malfunction of the motor and sensory systems, of peripheral nerve and muscle, have often attracted the major interest.

Psychiatrists, with their necessary concern with the total human condition, have come to find satisfactions in fields quite other than brain anatomy and physiology. Their indignant response to Griesinger ('mental diseases are brain diseases') still echoes down the years. Psychiatrists can be caught, moreover, in a trap of their own making — if they question too insistently the claims of psychodynamic theory their rebellion can be interpreted to them in a direct and personal manner! For a multitude of reasons psychiatrists came in the present century to focus their attention very little on the brain.

Thus, as successive generations of students have been recruited, we can see that the differences between neurologists and psychiatrists have tended to become intensified. Each scientific gain in neurology, each broadening of conceptions in psychiatry, has deepened the wedge between. In effect we would appear to have had polarising forces of steadily increasing intensity.

PRESENT-DAY NEUROLOGY AND PSYCHIATRY

This process, so clearly set in motion, could well have been predicted to continue on its course. The idea of a rapprochement between neurology and psychiatry may have come to seem remote, with common endeavour destined to remain a somewhat slender strand. Neurologists and psychiatrists shared certain clinical problems — dementia, epilepsy, hysteria — and were brought into occasional contact over questions of diagnosis and management. In the main, however, and except in a few special centres, they pursued their specialities in parallel and viewed one another from a considerable distance.

Yet Denis Hill foresaw, already a generation ago, that the status quo was changing, and that bridges would be built and strengthened. In fact, to an extent that is remarkable, events now appear to be turning full circle, and present-day neurologists and psychiatrists are finding themselves drawn ever closer together. They are often, indeed, united in common strategies and goals.

The reasons are not very far to seek. They hinge largely on the astonishing growth of the neurobiological disciplines which serve as underpinnings of clinical practice, and the windows these have opened up for both neurology and psychiatry. New understandings of brain physiology, biochemistry and pathology can be seen to have relevance for the origins of disturbed emotion and behaviour, not merely for disorders of motor control and sensation. In effect, psychiatry has begun over recent decades to turn attention once more to the working of the brain; cerebral physiology, previously discarded and overrun, has now evolved to the point when it seems that it can, after all, illuminate mental disorder.

Concurrently, and it must be admitted in part fortuitously, psychiatry has achieved a psychopharmacology which is quite as firmly established as neuropharmacology. This has brought undreamt of benefit to patients and facilitated the task of treatment for a large segment of the mentally ill. In consequence, the styles of practice of neurologists and psychiatrists now have an important element in common. Moreover, in the wake of pharmacotherapy psychiatrists have learned to dissect with unusual delicacy the phenomena their patients display. They have had to define and quantify with care, and to surmount the obstacles of strictly controlled comparisons in the realm of abnormal behaviour. What was once largely 'impressionistic' is now accessible, when necessary, to 'scientific method'.

The most recent unifying factor to appear on the scene has come from advances in techniques for imaging the brain. Here neurologists and psychiatrists watch every new development — CT scanning, magnetic resonance imaging, positron emission tomography — with equal expectation and with similar claims to hope for benefit for their disciplines.

Very significantly these advances of the past decades have proved their worth across a broad spectrum of psychiatric disorder — not just in relation to the obviously organic psychosyndromes, but with the so-called 'functional' illnesses as well. Neurochemical research is relevant to anxiety, pharmacology to depression, brain imaging to schizophrenia. Here it is also significant, and remarkable, to observe how closely the researches of neurologists and psychiatrists have come to converge at many points. Both are on the track of brain enzymes and transmitter systems — dopamine is relevant to Parkinson's disease and to the action of neuroleptics, the endorphins to pain control and to the addictions, acetylcholine to movement disorder and dementia. Similar strategies in PET scanning seem set to advance our understanding of the motor system and of schizophrenia. Such examples could be greatly multiplied.

These common endeavours have, of course, opened up a dialogue which might otherwise not have occurred. It has brought neurologists and psychiatrists into contact with one another in the laboratory, in scientific gatherings and, increasingly, in clinical practice. We now witness an exchange of ideas and a sharing of expertise to a degree that could scarcely have been foreseen.

Furthermore, and returning to the theme elaborated above, we can observe a blurring of the distinctions which once characterised the practitioners of neurology and psychiatry. Each type of specialist retains in large degree his 'personal style' and his chief sources of satisfaction, but there is now an overlap, more than a tenuous thread, which unites them indissolubly.

It cannot be doubted that it has been beneficial to the understanding of disorders of the brain and mind that we came to evolve these separate specialties, each with their particular approaches and orientations. But equally it seems clear that enormous value is destined to follow henceforward from close collaboration, mutual respect, and joint endeavours between the two.

REFERENCES

Abercrombie J 1828 Pathological and practical researches on diseases of the brain and the spinal cord. Edinburgh (quoted by Hunter R, Macalpine I 1963 Three hundred years of Psychiatry: 1586–1860. Oxford University Press, London)

Arnold T 1786 Observations on the nature, kinds, causes, and prevention of insanity, lunacy, or madness — II (quoted by Leigh 1961 — see below)

Bernheim H 1886 De la suggestion et de ses applications a la thérapeutique. Doin, Paris (quoted by Ellenberger H F 1970 The discovery of the unconscious. The history and evolution of dynamic psychiatry. Allen Lane, Penguin Press, London)

Critchley M 1949 Sir William Gowers (1845–1915): A biographical appreciation. William Heinemann, London

Critchley M 1979 Gordon Holmes: The man and the neurologist. In: The divine banquet of the brain. Raven Press, New York, p. 228–234

Freud S 1925 An autobiographical study. Translated by Strachey J, 2nd edn, 1946. Hogarth Press, London

Fritsch G, Hitzig E 1870 Uber dei elektrische Erregbarkeit des Grosshirns. Archiv für Anatomie, Physiologie und wissenschaftliche Medicin, p 300–332

Hecker E 1871 Die Hebephrenie. Archiv für pathologische Anatomie und Physiologie 52 (quoted by Zilboorg G 1941 — see below)

Kahlbaum K L 1874 Die Katatonie oder das Spannungsirresein. Berlin (quoted by Zilboorg G 1941 — see below)

Kahlbaum K L 1882 Über zyklisches Irresein, Irrenfreund, no 10 (quoted by Zilboorg G 1941 — see below)

Leigh D 1961 The historical development of British psychiatry. Vol I: 18th and 19th century. Pergamon Press, Oxford

Lewis A 1951 The twenty-fifth Maudsley lecture — Henry Maudsley: his work and influence. Journal of Mental Science 97: 259–277

Maudsley H 1867 Pathology of mind. MacMillan and Co, London

Purcell J A 1702 A treatise of vapours, or hysteric fits. Containing an analytical proof of its causes, mechanical explanations of all its symptoms and accidents, according to the newest and most rational principles: together with its cure at large. London (Quoted by Leigh 1961 — see above)

Walton H J 1969 Personality correlates of a career interest in psychiatry. British Journal of Psychiatry 115: 211–219

Whytt R 1765 Observations on the nature, causes, and cure of those disorders which have been commonly called nervous, hypochondriac or hysteric: to which are prefixed some remarks on the sympathy of the nerves. Edinburgh (quoted by Leigh 1961 — see above)

Zilboorg G 1941 A history of medical psychology. In collaboration with Henry G W. George Allen and Unwin, London

Structure and function in neurology and psychiatry

The antithesis between 'organic' and 'functional' disease states still lingers at the bedside and in medical literature, though it is transparently false and has been abandoned long since by all contemplative minds.

Kinnier Wilson 1940

Neurological practice is rooted in structure, in neuroanatomy and neuro-pathology. One of the primary objectives of the neurologist is to find the lesion. For this he has developed his skills in neurological examination and utilises increasingly sophisticated and costly investigative techniques. Neurological disorder is widely referred to as organic. Yet structural lesions produce their symptoms and signs by disturbing the function of the nervous system: by interruption, decrease, release or increase of function; by excitation, inhibition, instability or restoration of function. However, this disturbance of function in neurology is so often taught and practised as though it were a static or almost wholly 'reflex' neurophysiology — fixed lesions producing fixed defects in function. The neurological textbooks are littered with diagrams, figures and tables showing how a lesion at this or that site produces a clear-cut constellation of symptoms and signs based on a thorough knowledge of neuroanatomy and localisation of function. The reality for the observant neurologist is often rather different. Not all the expected symptoms and signs are present. Those that are present, whether motor, sensory, reflex, cognitive or behavioural, come and go or fluctuate in intensity over minutes, hours or days under a variety of intrinsic or extrinsic influences. Some are very intermittent, such as the seizures associated with a cerebral tumour or scar, or the migrainous headaches associated with an arteriovenous malformation. Furthermore, the symptoms and signs of a fixed structural lesion may be indistinguishable from those of functional disorders in the nervous system, e.g. the hemiparesis of a stroke and the Todd's paralysis following seizures. Psychological and social factors frequently clearly influence and interact with neurological symptoms and signs, but are often overlooked or ignored as though this was somehow part of 'psychiatry'.

Psychiatrists in general adopt an uncertain, even confused, approach to structure and function. Individually they may belong to very different schools of thought depending whether they are oriented to the neuropsychiatric or psychodynamic wing of the discipline (see Ch. 3). Some are concerned that they may be overlooking a structural lesion, something that really belongs to neurology! All recognise that various types of cerebral pathology produce mental symptoms which form part of the practice of psychiatry, so-called organic psychiatry or neuropsychiatry (Lishman 1978, Trimble 1981), which clearly has close links with neurology. At the very least it is borderline territory, the interface or bridge between the two disciplines. The main corpus of psychiatry is concerned with 'functional' disorder of the mind, self or psychic apparatus, brought about mainly by intra- and interpersonal forces of a psychological and social kind. Here the use of the word 'functional' is not physiological but psychological. The psychoses illustrate the dilemma, with the organic psychoses rooted in nervous system pathology and physiology, and the 'functional' psychoses conceived of in psychic formulations.

In recent years the conceptual dilemma for the psychiatrist has been made more acute by developments in the neurosciences, especially in psychopharmacology, neurochemistry and brain imaging techniques. More and more attention is being paid by psychiatrists to those developments, which have often revealed unsuspected structural or functional (in the neurological sense) disorders in their patients. For neurologists I would also argue that a wholly organic approach, which ignores or overlooks the impact of psychological and social factors in neurological disorders, is incomplete and, from the patient's point of view in particular, inadequate. The present widely held concept of neurology as organic and psychiatry as 'functional', with neuropsychiatry sitting uneasily in between, is unsatisfactory.

These contrasting views of structure and function by neurologists and psychiatrists have not come about by chance, but have been shaped by forces which have led to the separation of neurology and psychiatry as distinct disciplines with ill-defined borders. If we are to understand the present situation and to see our way forward to a more satisfactory and less confusing conceptual framework it is important to understand what these forces and developments were.

HISTORICAL BACKGROUND

In the beginning there were no neurologists or psychiatrists, but there were 'nervous diseases'. According to López-Piñero (1983), the concept of 'nervous diseases' emerged in Britain with Willis (1622–75) and Sydenham (1624–89). For example, both viewed hysteria and hypochondria as nervous diseases and not, as in the Galenic tradition, vapours emanating from the uterus or the spleen, liver and stomach. According to Willis (1682), hysteria 'the so-called uterine disease is primarily a convulsive disease caused by an alteration of the nerves and the brain'. The concept of nervous diseases was consolidated in the 18th century, when they also became fashionable, due to the influence of, among others: Cheyne (1733), whose treatise on the 'English malady' suggested that 'these nervous diseases being computed to make almost one-third of the complaints of the people of condition in England'; and of Whytt (1765), who expressed the opinion that 'all diseases may, in some sense, be called affections of the nervous system, because in almost every disease, the nerves are more or less hurt; and in consequence of this, various sensations, motions and changes are produced in the body'.

It is to Cullen (1710–90) that we owe the term 'neurosis'. William Cullen succeeded Robert Whytt to the Chair of the Practice of Physic at Edinburgh. For Cullen the word 'neuroses' was no more than a neologism for Whytt's 'nervous diseases'. Cullen was a lucid compiler rather than an original thinker and his nosological classifications of disease published in 1769 and 1777 were very influential. He recognised four classes of disease: three were general, i.e. I pyrexiae, II neuroses and III caquexiae; the fourth was local, i.e. IV locales. The class 'neuroses' were defined as 'affections of sense and motion without fever or evidence of local disease', i.e. they were general and functional affections of the nervous system and the presence of any local lesion would exclude them from the class. His classification of the neuroses into different orders is summarised in Table 5.1, where we see some disorders which belong to modern neurology (convulsions, paralysis, etc.) and some to modern psychiatry (hysteria, melancholia, etc.).

Table 5.1 Classification of neuroses (William Cullen 1777)

Comata e.g. apoplexy, paralysis
Adynamiae e.g. syncope, hypochondriasis
Spasmi e.g. convulsions, chorea, hysteria, tetany
Vesaniae e.g. melancholia, mania, impaired judgement

The concept of neuroses was taken up in France by Pinel (1725–1826) who translated Cullen's textbook. Pinel is better remembered today for his humanitarian than his nosological contributions, but the latter were very influential, coinciding as they did with the postrevolutionary development of the French clinicoanatomical method. He, too, described neuroses as alterations of sensitivity and motility which are not accompanied by fever, inflammation and structural lesion (Pinel 1798). His classification of the neuroses is summarised in Table 5.2 and, like Cullen's nosology, contains

Table 5.2 Classification of neuroses (Philippe Pinel 1798)

Neuroses of the senses .e.g. amaurosis, diplopia, deafness, tinnitus
Neuroses of cerebral function e.g. coma, hypochondria, amentia, catalepsy, melancholia, mania, hydrophobia
Neuroses of locomotion and voice e.g. convulsions, chorea, palsy, tetanus, aphonia
Neuroses of nutrition e.g. dyspepsia, asthma, palpitations, colic, anorexia
Neuroses of sexual function e.g. priapism, hysteria

a mixture of modern neurology and psychiatry, as well as some general medical disorders undoubtedly influenced by the nervous system. The clinico-anatomical method set limits to what could be included under the class neurosis. As the discovery of any structural lesion by definition excluded a disorder from this category, the stage was now set for the systematic contraction of the neuroses. More and more disorders were eliminated by the progressive triumphs of French and other European neuropathologists and cerebral localisers throughout the 19th century, culminating in the great achievements of Charcot (1825–93) at the Salpêtrière. At the same time rearrangements of the classification of the neuroses on anatomical principles were introduced, such as that of Jaccoud (1872) (Table 5.3). The point remained, however, that these were all functional disorders of the nervous system for which there was no known structural pathology. If structural pathology was discovered in a neurosis it was either reclassified or sometimes a certain ambiguity crept in with the use of such phrases as 'symptomatic neurosis', e.g. idiopathic and 'symptomatic' epilepsy.

Table 5.3 Classification of neuroses (Sigismond Jaccoud 1872)

Brain neuroses e.g. mental diseases
Cerebrospinal neuroses e.g. epilepsy, hysteria, catalepsy
Brainstem neuroses e.g. chorea, tetanus, paralysis agitans
Peripheral neuroses e.g. anaesthesias, neuralgias, hyperkinesias

The same forces in the 19th century which were leading to the contraction of the neuroses were also leading to the growth of neurology as an independent scientifically based discipline. Thus the first textbook of neurology from Germany by Romberg, which appeared in parts between 1840 and 1846, was based on physiological or functional principles. There were no illustrations and no pathological classifications. Romberg owed a debt to Cullen. Nervous diseases were classified into two main divisions: neuroses of sensitivity and neuroses of motility. However, by the end of the century neurological textbooks were firmly rooted in the new anatomy and pathology and to a much smaller extent on physiological principles, i.e. on structure rather than function. For example, Gowers' *Manual of Diseases of the Nervous System* published in 1886 illustrates the many new neurological diseases that had been discovered and classified on the basis of the new principles of neuropathology and localisation of function. The new neurophysiology was, however, of a rather static kind with lesions interrupting activities or pathways, with fixed functions. Neurological textbooks, such as Gowers, still included functional disorders (i.e. neuroses), but exemplified the great reduction that had taken place in the number of neuroses of sensation and motility since Cullen, Pinel and Romberg.

Before turning to parallel developments in 19th century psychiatry, it is appropriate to refer to the views of Hughlings Jackson (1835–1911). Although he did not produce a neurological textbook he was very influential both in Britain and abroad. He was greatly admired, for example by Charcot, who introduced the term Jacksonian epilepsy. He accepted that some disorders of the nervous system were functional, i.e. neuroses, including some insanities, which he linked to current evolutionary theories, proposing the concept of dissolution of nervous system function. However, his view of functional neurological disorder had another unique quality. Jackson recognised two kinds of abnormal function. As the normal function of nerve tissue was to 'store up and expend force' so abnormal function could be either 1) loss of function (i.e. reduced or absent storage and expenditure), or 2) overfunction (i.e. increased storage and expenditure), the latter also contributing to *instability* of function. The former could lead to palsies and anaesthesias, the latter to epilepsies, chorea and tetanus, for example. He believed that both had a pathological basis. However, although the 'destroying lesions' responsible for the former were usually readily enough apparent to the pathologist, this was often not the case for his 'discharging lesions', for which he had to invoke 'morbid nutrition', e.g. in idiopathic epilepsy. Jackson emphasised that he was not using the word functional in the conventional 19th century way of 'absence of or undetected brain pathology' (Jackson 1873).

Just as the number of neurological neuroses, i.e. functional disorders of the nervous system, was diminishing towards the end of the 19th century, a wholly new concept of the neuroses arose in the evolving discipline of psychiatry. Psychiatry has a longer history than neurology as Denis Hill (1964) (see Ch. 3), among many others, has described. In the 19th century the medical profession and humanitarians came together to throw off the earlier grip of theologians, philosophers, moralists and public prosecutors, the era of psychiatry without doctors. The main medical groupings were the alienists in charge of new mental institutions and the neuropsychiatrists in the tradition of Willis, Sydenham, Cullen and Pinel. Especially prominent throughout the 19th century were the German and Austrian schools of neuropsychiatry, illustrated by Griesinger (1817–68), a contemporary of Romberg in Berlin, and Meynert (1833–92) in Vienna. For them mental diseases were brain diseases. Meynert (1884) subtitled his psychiatric text book 'Diseases of the forebrain'. Neurosyphilis and general paralysis of the insane (GPI) was the model. The French clinicoanatomical method was applied as vigorously to mental diseases as it was being applied to neurological diseases, although with less satisfactory results. Kraepelin (1856–1925), whose nosology has been so influential in 20th century psychiatry, belonged to this tradition, and so did Freud (1856–1939). Freud was well grounded in the new neuroanatomy, neuropathology and neurology, but he found these an incomplete explanation of the clinical phenomena he was observing, as his studies on aphasia made clear (Freud 1891). As a young man he spent several months of 1885–1886 at the Salpêtrière in Paris where he was greatly influenced by the famous Charcot, some of whose works he translated into German. Charcot was coming to the end of his distinguished career and was now studying hysteria and hypnosis, which led him to suspect the presence of subconscious and psychological mechanisms. Once again hysteria was to have a profound effect on the history of neurology and psychiatry. On his return to Vienna Freud became more interested, not so much in how his patients spoke, but in what they said! With his and other discoveries of the unconscious the subjective became the province of the new psychiatry. Previously the neuropsychiatrists had studied the objective behaviour of their patients and tried to relate their clinical findings to brain mechanisms in terms of anatomy, pathology and physiology. Now the field of study was patients' feelings, motives, beliefs and interpersonal relationships; instead of brain disease, disorder of the psychic apparatus, to be understood and explained in relation to the new disciplines of psychoanalysis, psychology and sociology. Thus was born 20th century dynamic psychiatry, which for the most part has tended to dominate 20th century neuropsychiatry. This is illustrated by what has happened to the neuroses. With Freud and the dynamic psychiatrists appeared a whole new range of disorder and meaning — the PSYCHOneuroses, i.e. anxiety neurosis, obsessional neurosis, depressive neurosis, etc. No longer disorders of sensation and motility to be understood on the basis of disturbance in nervous system physiology, but a disorder of the psychic apparatus to be interpreted in terms of unconscious motivation or maladaption to psychological or social pressures or conflicts. Thus the words 'neurosis' and 'functional' were taken over by the dynamic psychiatrists with a new meaning. The growing numbers of neurologists and diminishing numbers of neuropsychiatrists were left with the word organic.

In retrospect it is surprising that neurologists allowed psychiatrists to hijack the words neurosis and functional and invest them with new meaning, without a protest. Perhaps they felt that the flourishing and successful discipline of neurology could do without them. After all, most of the neurological neuroses of Cullen, Pinel and Romberg had evaporated by the end of the 19th century as a result of the successful application of the clinicoanatomical method, which reclassified them as neurological diseases with a recognisable neuropathology. Perhaps they felt that the remaining neuroses would eventually succumb to the same relentless process, or if not, psychiatrists might as well have them anyway! If so, they may have been mistaken. At least one outstanding 20th century neurologist implied so.

Kinnier Wilson (1878–1937) is distinguished, among other reasons, for the discovery of the disease which bears his name and for his textbook of neurology which was published in two volumes in 1940 after his death. He was the last British neurologist to include a section on 'the neuroses' in a textbook of neurology (Table 5.4). In keeping with 19th century neurological tradition, he recognised motor, sensory, reflex, and psychoneuroses. Although he does not discuss psychoneuroses, as these belong to psychiatry, he does protest that 'to equate "psychoneurosis" and neurosis is to take a

Table 5.4 Classification of neuroses (Kinnier Wilson 1940)

Motor neuroses	e.g. tics, rhythmias, myospasms, myotonia, torticollis, occupational
Sensory neuroses	e.g. neuralgias (e.g. trigeminal), causalgia, acroparaesthaesias
Reflex neuroses	e.g. eneuresis, retention
Psychoneuroses	e.g. obsessional, anxiety

part for the whole'. He goes on to maintain that 'no radical distinction can exist between a "neurosis" and any other type of nervous syndrome. In theory and by etymology it should denote disturbance of the intrinsic function of nerve tissue'.

Kinnier Wilson understood that current neurological opinion took the word neurosis to signify a disorder of nervous function for which, as yet, no underlying structural basis had been found. However, he pointed out that 'molecular change must accompany all reactions whether those of a neurosis or of structural disease and, if on the one hand it induces lesions that can be seen and in the other not, no fundamental separation between them is thereby affected. He argues persuasively for the retention of the words neurosis and functional in the neurological camp. For him neurological symptoms, whether in the presence of structural disease or not, exhibit a dynamic quality which can only be explained by a dynamic neurophysiology, a functional disturbance in the nervous system which owes something to Jackson's views, as well as newer concepts of excitation and inhibition. Psychiatrists can have their psychoneuroses and explain them as they wish, but if they take over the words neurosis and functional completely then presumably new words would have to be invented to describe the disturbances in nervous system function observed and treated by neurologists. He would have been disappointed to learn that the antithesis between 'organic' and 'functional', which he regarded as false, is even more deeply rooted today, as Trimble (1982) has also deplored.

THE PRESENT SCENE

In the preceding section I have described how two processes in particular led to the progressive evolution of neurology and psychiatry as distinct independent disciplines. On the one hand, in the 19th century the triumphs of neuropathology and the clinicoanatomical method culminated in the progressive replacement of the earlier functional neurology, i.e. disorders of sensation and motion, by a structurally based discipline associated with a rather fixed functional localisation. On the other hand, in the late 19th century and for most of this century the evolution of dynamic psychiatry took with it the concepts of functional disorder and neuroses (nervous diseases) and gave them a new meaning within the conceptual framework of a psychic apparatus either separated from or only obscurely linked to the nervous system. Two consequences of these developments have been that 1) psychiatry has tended to split into two camps with its neuropsychiatric wing having common roots and links with neurology, and 2) neurologists have tended either to overlook those complex disorders of function in the nervous system, which did not seem to fit into their more simplified views of functional localisation, or even to pass them off as in some way 'psychiatric'.

Two modern trends highlight the difficulties posed by a predominantly organic, structurally based and functionally localised neurology and a predominantly 'functionally' based psychiatry: 1) in neurology there is growing evidence that the disorders of function in the nervous system associated with structural disease, or even unassociated with structural disease, are much more complex and dynamic than hitherto understood, 2) in psychiatry the discovery of structural lesions by modern imaging techniques are proving very difficult to integrate into 'functional' disorders.

DISORDER OF FUNCTION IN NEUROLOGY

Excitability of the cerebral cortex

Function within the nervous system is achieved by 'transient electrical potentials travelling the fibres of the nervous system' (Sherrington 1941). Some insight into the functioning of the human cerebral cortex in health and disease was gained by Penfield's studies of cortical stimulation in patients with epilepsy undergoing evaluation for surgery (Penfield 1958, Penfield & Jasper 1954). He showed that functional activity in the cortex was not simple, repeatable and fixed but complex, variable and *dynamic*. As in animals, functional localisation does not exist in 'centres' or 'points' but in areas and patterns that extend into various regions of the brain. Although the order of cortical representation of function across, for example, the motor or sensory cortex may be consistent from patient to patient, the site and size of representation may not only vary between patients but even within patients at successive explorations. As also noted by Grunbaum & Sherrington (1901, 1903) in anthropoids there are considerable spontaneous variations in cortical stimulability. Some variation is due to the phenomena of either facilitation or extinction, depending on the time interval between successive stimulations. However, the character and intensity of a response are also influenced by antecedent stimulation of adjacent points, implying that response will vary with the internal or external environment. Instability of response is a characteristic of the human cortex (Penfield and Welch 1949). A motor or sensory response can be displaced into a previously unresponsive territory by advancing stimulations. Sometimes motor responses can be elicited from the sensory cortex or sensory responses from the motor cortex.

Seizure discharges often sensitise the cortex ('epileptic sensitisation') so that evidence of the functional activity of a particular area may be elicited by electrical stimulation, where usually no response would be found. For example, the temporal cortex, which ordinarily gives no psychical response to stimulation may, in the case of an epileptic patient, produce hallucinations or illusions, but only when that part of the cortex has been the seat of epileptic discharges. This activation does not necessarily apply only to patterns of response which appear in the patients' seizures, but can involve neighbouring elements of the cortex and other patterns of response. On other occasions after a seizure the cortex may be in a refractory state and this may be associated with displacement of responses to other areas of cortex. Depression of stimulability of one area may be associated with hyperstimulability of another area.

Disorder of function in epilepsy

The study of epileptic patients provides other evidence of dynamic disorder of function in neurological disease. Even in the presence of an obvious cerebral lesion it has to be asked why seizures occur in some patients, but not in others, and why seizures occur in an individual patient at particular times and not at other times? It is often apparent that provocative factors, especially of a sensory or emotional kind, are playing a triggering role. Sometimes it is the summation of several factors that triggers an individual attack: anything that may increase the instability around Jackson's 'discharging lesion', e.g. change in level of alertness or sleep, physical or emotional stress or fluctuation in hormonal pattern associated with menstruation, may precipitate a seizure.

Other considerations relating to the effects of individual seizures on brain function may also be important. It is apparent that most epileptic patients are well controlled on treatment or go into spontaneous remission (Reynolds et al 1983). About one-quarter, however, go on to develop chronic epilepsy apparently resistant to currently available medication. How does this come about? Certain factors increase the risk of chronic epilepsy with a poor prognosis, such as brain damage, neurological, psychological and social handicaps. In addition, the longer seizures continue after the start of treatment the less likely they are to go into remission (Elwes et al 1984). This is in keeping with Gowers' (1881) hypothesis that seizures beget further seizures, that each seizure may increase the predisposition to the next one. The natural history of untreated epilepsy is largely unknown, but in a retrospective study of new referrals with between two and five untreated tonic-clonic seizures it was remarkable that, in most patients, the time interval between successive seizures was shortening, suggesting that processes were going on in the brain leading to an escalation of epilepsy (Elwes et al 1988). All this suggests that early effective treatment may be important to prevent the evolution of chronic epilepsy (Reynolds 1987). Epilepsy should perhaps be viewed not as a random succession of seizures but as a process — a process in which important events occur in the brain in between seizures and in which the early course of the disease influences the later prognosis (Reynolds et al 1983, Shorvon & Reynolds 1986). It should clearly be understood that there are processes in the brain which lead to *remission* of epilepsy as well as escalation of the disorder.

Kindling

An experimental model which is to some extent relevant to Gowers' view of seizures begetting seizures and Penfield's observations on 'epileptic sensitisation' of the cortex, is that of kindling (Goddard 1967, Wada 1976, 1981). In this model the repeated application of subthreshold electrical or chemical stimuli produces a progressive increase in convulsive response eventually culminating in a seizure. The subsequent application of a single subthreshold stimulus will again evoke a seizure. Eventually chronic seizures can be produced *without evidence of tissue damage*. There are variations in the model depending on the species, the nature of the stimulus and the area of the brain to which it is applied, but a central feature is that every one of the stimuli are necessary to kindle the seizure, provided they are applied at sufficient intervals of time. In other words each stimulus leaves its mark on the brain, but the nature of this mark has so far eluded detection. If a subthreshold stimulus can change brain function, why not a seizure itself? Indeed it is certain that some functional change takes place as evidenced by the clinical effect of convulsive therapy in depression.

The mirror focus

Another model which remarkably illustrates the remote functional effects of a structural lesion in the brain is the mirror focus (Morrell 1969). The mirror focus is a new epileptogenic focus in an area of brain contralateral and homotopic to an original focus. The secondary focus is induced by and can become completely independent of the original epileptogenic focus. Again the time scale of the phenomenon varies in different species and is longest in man. Morrell (1985) has marshalled the evidence, derived from studies of patients evaluated and treated surgically for unilateral temporal lobe lesions, that the phenomenon occurs in man. Successful temporal lobectomy may be undertaken in patients with a unilateral structural lesion despite bitemporal epileptogenic EEG discharges if the contralateral discharges have not yet become independent.

The influence of environment and social factors on cerebral activity and structure

Aggressive behaviour can be studied in animals by means of electrical stimulation of cerebral activity. Offensive-defensive reactions have been related to many subcortical structures, extending almost continuously from forebrain to brain-stem and involving ventral septum, preoptic area, amygdala, stria terminalis, anterior and posterior hypothalamus, posteroventral nucleus of the thalamus, tectal area, central gray, reticular substance and spinothalamic tract (Delgado 1967). There is, however, much that is uncertain in the anatomical and functional relationships of these various areas. Furthermore, many of the studies have been in lower animals in restrained (e.g. caged) situations and without regard to social situations. Delgado (1967) and Delgado & Mir (1969) have overcome many of these limitations by studying monkeys equipped with intracerebral electrodes in whom stimulation was achieved by means of radio stimulators. The animals formed part of an established colony with three or four other monkeys, so that individual and group behaviour could be studied in various free-ranging and social situations. The full pattern of well organised, purposefully orientated aggression, adapted to changes in the environment and related to the animals past experience, was evoked by stimulation of the nucleus ventralis posterolateralis of the thalamus and the pedunculus cerebellaris medius. Of particular interest is that this full effect was only evident when the social rank of the stimulated monkey was high and disappeared when the animal was in a subordinate position. Thus,when a monkey's social status was low, brain stimulation induced only increased motor activity and occasional threats, which provoked attacks against it. As social rank improved stimulated attacks against other animals increased. The effect of stimulation of the same cerebral point therefore differed in degree and had opposite social consequences, depending on hierarchical position. Like the studies of epilepsy previously described, these findings indicate that functional representation in the brain should not be expressed in absolute terms, but cerebral activity is in a dynamic state modified by environmental and social inputs.

Environmental factors not only modify the function of the brain but may also alter its *structure*. The infant or immature brain is especially vulnerable to such modification. Experimental studies have shown that early loss of visual stimulation in one eye, or disruption of the usual binocular stimulation, will lead to permanent change in the architecture of the occipital cortex (Wiesel & Hubel 1965, Blakemore & Cooper 1970). The clinical counterpart is the child with uncorrected strabismus. To avoid diplopia, visual impulses from the weak eye are suppressed and permanent blindness develops. This does not happen in the adult or mature nervous system. Similar effects of sensory deprivation have been described in other areas of the brain, and conversely an enriched and stimulating environment enhances the branching of cortical dendrites and the development of dendritic spines (Bennett et al 1964, Volkmar & Greenough 1972). These observations are probably relevant to the effects of early emotional and social deprivation on later mental health and behaviour, as illustrated in the early infant deprivation studies in monkeys (Harlow et al 1971) and the behavioural imprinting investigations of ethologists (Lorenz 1970).

The neurological examples described above illustrate that whether or not structural disease is present, disorder of function in the nervous system is much more complex and dynamic than is usually envisaged by such phrases as 'functional localisation'. In particular, cerebral activity, whether local or more general is influenced by a wide range of internal and external factors, including psychological and social influences. Especially in the less mature nervous system prolonged disturbance of function may even lead to changes in structure.

STRUCTURAL DISEASE IN PSYCHIATRY

CT scanning in schizophrenia

There is no doubt that in the last decade there has been a remarkable rekindling of interest in structural brain disease in psychiatric disorders, stimulated by the development of non-invasive, increasingly sophisticated imaging techniques. Most attention has focussed on schizophrenia, especially the chronic disease. Since the report by Johnstone et al (1976) many CT scan studies have confirmed significant lateral ventricle enlargement and increased ventricle to brain ratio (VBR) in chronic schizophrenia compared to various control groups (Reveley 1985 and Ch. 15, Owens et al 1985), so much so that Farmer et al (1987) felt able to say that this finding 'may now be regarded as probably the most replicable biological feature which investigations of the condition have yet revealed'. Even so, doubts and uncertainties remain. Not all studies have confirmed the finding. Smith & Iacono (1986) have compared the data in 14 positive studies and 7 negative studies. The VBR was much the same in the schizophrenic patients in all the studies, but the VBR was significantly lower in the control groups from the positive studies than in the controls from the negative studies. They concluded that the differences between the studies had more to do with the choice of controls than schizophrenic patients. Owen & Lewis (1986) have also analysed the choice of controls and suggest that some differences between control values can be accounted for by the fact that sometimes patients with conditions known to be associated with ventricular enlargement have been used, whereas in others there has been a selection bias against controls with large ventricles. Even if it is accepted that the association of ventricular enlargement with schizophrenia is a reliable finding it is certain that it is not specific for the disorder as similar observations have been reported in manic-depressive illness (Pearlson & Veroff 1981, Standish-Barry et al 1982).

The significance of ventricular enlargement in schizophrenia is an even more contentious issue. At first it was suggested that ventricular enlargement might be related to cognitive impairment ('the dementia of dementia praecox') or the 'negative' clinical features of a 'type 2' syndrome (Johnstone et al 1978; Crow 1980) but subsequent studies have not supported this hypothesis (Owens et al 1985; Kalakowska et al 1985; Farmer et al 1987). Others have suggested a relationship to different clinical subtypes, e.g. paranoid schizophrenia (Nasrallah et al 1982), but again this has not been confirmed (Farmer et al 1987). The latter authors reported an association with Schneider's first-rank symptoms and a complex relationship with Feighner diagnostic categories. Several studies have examined the relationship between enlarged ventricles and the genetic background of schizophrenia. Reveley et al (1982, 1984) reported that, in monozygotic twins discordant for schizophrenia, the schizophrenic probands had significantly larger ventricles than the unaffected control twins. Furthermore, large ventricles were associated with the absence of a family history of 'psychiatric disorder'. The authors therefore suggest that schizophrenia can be categorised into a familial form with normal ventricles and a presumed genetic aetiology, and a non-genetic form associated with enlarged ventricles due to environmental insults to the brain. However several non-twin studies have cast doubt on the proposed inverse relationship between enlarged ventricles and a positive family history of schizophrenia (Nasrallah et al 1982, Owens et al 1985, De Lisi et al 1986, Farmer et al 1987). This issue is discussed by Reveley in Chapter 15, who points out that such a relationship is more likely to be revealed in twin studies.

Other uncertainties remain. Do the reported CT abnormalites antedate or postdate the onset of schizophrenia? Are they static or do they evolve in parallel with the clinical picture? Do they predispose to schizophrenia? Are they an intrinsic aspect of the disorder or are they the result of schizophrenia and its treatment? Such questions can only be clarified in the light of longitudinal imaging studies over many years, which have not yet been adequately undertaken (Nasrallah et al 1986). Do patients with CT abnormalities represent a subgroup with so-called organic as opposed to 'functional' schizophrenia? Kalakowska et al (1985) looked specifically at indices of 'organic dysfunction' in schizophrenia and found no correlation even between the indices themselves, i.e. enlarged ventricles, cognitive impairment and 'soft' neurological signs. Neurological signs were related to a history of developmental abnormalities, cognitive impairment to higher doses of current medication, and large ventricles to neither of these variables. This suggested that the three signs may be determined by different sets of factors. Furthermore there were no clinical differences between those with and without organic signs, but only evidence of a more unfavourable outcome in the latter (Williams et al 1985).

Where in the brain is schizophrenia?

In addition to the more general and widespread abnormalities suggested by the CT findings discussed above, many other studies of a structural (CT, MRI, neuropathology) or functional (cerebral blood flow, psychometry, evoked potentials, PET and SPECT) kind have focussed interest on specific brain regions as the site of the lesion or dysfunction in schizophrenia, e.g. the frontal lobes, the temporal lobes and limbic system, the left hemisphere, the basal ganglia, the corpus callosum, the hypothalamus, diencephalon and even the cerebellum. Much of this is discussed by Reveley in Chapter 15 and in the monograph edited by Andreasen (1986) and need not be repeated here. Indeed we are in the midst of an explosion of interest in studies of this type. It seems that many authors regard the seat of the lesion or dysfunction in this disorder as one of the several sites described above on which they have focussed their attention and investigations. By way of illustration Weinberger et al (1986) and Berman et al (1986) have summarised their own and other evidence implicating the frontal lobes in schizophrenia and suggesting a physiological dysfunction of the dorsolateral prefrontal cortex to account for both the 'negative' and 'positive' features of the disease. A recent MRI study is said to be in keeping with the 'hypofrontality hypothesis' (Andreasen et al 1986).

The number and variety of attempts to localise schizophrenia in this or that region of the brain emphasises their implausibility, which stretches the credulity of a neurologist, who is used to seeing many patients with lesions in the incriminated regions of the brain without schizophrenia. These attempts to localize schizophrenia are in part based on what some psychiatrists view as a rediscovery of the writings and wisdom of 19th century neurologists with their emphasis on functional localisation. This renewal of interest in localized function in psychiatric disorders is sometimes referred to, especially in the USA, as behavioural neurology (Pincus & Tucker 1985). However, as I have illustrated in the preceding section, disorder of function in the nervous system is now seen to be much more complex and dynamic than envisaged by even these great 19th century pioneers. For example, I have described the many different areas of the brain which may be involved in the relatively circumscribed function of aggression or offensive-defensive reactions. Is it conceivable that the complex disorders of neurological/psychological function which occur in schizophrenia can be understood in terms of only one system such as the dorsolateral prefrontal cortex? It is probably much more complex and subtle than that.

CONCLUSIONS

In this chapter I have described the historical evolution of neurology from a wholly functionally based discipline to one which is now widely viewed as structurally and organically based and associated with concepts of functional localisation. At the same time the evolution of psychiatry as a separate discipline has taken with it the word functional and converted it into a psychological concept, the very antithesis of organic, with neuropsychiatry sitting somewhat uneasily in the middle. Two modern developments suggest the possibility of reconciling these logically confusing, if practically convenient, diverging trends in neurology and psychiatry.

The current widely held view that neurology is wholly organic and somehow synonymous with structural disease of the nervous system is fallacious. Neurological patients have complex dynamic disorders of function in the nervous system, whether or not they have structural disease. These disorders of function cannot be understood wholly in terms of oversimplified notions of functional localisation. A single structural lesion may have remote functional effects far from the pathological site. Cerebral function is profoundly influenced by psychological and social factors.

In psychiatry the renewed interest in and discoveries of cerebral pathology with modern imaging techniques are proving difficult to integrate because they are being inappropriately linked to outdated 19th century concepts of functional localisation. It is very doubtful that the complex clinical disorders of function which occur in schizophrenia, for example, can be linked to a lesion or dysfunction at a single site in the nervous system. Nor need it be expected, as seems to be a common view, that such hypothetical lesions or dysfunctions will be found in all cases of schizophrenia. Like epilepsy, schizophrenia may or may not be associated with cerebral pathology which may sometimes influence the course and prognosis. This need not lead to separate categories of organic and functional in the psychological sense. Both, however, remain functional disorders of the nervous system (neuroses) in the older neurophysiological sense of the word, whether or not detectable pathology is present. Both are influenced by psychological and social factors. Why should one (epilepsy) be viewed as organic and the other (schizophrenia) as functional? Nor is the answer to reclassify schizophrenia as organic as some demand. Psychiatrists might profitably spend less time taking sides in inappropriate conflicts between false dichotomies, and neurologists might profitably spend more time studying the influence of psychological and social factors on brain function and on their patients' disabilities.

In the 18th and 19th centuries neurology was conceived in terms of disorders of 'sensation and motion', i.e. a functional discipline. The difficulty at that time, for many historical reasons, was to know where to place disorders of the 'mind' in this scheme of things. In the event they were split into 'neuropsychiatry' and 'psychodynamic psychiatry' (Hill 1964). It is not difficult today to envisage the mind with its varied activities (attention, memory, mood, etc.) as a function of the brain, like sensation and motion. This in no way undermines the importance of psychological, social or psychodynamic factors in either psychiatric or neurological disorders, but it does profoundly alter our conception of both types of disorder and the relationship of the two disciplines.

REFERENCES

Andreasen N C (ed) 1986 Can schizophrenia be localized in the brain? American Psychiatric Press, Washington

Andreasen N, Nasrallah H A, Dunn V et al 1986 Structural abnormalities in the frontal system in schizophrenia: a magnetic resonance imaging study. Archives of General Psychiatry 43: 136–144

Bennett E, Diamond M C, Krech D, Rosenzweig M R 1964 Chemical and anatomic plasticity of the brain. Science 146: 610–619

Berman K F, Zec R F, Weinberger D R 1986 Physiologic dysfunction of dorsolateral prefrontal cortex in schizophrenia. II. Role of neuroleptic treatment, attention, and mental effort. Archives of General Psychiatry 43: 126–135

Blakemore C, Cooper G F 1970 Development of the brain depends on the visual environment. Nature 228: 477–478

Cheyne G 1733 The English malady: or, a treatise of nervous diseases of all kinds, as spleen, vapours, lowness of spirits, hypochondriacal and hysterical distempers. Strahan and Leake, London

Crow T J 1980 Molecular pathology of schizophrenia: more than one disease process. British Medical Journal 280: 66–68

Cullen W 1769 Apparatus ad Nosologiam Methodicam, seu synopsis nosologiae methodicae in usum studiosorum. Edinburgh

Cullen W 1777 First lines of the practice of physic. Creech, Edinburgh

Delgado J M R 1967 Aggression and defense under cerebral radio control. In: Clemente C D, Lindsley, D (eds) Aggression and defense, neural mechanisms and social patterns. UCLA forum in Medical Science, no 7, vol V. University of California Press, Berkeley, p 171–193

Delgado J M R, Mir D 1969 Fragmental organization of emotional behavior in the monkey brain. Annals of New York Academy of Science 159: 731–751

DeLisi L E, Goldin L R, Hamovit J R, Maxwell E, Kurtz D, Gershon E S 1986 A family study of the association of increased ventricular size with schizophrenia. Archives of General Psychiatry 43: 148–153

Elwes R D C, Johnson A L. Shorvon S D, Reynolds E H 1984 The prognosis for seizure control in newly diagnosed epilepsy. The New England Journal of Medicine 311: 944–947

Elwes R D C, Johnson A L, Reynolds E H 1988 The course of untreated epilepsy. British Medical Journal 297: 948–950

Farmer A, Jackson R. McGuffin P, Storey P 1987 Cerebral ventricular enlargement in chronic schizophrenia: Consistencies and contradictions. British Journal of Psychiatry 150: 324–330

Freud S 1891 Zur Auffassung der Aphasien. Wien (Authorised translation with an introduction by E. Stengel. Imago Publishing Company, London 1953)

Goddard G V 1967 Development of epileptic seizures through brain stimulation at low intensity. Nature 214: 1020–1021

Gowers W R 1881 Epilepsy and other chronic convulsive disorders: their causes, symptoms and treatment. Churchill, London

Gowers W R 1886 Manual of disorders of the nervous system, 2 vol. Churchill, London

Grunbaum A S F, Sherrington C S 1901 Observations on physiology of the cerebral cortex of some of the higher apes. Proceedings of the Royal Society, London 69: 206

Grunbaum A S F, Sherrington C S 1903 Observations on physiology of the cerebral cortex of anthropoid apes. Proceedings of the Royal Society, London 72: 152

Harlow H F, Harlow M K, Suomi S J 1971 From thought to therapy; lessons from a primate laboratory. How investigation of the learning capability of rhesus monkeys has led to the study of their behavioral abnormalities and rehabilitation. American Science 59: 538–549

Hill D 1964 The bridge between neurology and psychiatry. Lancet i: 509–514

Jaccoud S 1872 Traité de Pathologie Interne, 2nd edn, 2 vols. Delahaye, Paris

Jackson H J 1873 On the anatomical, physiological, and pathological investigation of epilepsies. Reports of the West Riding Lunatic Asylum 3: 315–339

Johnstone E C, Crow T J, Frith C D, Husband J, Kreel L 1976 Cerebral ventricular size and cognitive impairment in chronic schizophrenia. Lancet ii: 924–926

Johnstone E C, Crow T J, Frith C D, Stevens M, Kreel L, Husband J 1978 The dementia of dementia praecox. Acta Psychiatrica Scandinavica 57: 305–324

Kalakowska T, Williams A O, Ardern M et al 1985 Schizophrenia with good and poor outcome. 1: Early clinical features, response to neuroleptics and signs of organic dysfunction. British Journal of Psychiatry 146: 229–246

Kinnier Wilson S A 1940 Neurology, 2 vols. Arnold, London

Lishman A W 1978 Organic psychiatry: the psychological consequences of cerebral disorder. Blackwell Scientific Publications, Oxford

López-Piñero J M 1983 Historical origins of the concept of neurosis (translated by D Berrios). Cambridge University Press, Cambridge

Lorenz K 1970 Studies in animal and human behaviour, vol 1 (translated by Robert Martin). Methuen, London

Meynert T 1884 Psychiatrie: klinic der erkrankungen def vorderhirns. W Braumüller, Vienna

Morrell F 1969 Physiology and histochemistry of the mirror focus. In: Jasper H H, Ward A A, Pope A (eds) Basic mechanisms of the epilepsies. Little Brown, Boston, p 357–370

Morrell F 1985 Secondary epileptogenesis in man. Archives of Neurology 42: 318–335

Nasrallah H A, Jacoby C G, McCalley-Whitters M, Kuperman S 1982 Cerebral ventricular enlargement in subtypes of chronic schizophrenia. Archives of General Psychiatry 39: 774–777

Nasrallah H A, Olson S C, McCalley-Withers M, Chapman S, Jacoby C G 1986 Cerebral ventricular enlargment in schizophrenia. Archives of General Psychiatry 43: 157–159

Owen M J, Lewis S W 1986 Lateral ventricular size in schizophrenia. Lancet ii: 223–224

Owens D G C, Johnstone E C, Crow T J, Frith C D, Jagoe J R, Kreel L 1985 Lateral ventricular size in schizophrenia; relationship to the disease process and its clinical manifestations. Psychological Medicine 15: 27–41

Pearlson G D, Veroff A E 1981 Computerised tomographic scan changes in manic depressive illness. Lancet ii: 470

Penfield W 1958 The excitable cortex in conscious man. The Sherrington lectures. Liverpool University Press. Liverpool

Penfield W, Welch K 1949 Instability of response to stimulation of the sensorimotor cortex of man. Journal of Physiology 109: 358–365

Penfield W, Jasper H 1954 Epilepsy and the functional anatomy of the human brain. Churchill, London

Pincus J H, Tucker G J 1985 Behavioral neurology. Oxford University Press, Oxford

Pinel P 1798 Nosographie philosophique, ou la methode de l'analyse appliquée a la médicine. Brosson, Paris

Romberg M H 1840–1846 Lehrbuch der nervenkrankheiten des menschen. 2 vols. Duncker, Berlin

Reveley M A 1985 Ventricular enlargement in schizophrenia: The validity of computerised tomographic findings. British Journal of Psychiatry 147: 233–240

Reveley A M, Reveley M A, Clifford C A, Murray R M 1982 Cerebral ventricular size in twins discordant for schizophrenia. Lancet i: 540–541

Reveley A M, Reveley M A, Murray R M 1984 Cerebral ventricular enlargement in nongenetic schizophrenia; A controlled twin study. British Journal of Psychiatry 144: 89–93

Reynolds E H 1987 Early treatment and prognosis of epilepsy. Epilepsia 28: 97–106

Reynolds E H, Elwes R D C, Shorvon S D 1983 Why does epilepsy become intractable? Prevention of chronic epilepsy Lancet ii: 952–954

Sherrington C S 1941 Man on his nature. The Gifford lectures, Edinburgh 1937–38. Cambridge University Press, Cambridge

Shorvon S D, Reynolds E H 1986 The nature of epilepsy: evidence from studies of epidemiology, temporal patterns of seizures, prognosis and treatment. In: Trimble M R, Reynolds E H (eds) What is epilepsy? Churchill Livingstone, Edinburgh, p 36–45

Smith G N, Iacono W G 1986 Lateral ventricular size in schizophrenia and choice of control group. Lancet i: 1450

Standish-Barry H M A S, Bouras N, Bridges P K, Bartlett J R 1982 Pneumoencephalographic and computerised axial tomography scan changes in affective disorder. British Journal of Psychiatry 141: 614–617

Trimble M R 1981 Neuropsychiatry. Wiley, Chichester

Trimble M R 1982 Functional diseases. British Medical Journal 285: 1768–1770

Volkmar F R, Greenough W J 1972 Rearing complexity affects branching of dendrites in visual cortex of rats. Science 176: 1445–1447

Wada J A (ed) 1976 Kindling. Raven Press, New York

Wada J A (ed) 1981 Kindling 2. Raven Press, New York

Weinberger D R, Berman K F, Zec R F 1986 Physiologic dysfunction of dorsolateral prefrontal cortex in schizophrenia. I. Regional cerebral blood flow evidence. Archives of General Psychiatry 43: 114–124

Whytt R 1765 Observations on the nature, causes and cure of those disorders which are commonly called nervous, hypochondriac or hysteric. Becket and Du Hondt, Edinburgh

Wiesel T V, Hubel D H 1965 Extent of recovery from the effects of visual deprivation in kittens. Journal of Neurophysiology 28: 1029–1040

Williams A O, Reveley M A, Kolakowska T, Ardern M, Mandelbrote B M 1985 Schizophrenia with good and poor outcome. II. Cerebral ventricular size and its clinical significance. British Journal of Psychiatry 146: 239–246

Willis T 1682 Opera omnia. Wetstenius, Amstelodami

On states of consciousness*

The title of this chapter assumes that there are different states of consciousness, as well as different degrees of it. I make the assumption that there are qualitative differences as well as quantitative ones. To substantiate this I can draw your attention to the differing states of full conscious attention, reverie, dreaming sleep, hypnotic trance and transcendental meditation.

It is necessary that I should describe or define what I mean by consciousness. For centuries, in the hands of philosophers, consciousness was coterminous with Mind with a capital M. Mental events were those events, and only those events, which occurred in consciousness and consciousness was experience. Mental events outside consciousness then by definition could not occur. In this view, logical, purposive, adaptive behaviour was dependent upon consciousness and without it could not occur. The idea that this consciousness was something incorporeal and extracerebral was finally given credence by Descartes (1596–1650) who removed Mind from physiological consideration and put it on the other side of the pineal bridge, unextended in space but extended in time. Mind or consciousness then became the 'ghost in the machine' — the otherwise bodily automaton, to which Gilbert Ryle (1949) took such exception. We now know with some certainty that this is not how things are and that consciousness, at least in many of its aspects, is dependent upon brain mechanisms. This is not of course a final refutation of psychophysical dualism.

In defining what I mean by consciousness, I am following Karl Jaspers (1962) fairly closely. Firstly, consciousness involves awareness of events, and this is a primary irreducible datum of human experience. We are aware of events in the environment and also of events in our minds. Consciousness also involves another awareness, equally irreducible, the awareness of the 'I' or 'me'; this is also a primary datum of experience. To deny it is to deny that one exists — the famous Cartesian 'cogito'. To deny it, as A. J. Ayer is alleged to have said, is to pretend that one is anaesthetised (Armstrong 1968). But this awareness of one's self-hood has been put in various ways.

*Based on the Litchfield lecture given at Oxford, 5 May 1981, and the Sandoz lecture given at Edinburgh, 17 June 1981.

Some would say, with the 18th century philosopher David Hume (1711–76) that the question of a 'substantial' self is highly problematical. For Hume, as for others since his time, the awareness of self is only the awareness or memory of a 'bundle' or collection of past experiences. According to this view, memory of the past is essential to awareness of the self and this is all it is. Is there, however, a situation, perhaps one drawn from medical knowledge, in which there is no memory of the past, but nevertheless awareness of self-identity? Is awareness of the self more than the memory of past experiences?

Introspection tells us that the self is an active, indeed a very active, self — that it has wants and wishes, that it computes and predicts and that it has some degree of freedom of choice. Or so it seems. Many have believed that to follow this argument is to be forced towards dualism. Karl Popper (Popper & Eccles 1977), the most contemporary and distinguished philosopher of neo-Cartesian dualism, put it this way, speaking of self:

> Like a pilot it observes and takes action at the same time. It is acting and suffering, recalling the past and planning and programming the future; expecting and disposing. It contains in quick succession, or all at once, wishes, plans, hopes, decisions to act and a vivid consciousness of being an acting self, a centre of action.

Popper & Eccles (1977) regard consciousness and self-conscious awareness as the highest development yet of biological evolution, the results of natural selection.

The words 'mind' and 'mental events' are now antique, but it is difficult not to use them. If mental events require awareness, then without consciousness they cannot occur. But purposive, logical adaptive behaviour, involving reasoning and choices, does in fact occur in the absence of awareness. Leaving aside for the moment this everyday experience, the well-known experiments of Sperry and his colleagues (Sperry 1966) on patients with total transection of the corpus callosum demonstrated this. In these patients the right non-dominant hemisphere could respond logically to perceptual stimuli, make choices based upon reasoning, indicate thereby the access of the system to memory and perform in fact as an independent brain. Yet, separated from the left dominant hemisphere, none of this activity entered conscious awareness. The self was unaware of what its right hemisphere was doing — which was responding 'as if consciously' to tasks it was given. Consciousness, and consciousness of the self and what it is doing, is somehow tied to the activities of the left dominant cerebral cortex — the one concerned with language.

From an entirely different point of view, it was evident to psychologists and clinicians, long before Freud, that there are human mental activities which are unconscious, of which the individual is unaware, but which nevertheless can profoundly influence behaviour and consciousness. Although still unconscious they are events determined by meaning, reliant on memory, even upon prediction. They are similar in these respects to the work of the separated non-dominant hemisphere investigated by Sperry. They are events which can be described as thinking but without thoughts, for they do not use language which is not available to them.

It was Francis Galton (1907) at the beginning of the century who demonstrated, by experiments upon himself how narrow is the field of consciousness at any one time. To quote him:

> . . . many investigations concur in showing the vast multiplicity of mental operations that are in simultaneous action of which only a minute part falls within the ken of consciousness.
>
> Perhaps the strongest impressions left by these experiments regards the multifariousness of the work done by the mind in a state of half-unconsciousness, and the valid reason they afford for believing in the existence of still deeper strata of mental operations, sunk wholly below the level of consciousness, which may account for such mental phenomena as cannot otherwise be explained.

Galton gave us his famous idea that as he said: 'there seems to be a presence chamber in my mind where full consciousness holds court'. He was referring to what we would now call the focus of attention. The corollary is that awareness is a variable; it is a matter of degree.

I propose to discuss only three of what I regard as fundamental aspects of consciousness. First there is the dimension of vigilance, a readiness to attend. Secondly consciousness involves awareness, not only of the 'here and now', but also of the anticipated future. Thirdly, consciousness also involves awareness of being a 'self' — the 'I' or 'me'. Each of these, vigilance and awareness in its several aspects, is subject to variability — each is a matter of degree and each can operate almost independently of the other two. Later I shall refer to how these elements are disturbed in clinical disorders.

Man ascribes immense importance to awareness of himself, to his sense of continuity and reality. It is evident that the loss of that awareness, or the threat of it, called loss of self-identity, is one of the most frightening experiences there is. A remarkable fact is that this self awareness has a continuity and a sameness which survives sleep, unconsciousness and coma, and the extreme perturbations of cerebral activity which occur in, for example, the epileptic fit.

The self is an elusive entity, pursued by mystics by techniques either to focus down upon the inner reality of personal being, or to try to expand consciousness of self in order to submerge individuality into a hypothesised universal consciousness. This is not my subject, but artists, writers, scientists and philosophers, without mystical aspirations, have shown their belief in the realisation of self as the ultimate goal of the evolutionary process. Bernard Shaw, a reluctant follower of Darwin, believed in a universal life force, which has reached its ultimate expression so far in man. Karl Popper's position is very similar. Shaw, in the famous scene in Hell in the third act of *Man and Superman*, made his hero say:

I tell you that as long as I can conceive something better than myself, I cannot be easy unless I am striving to bring it into existence or clearing the way for it. That is the working within me of Life's incessant aspiration to higher organisation, wider, deeper, intenser self-consciousness and clearer self-understanding.

Shaw paraphrased Freud when he made his hero say:

So far, the result of Life's continual effort not only to maintain itself, but to achieve higher and higher organisation and completer self-consciousness is only at best a doubtful campaign between its forces and those of Death and degeneration.

A NEUROBIOLOGICAL APPROACH

A neurobiological approach to consciousness, awareness and self is that of the French psychiatrist-philosopher Henri Ey. I owe my understanding of his theoretical position largely to Dr Philip Evans who spent four months with Ey, studying his ideas and his writings (Evans 1972). Ey accepted that consciousness is far more than vigilance, a watchfulness of what is going on. It is the basis of relational life between the individual and others. It has a vivid reality, awareness of self, intentionality and some freedom of choice. Consciousness then is an activity related to purpose. But Ey was not a Cartesian dualist and certainly not a behaviourist. For him consciousness is not simply the 'clarity which illuminates psychic life', though to be fully conscious is to be lucid. Consciousness is concerned with organising experience. For Ey, consciousness has two dimensions — the transverse section of conscious existence is the here and now experience of the present; and the longitudinal section, involving awareness of the past which is the personality in its historical construction. Experienced from the inside, it is the self.

Ey developed his so-called organodynamic theory of consciousness from, on the one hand, an acceptance of the evolutionary principles of organisation and disorganisation of the nervous system of Hughlings Jackson, and, on the other, an acceptance of the basic principle of unconscious 'mental' activity of Freud. Following Jackson and Freud he accepted the idea of control of higher levels of organisation over lower levels and the notion of escape of lower levels from control under certain circumstances. Following Freud he accepted that much of 'mental' activity is unconscious, and therefore much of the activity of the self is so.

Moreover, there is an essential opposition between higher and lower levels, between conscious and unconscious activity. Ey considered that repression was Freud's greatest discovery. Based on Jacksonian hierarchical structure, consciousness develops ontogenetically; there is none in the newborn baby. Consciousness gradually develops out of unconscious activity with maturation of the nervous system and the impact of experience, which in course of time provides the phenomenal field of personal life as one knows it — and finally the awareness of being a self, a personal identity. The views of Popper & Eccles (1977) are very similar. To quote Evans (1972):

> A well-balanced field of consciousness exercises a mastery over time and holds at bay an intemporal unconscious which would otherwise drag the present into the fatality of the past, or into the omnipotence of the future. The highest level of organisation of consciousness and its degree of maturity is represented by its power of integrating the present situation. . . . changes in awareness are part of the activity of consciousness . . . pathology begins when this ability is lost.

For Ey then *pathology begins* when the controlling, directing power of full consciousness is lost, the power to maintain order over disorder. For him the unconscious is an automaton with vegetative roots; it is the infrastructure of consciousness, continually threatening it, but controlled by the function of repression.

When pathology occurs, the Jacksonian ideas of disorganisation and decontrol are very similar conceptually to Freud's regression. Jackson emphasised that the higher centres are less rigidly organised than the lower, more complex, less automatic and most voluntary. They are also more vulnerable, being, for example, the first to be affected by alcohol and other toxic substances. We also find in Ey the same mystical assertion as that of Popper, Freud, Shaw and other artistic evolutionists that the highest purpose of man is the development of full consciousness and full awareness of the self with which is associated creativity and originality and, above all, *freedom*, in some degree. The loss of that freedom, or the failure even to develop it, is for Ey the basis of mental disorder.

When it comes, however, to the application of the general theory to therapy, it is evident that there is a marked contrast, indeed an antithesis, between the position of Ey on the one hand and Freud on the other. For Ey, treatment consists of enhancing the power of consciousness over deeper levels of the mind by increasing control over them. In this way, by whatever means are adequate to provide it, freedom is restored or enhanced. I believe this is in accord with much of contemporary psychiatric treatment, whether it be physical or social. On the other hand Freud saw psychoanalytic treatment, even from its earliest beginnings when hypnosis was used or when free-association was developed, as increasing the power and range of consciousness at the expense of the unconscious, by making the latter conscious, by diminishing rather than enhancing repression. 'Where Id was, there shall ego be', he is quoted as saying.

Psychoanalysis, certainly until recent years and certainly in the hands of its founder, was primarily a study of unconscious activity. Freud has little to say about the structure or functions of consciousness, although he regarded them as biological. He regarded consciousness as an 'inner eye', rather similar to vigilance. At the end of his life he wrote that 'the question of the relation of the conscious to the psychical may now be regarded as settled: consciousness is only a *quality* or attitude of what is psychical, and moreover an inconstant one' (Freud 1964). But in the *Outline of Psychoanalysis*, published posthumously (1940), he seems to have contradicted this for he declared (Freud 1966) 'that the starting point of the investigation into the structure of the psychical apparatus is provided by a fact without parallel, which defies all explanation or description, the fact of consciousness'; and he berates behaviourism for trying to construct a psychology which disregards this fundamental fact! His translator, James Strachey, said of this: 'It would be perverse indeed to seek to impute a similar disregard to Freud himself'.

At this point it may be helpful to recapitulate. I am not concerned with the ultimate nature of consciousness, nor with philosophical issues about mind-brain relationships. Nor, although many of the phenomena of consciousness are dependent obviously on neural mechanisms, what the relation is between the activities of neurones and the activities of consciousness. I shall, however, discuss the effects on consciousness which we observe in some neurological and psychiatric disorders and the relation these may have to major brain systems. Having proposed a broad descriptive definition of consciousness as comprising vigilance, awareness and self-awareness, I will now examine in more detail each of these elements.

VIGILANCE

Vigilance is watchfulness, an alertness to potential events; it involves the readiness to attend. In neural terms it is dependent upon a degree, a sufficient but not an excessive degree, of physiological arousal of the cerebral cortex. Excessively aroused, as occurs in panic, vigilance fails, and it does so of course when arousal is severely diminished, as in stupor, and is absent in coma. The neurophysiological basis of vigilance is, on the one hand, tied therefore to the arousal mechanism and, on the other, to whatever mechanism there is for focussing attention and shifting it at a moment's notice. Vigilance is therefore probably maximal around the middle range of the EEG cortical frequency spectrum, that area where the alpha rhythm is at its greatest readiness to respond to stimuli.

Despite the philosopher Kant's warning that mind exists only in time and not in space, many have spoken of a location for consciousness. The last of these is probably the proposal of Popper & Eccles (1977) that it resides in or is closely associated with the cortex of the dominant language hemisphere. But over 20 years ago Wilder Penfield (1957) proposed a centrencephalic centre for consciousness and the evidence for this was that destructive lesions throughout the core of the brain stem, from the pons to the third ventricle resulted in both man and animals in loss of vigilance and unresponsiveness. In man, if the lesion was extensive and in certain parts of the system, coma would be permanent.

The story of the so-called reticular activating system, now so familiar a concept began in 1935 with the work of Frederick Bremer in Brussels, who transected the brain stem of the cat to isolate either the whole brain from the periphery, or to isolate it at the mid-brain level. In the former the cat could be aroused by appropriate stimulation of sensory cranial nerves, at the latter level the animal was permanently non-arousable. The concept of a neural net of great phylogenetic antiquity extending from the pons, ventral to the aqueduct, up to the posterior hypothalamus and thence upwards in the walls of the third ventricle, to be relayed to the cortex by certain non-specific thalamic nuclei has been widely accepted. This system, responsible for arousal, is envisaged as lying between the main sensory and motor pathways, but having intimate association with both and regulating them. This opened the way to better understanding of many normal and pathological phenomena associated with consciousness, and particularly vigilance, sleep, stupor and coma.

Under conditions when lesions affect either the afferent inputs to the reticular system or its onward-going pathways (Walton 1969), vigilance can exist, or appear to exist, in an extremely attenuated form. An example is 'coma-vigil', possibly identical with akinetic mutism in which the patient shows general muscular relaxation as in sleep, is mute and motionless but the eyes are open and watchful. In the famous case of epidermoid cyst of the third ventricle reported by Cairns et al (1941), it was shown that it was pressure on the ventricular walls which produced the condition and aspiration of the cyst relieved it. The eyes of the patient regarded the observer steadily and would follow moving objects and they might be diverted by sound. There was therefore a vestigial capacity for attention. The patient might even answer questions in whispered monosyllables, but there was no spontaneous speech, movement or reaction to pain. Despite the evidence, therefore, that a low level of what is commonly called consciousness existed, there was subsequently a complete and dense amnesia for the duration of the episode. Depressive and catatonic stupor, which bear some resemblances to this condition, may also be followed, according to Joyston-Bechal (1966), by subsequent amnesia in about 50% of cases, although I believe more commonly in the catatonic group.

Jennett & Plum (1972), in describing what they call a 'persistent vegetative state', reported that after severe brain damage from trauma or ischaemia, the patient who will never recover recognisable mental functions, may nevertheless recover from a sleep-like coma in that there are periods of wakefulness when the eyes are open and move. The severe pathology in these cases may be in the cerebral cortex itself, in subcortical structures or in the brain stem, or in all three.

Attention

I will now turn to the subject of attention, the capacity for which is dependent again upon a sufficient degree, but not an excessive degree of arousal, i.e. vigilance. Normally attention proceeds in awareness, but from the work on the bisected brain, attention can occur in the absence of it. Attention may have a wide span in which case there is no focus of concentration, just a general vigilance, ready to focus on this or that; or there is a narrow span when attention is focussed down intensely upon some external event, or some internal event, image or memory, or on to the self itself, to the exclusion of all else. There is also the capacity to shift the focus hither and thither, upon external space, upon the body or upon internal events in the recent or remote past. It is evident that in many mentally ill patients the capacity to focus attention, to shift it or to divert it — say from the self — is impaired or even lost.

Long ago Adrian (1944) postulated that there must be some subcortical central mechanism for these functions and Mountcastle (1978), in his Sherrington lecture, reiterated this view. Nevertheless he produced evidence that, in the case of attention to body parts, the mechanism lies in the parietal cortex and its systems. The awareness of choice of what we shall attend to, the choice itself and our capacity to sustain attention remain a mystery. It is certainly not dependent upon environmental stimuli.

Adaptive unconscious behaviour

Vigilance and attention can be, and often are, dissociated. What a lot we can do unconsciously to pursue our own ends in that state. Driving a car provides an example. On a very familiar route, but complicated and with many turns, junctions and traffic signals, and perhaps in dense traffic, one can successfully negotiate the journey without much recollection of having attended to it; instead one has attended perhaps with concentration to something else, to a recollection of a previous event, to a contemporary problem or so on. At any moment, however, attention can be immediately redirected to the immediate scene. Throughout the journey vigilance has protected the driver from disaster and purposive and meaningful actions and choices have been made without awareness or recollection of them.

But driving a car in dense traffic, in unfamiliar streets, finding the way, is another matter. Vigilance is high and there is a wide span of attention to the immediate environment, ready to focus at a moment's notice to one event after another or several at the same time.

AWARENESS

I come now to awareness, the second aspect of consciousness which I have suggested. This, which involves attention to something, can be divided into two aspects — awareness of the present environment, of the body, of the past and of the predicted future — and secondly awareness of the self — the 'I' or 'me' which I will discuss later. How do pathological cerebral states affect these aspects of awareness?

If for any reason, normal or pathological, vigilance is low and attention unfocussed on the environment, there is a tendency, as Galton (1907) first pointed out, to engage in reverie, in phantasy. Extreme fatigue and exhaustion, deprivation of sleep, toxicity and many pathological conditions illustrate this. But there is a surprising and important consequence, which is that the content of reverie tends to be projected, to be hallucinated, particularly in the auditory and visual modalities. This occurs in many confusional and delirious states, irrespective of cause and without any evidence of localised cerebral pathology. But in the absence of obvious confusion, with clear orientation and memory, projection and hallucination may also occur with localised cortical lesions in the receptor areas and also when the main pathways for sensory perception are suddenly interrupted. For example, about 20% of recently blinded people, as a result of lesions anywhere from the retina to the occipital cortex, experience visual hallucinations (Fitzgerald 1970). Following infarction of the occipital lobe from vascular disease, some patients report vivid moving visual hallucinations, often of animals or people and confined to the blind hemianopic visual field (Lance 1976). None of Lance's patients were deluded, that is they had no belief in the reality of their experiences, which they often found amusing. A totally blind patient who had been treated for neurosyphilis described to me hallucinated scenes of hell-fire and devils with pitchforks casting the damned into the fire. I discovered later that the hospital chaplain had just previously read to him from the Book of Revelation in the Bible. It was Freud of course who first drew attention to the role of projection in normal and abnormal mental life.

Normal awareness of the here and now depends, then, not only on vigilance and the capacity to attend and to shift attention, but also upon the integrity of the perceptual apparatus. There may be difficulty otherwise in discriminating between the reality of external and internal events. Sensory isolation experiments (Lilly 1956) on normal subjects provided further evidence of this phenomenon, but they also indicated the extreme need of the isolated individual to experience true sensations and perceptions, by making any little movement of a limb that he could. To be in relationship with the world around us through the perceptual apparatus and to be able to attend to it is a requirement of normal awareness of the here and now.

Sleep

Sleep and its disorders, which are related to the integrity and functions of the reticular activating system, also provide evidence of unusual states of awareness. It is generally believed that cataplexy, sleep paralysis and hypnagogic hallucinations are the consequences of the differential activation of separate parts of the sleep mechanism. Cataplexy and sleep paralysis are seen as activation separately of the descending pathways which inhibit motor action, and hallucinations to activation separately of the REM system of dreams, without the rest of sleep. All these phenomena occur in full awareness, but the hallucinations, particularly when associated with motor paralysis, occupy the patient's full attention and can be very frightening. Subsequently they are appreciated as having been unreal, unlike the schizophrenic.

Memory

The awareness of the past, memory, is of great importance to us; some would say, with Hume, that it is the structure of the self. It is evident that the capacity to recall the past is a variable at different times and between different subjects. It can be grossly impaired by cerebral disease. The memory store is almost certainly a selective one. Probably it only contains events which were themselves previous conscious events. The phenomenon of repression, the recall of memories under hypnosis or free-association suggest that these are of previous events, once conscious, which are now outside voluntary recall. Consideration of the evidence suggests to me that there is no fixed barrier between the conscious and the unconscious, and that the capacity to recall is a variable, changing from time to time, and is of course much affected by many mental illnesses.

What happens when an individual, who has normal vigilance and attention and is fully aware of the here and now, is suddenly deprived of his memory to recall the past? In 1958 Fisher & Adams at Harvard described transient global amnesia, a condition well recognised and reported by many others since then. Previously these cases had been regarded as hysterical. Due probably to temporary ischaemia of both hippocampi from interference with the vertebrobasilar origin of their blood supply, the patient, usually middle-aged or older, suddenly finds he has no memory of the past; he does not know what has happened to him, cannot understand why he is where he is, and his dense retrograde amnesia may go back even for many years. He recovers fully in a matter of hours or days, but retains total amnesia for that period.

The patient is extremely alarmed and asks constantly for reassurance on why he is where he is, what has happened and whether he is going mad because he cannot remember anything. But many such patients have been reported, shortly after the abrupt onset, to have carried out skilled and complicated activities, such as driving the car home and going to bed, or cooking dinner and eating it. Above all, the patient, unlike the hysteric, is aware of his personal identity; he retains the awareness of being himself, although the memory of events related to himself has ceased perhaps many years before. He is vigilant, able to attend and to relate appropriately and socially to people around him whom he recognises. There are no neurological deficits and the only disorder is the profound retrograde amnesia.

Can we infer from this that awareness of self, or individuality, is not dependent upon the awareness of the record of past experience?

AWARENESS OF THE SELF

I now, therefore, turn to awareness of the self, the actuality and reality of which has been so well described by Popper. Most of the time we are unaware of nearly all that happens in the environment, but we negotiate it and are unaware of doing so. Equally, most of the time we are unaware of our bodies and the position of our limbs in space, but unconsciously we carry out many skilled motor actions depending on the task in hand. Equally also we are most of the time unaware of past events, personal or impersonal, but we often act in ways which make clear that past events are influencing us. Much of behaviour, logical and adaptive is outside conscious awareness. It seems to us that by an act of will we can bring any of them or most of them into awareness — into that 'chamber of mind' where, as Galton said, consciousness holds court.

We are certainly not aware of ourselves all the time, in fact only on occasion. Yet the potentiality for that awareness exists throughout life — probably, Piaget suggested, after the age of 7 or 8 years. I must again emphasise the remarkable durability of this awareness of self, its survival despite loss of memory, and if recovery occurs after the most extreme perturbations of cerebral activity, after the most extreme degree of loss of metabolic function. It also survives major surgery when large parts of the brain are removed — lobectomy, hemispherectomy and transection of the corpus callosum. Provided the vigilance and attention functions, which are dependent on subcortical mechanisms (and also of course some cerebral cortex), are maintained, awareness of the self is possible.

Let me turn briefly to those different state of consciousness of which the normal individual is capable. In sleep the metabolic activity of the brain is not much decreased, in fact at times the contrary. In dreaming or REM sleep cerebral blood flow is markedly increased and there is a specific altered pattern of cortical electrical activity, profound physiological changes in the body and probably hormonal associations. The dream itself is a very restricted state of awareness, with a narrow attentive span and the experience is hallucinated, usually visual, occasionally auditory. The dreamer is usually a spectator, but the experience has a shadowy but nevertheless complete reality of its own. On waking it is recalled, but immediately its unreality is recognised. It has a transitory existence — few dreams enter the record of past experience, are built into the structure of awareness of the self. In the dream there is little or no awareness of the whole integrity of the self — or a great restriction or narrowing of that awareness. But it is of interest that if on waking one tells one's dream to another or writes it down, i.e. we have described it in words, we tend to remember it.

The neurophysiological accompaniments of the hypnotic trance are unknown to us, but from what we do know they do not appear to be different from the waking state. Yet in so-called deep hypnosis the subject on command may have control over autonomic functions which in the normal conscious state he has not got.

In transcendental meditation, as in hypnosis and also in dreaming sleep, there is a narrowing, a focussing down of conscious attention to an extreme degree. In meditation the physiological state is said to be held at the threshold between sleep and wakefulness. In all three there is apparent obliteration of self-awareness. In hypnosis the subject's attention is first focussed down on a single object, then on the operator's voice, to the exclusion of all the sensory stimuli, including pain, which may be 'blocked off', as are all other aspects of awareness, including time sense. Jaynes (1976) has drawn attention to the induction method: the concentration of a single visual object and then the commands to attend only to the operator's voice — 'all you hear is my voice, you are getting sleepier and sleepier, deeper and deeper', and so on. It can be said that in hypnosis the controlling self-observing state of consciousness is taken over by another, but only if the individual is compliant for this to happen.

Depersonalisation

To conclude this lecture I will refer to one phenomenon in which awareness of the self is specifically altered — depersonalisation. Depersonalisation has fascinated psychiatrists for over 100 years and became the subject of many enquiries in the 1950s and 1960s. Surveys of normal student populations (Dixon 1963, Roberts 1960) have shown that up to 50% of young adults occasionally experience it transiently. When it occurs in mental illness, the experience is more profound, more unpleasant, more frightening and more lasting. It is common in all mental illness, with the possible exception of paranoid and manic states, but occurs particularly in depression and schizophrenia. It is not, however, diagnostic of any particular condition. It has not, I believe, been reported in children under the age of 10. Essentially it is that the awareness of the self has been lost or the self has become unreal. This may refer to the bodily self, parts of it, or to the inner mental self. It is often, but not invariably associated with an altered perception of the external world which also has become unreal (derealisation).

Aubrey Lewis in his classical monograph on depression (1934) quoted patients as saying: 'My body is dead, no feeling in it. I feel all dead.' Another: 'I am losing my personality. I do things mechanically. My inside is stiff.' Another: 'My hands and legs don't belong to me. My voice isn't mine. I am changed.' Another: 'I have a dreadful feeling I am not real. I don't feel real. It's not I that's talking.'

In his Manson lecture (1949) Lewis quoted another patient as saying: 'I am a stranger to myself. I have stopped being. I am not the same person that I was before.'

Schilder (1935) gave a clear description:

> The individual feels totally different from his previous being; he does not recognise himself as a person. His actions seem automatic. He behaves as if he were an observer of his own actions. The outside world appears to him strange and new and it has lost the character of reality. The 'self' does not behave any longer in its former way.

Lewis, like many others, considered that the degree and range of consciousness at any one moment is slight, but that it is the capacity of consciousness to range over past events which gives continuity and integration — the awareness of 'one-ness' of the self. Yet, as we have seen in transient global amnesia when retrograde amnesia may be profound and of very long duration, awareness of the self is not apparently altered.

There is evidence that when depersonalisation is transiently experienced by normal subjects, it is commonly in states of fatigue, in the hypnogogic state, in toxic illness, or after sleep deprivation. It also occurs in sensory isolation experiments and is experienced by those taking psychotomimetic drugs, the first reported being mescaline, then LSD. All this was ably reviewed by Sedman (1970).

Occurring in normal or neurotic subjects, depersonalisation has an 'as if' quality, the subject knowing it to be a symptom, something wrong, and it is unpleasant. In psychotic subjects it has a delusional quality and the 'as if' quality is lost, but it is certainly unpleasant. In patients with temporal lobe epilepsy, depersonalisation and derealisation occur as sudden, extremely intense experiences of short duration, even seconds. It has been known since the time of Hughlings Jackson that the pathology in such cases lies in the amygdala-uncal-hippocampal region. Some have the brief experience of deja vu, of an extreme sense of familiarity with some new event, a disorder of the normal segmental ordering of events in time, between the past and the present, a form of 'temporal disintegration' (Freeman & Melges 1977). There is a great variety of altered states of experience and awareness in these patients — nearly all the symptomatology of the major functional psychoses being witnessed as in a tachistoscope. Denis Williams (1968) suggested that these phylogenetically ancient parts of the brain — the parietotemporal cortex and the subjacent limbic lobe — are concerned with the final integrative mechanisms normally responsible for the experience of self — the discrimination between 'I am' and 'I am not', the complete expression of which is unconsciousness, amnesia, automatism — and the partial expression of it in the dreamy state, depersonalisation, hallucinations of the bodily self (autoscopy), and seeing the self from the outside. Epileptic memories are always intimately concerned with the self, and this was a common characteristic of those relived experiences which Penfield & Perot (1963) evoked by electrical stimulation of the temporal cortex of conscious epileptics at operation. The patients, while vividly experiencing themselves in the past, at the same time retained their awareness of themselves in the present, knowing they were on the operating table in Montreal.

Theories about the mechanism of depersonalisation have abounded for years. Many have proposed an association with some lowering of conscious awareness (i.e. arousal), and this is evident in toxic and confusional states, and in normal people when isolated or exhausted, but there is no such evidence for the chronic condition in neurotic and psychotic patients (Sedman 1970). Whenever, and under whatever conditions it occurs, descriptions by patients have an essential similarity. Mayer-Gross (1935) proposed an inbuilt 'preformed mechanism' in the nervous system, similar for example to epilepsy and catatonia. This follows the Jackson-Ey concept of disorganisation and decontrol of higher centres over lower ones to which I have referred. Possibly, as Roth & Harper (1962) suggested, this occurs in response to some external threat of great disaster and could serve a protective function. Some psychoanalytic writers on the other hand, see the threat as coming from inside — the upsurge of instinctual aggression threatening the ego. More formal psychometric studies indicate a relation to anxiety and depressive mood, to obsessionality and to Eysenck's introversion (Sedman 1970).

DISCUSSION

Following Karl Popper I have suggested that consciousness in the sense in which I have defined it, is evolution's greatest achievement, and some aspects of it man no doubt shares with higher mammals. Nevertheless self-conscious awareness, self-hood or identity, which involves some sense of control, is man's most precious possession. The threat of losing it, or of its disintegration is one of man's greatest fears. He has many means of coping with this and is prepared to suffer much to defend it.

After recent hemiplegia from vascular accident there are unconscious inbuilt mechanisms for denying the existence, or loss of function, of half the body (anosognosia). Thus the awareness of the 'wholeness' or 'one-ness' of the bodily self is preserved. I suggest that so too there are unconscious inbuilt mechanisms to deny or to exclude from awareness mental events and experiences which threaten the awareness of self-hood or self-identity. There is, however, the obverse of this, when instead of exclusion or denial of threat or defect, there is an unremitting intense focussing down of attention upon the defect or altered state. This occurs in the example I have given of visual hallucinations in the recently blinded, but it is self-evident in depersonalisation; attention can hardly be diverted to anything else, and this also occurs in patients with obsessive anxiety and hypochondriasis.

Finally and speculatively, one can ask whether this approach to consciousness has any relevance to understanding schizophrenia, the condition above all in which awareness of the self is altered or threatened. We have been taught, and indeed teach, that schizophrenia occurs in 'clear consciousness' and without that the diagnosis is incorrect. Yet for decades there have been numerous reports of cognitive defects in the disorder. A reduced attention span, high or low arousal, increased or decreased vigilance have all been implicated. Frith (1979) recently, from the point of view of systems theory, has suggested that schizophrenia is a basic disorder of consciousness, but one in which there is an *excessive* not a diminished selfawareness. In this the self is overwhelmed by information because there is a defect in the sensory and internal filtering systems, an idea originally proposed by Payne et al (1959). If so the individual is no longer 'free', as Henri Ey put it, because he has become aware of too much of what normally goes on automatically at a subconscious level.

In this text I have examined the phenomena of consciousness from the point of view of experience, rather than behaviour. I have suggested that there are three aspects of consciousness which, though interdependent, may nevertheless be examined separately. Each I have suggested is itself a variable, potentially independent of the other two, and each is a matter of degree. I have laid particular emphasis on the awareness of self and suggest that this, like the other aspects of awareness, can be encompassed in a general theory of the hierarchical structure of the nervous system. We are still ignorant of the fundamental arrangements which make awareness of the self possible. Yet I believe that the concept of self is fundamental to psychology, and particularly to psychiatry. We cannot do without it.

REFERENCES

Adrian E D 1944 Brain rhythms. Nature 153: 360
Armstrong D M 1968 A nationalist theory of the mind. Routledge and Kegan Paul, London
Bremer F 1935 Cerveau 'isole' et physiologie du sommeil. Comptes rendus des séances de la Société de biologie 118: 1234–1241
Cairns H, Oldfield R C, Pennybacher J B, Whitteridge D 1941 Akinetic mutism with an epidermoid cyst of the third ventricle. Brain 64: 273–290
Dixon J C 1963 Depersonalisation phenomena in a sample population of college students. British Journal of Psychiatry 109: 371–375
Evans P 1972 Henri Ey's concepts of the organisation of consciousness and its disorganisation: an extension of Jacksonian theory. Brain 95: 413–440
Fisher C M, Adams R D 1958 Transient global amnesia. Transactions of the American Neurological Association 83: 143–145
Fitzgerald R G 1970 Reactions to blindness: An exploratory study in adults with recent loss of sight. Archives of General Psychiatry 22: 370–379
Freeman A M, Melges F T 1977 Depersonalisation and temporal disintegration in acute mental illness. American Journal of Psychiatry 134: 679–681
Freud S 1964 The complete psychological works of Sigmund Freud, vol 23 (1937–1939). p 282–286
Freud S 1966 The complete psychological works of Sigmund Freud, vol 1 (1940). p 293
Frith C D 1979 Consciousness, information processing and schizophrenia. British Journal of Psychiatry 134: 225–235
Galton F 1907 Enquiries in human faculty and its development. Everyman's Library, Dent, London

Jaspers K 1962 General psychopathology. Trans: Hoenig J, Hamilton M W. Manchester University Press, Manchester

Jaynes J 1976 The origin of consciousness in the breakdown of the bicameral mind. Houghton Mifflin, Boston

Jennett B, Plum F 1972 Persistent vegetative state after brain damage. Lancet i: 734–737

Joyston-Bechal M P 1966 The clinical features and outcome of stupor. British Journal of Psychiatry 112: 967–981

Lance J W 1976 Simple formed hallucinations confined to the area of a specific visual field defect. Brain 99: 719–734

Lewis A J 1934 Melancholia: a clinical survey of depressive states. Journal of Mental Science 80: 277–378

Lewis A J 1949 Philosophy and psychiatry. Philosophy 24: 99–117

Lilly J C 1956 In: Research techniques in schizophrenia. Psychiatric Research Report no 5, American Psychiatric Association

Mayer-Gross W 1935 On depersonalisation. British Journal of Medical Psychology 15: 103–122

Mountcastle V B 1978 Brain mechanisms for directed attention. Journal of the Royal Society of Medicine 71: 14–29

Payne R W, Matussek P, George G I 1959 An experimental study of schizophrenic thought disorder. Journal of Mental Science 105: 627–652

Penfield W 1957 Consciousness and centrencephalic organisation. Montreal Neurological Institute, reprint no 571

Penfield W, Perot P 1963 The brain's record of auditory and visual experience. Brain 86: 596–696

Popper K, Eccles J C 1977 The self and its brain. Springer International, New York

Roberts W W 1960 Normal and abnormal depersonalisation. Journal of Mental Science 106: 478–494

Roth M, Harper M 1962 Temporal lobe epilepsy and the phobic anxiety-depersonalisation syndrome. Comprehensive Psychiatry 3: 215–226

Ryle G 1949 The concept of mind. Hutchinson, London

Schilder P 1935 The image and appearance of the human body. Kegan Paul French and Trubner, London

Sedman G 1970 Theories of depersonalisation: a reappraisal. British Journal of Psychiatry 117: 1–14

Sperry R W 1966 Brain bisection and consciousness. In: Eccles J C (ed) Brain and conscious experience. Springer, Berlin, p 298–313

Walton J 1969 In: Brain's diseases of the nervous system, 7th edn. Revised by Brain and Walton. Oxford University Press, Oxford

Williams D 1968 Man's temporal lobe. Brain 91: 639–654

Sleep and its disturbances

Complaints about the quality and amount of sleep are commonly presented by patients to general practitioners and frequently lead to the prescription of 'sleeping pills'. The vast majority of such complaints seem to have a psychosomatic basis. Others experience impairment of their sleep, do not specifically seek help, but may yield the information within a medical consultation. In this respect such disturbances may resemble the experience of pain where Merskey (1975) has shown that about half of all 'psychiatric' patients will complain of it if asked.

This article addresses some aspects of the interface between human, social and biological processes and its experiential psychological and somatic expressions with reference to sleep. The author's interest in sleep stems from the work on the impact on the body of the kinds of starvation that can accompany the state of anorexia nervosa. During the last 15 years he and his colleagues have also operated a sleep laboratory and, more recently, a general sleep disorders clinic. During this time they have borne in mind the recent classification of sleep disorders (Roffwarg 1979) and have attempted to relate it to their own work. This chapter addresses a few of these issues drawing upon some of the research findings of the author and his colleagues and focusing ultimately on the psychoneurotic elements of two categories of sleep disorder with which the clinic and laboratory have been particularly concerned.

THE NATURE OF SLEEP

Sleep normally occurs rhythmically, alternating with wakefulness/activity. Activity, associated with food seeking and ingestion, alternating with inactivity/rest and synthesis are properties of the simplest organisms. Perhaps sleep is the optimal condition and wakefulness the interlude during which it is essential to ingest and sooner or later reproduce before returning to it! Our activity/sleep rhythm is linked to the 24-hour light/darkness cycle but, if isolated from such constraints, most people begin to cycle on a slightly longer rhythm with about a 25-hour length. It has been suggested that this more primitive rhythm relates to our oceanic origins when the moon and the tides had greater influence on biological systems. This underlying propensity may therefore be one disruptive influence on present day man's habitual sleep. Meanwhile, Gagnon et al (1975) have emphasised the existence of a potentially intrusive underlying 12-hour cycle of episodes of slow wave sleep (SWS) and suggests that rhythms also exist with roughly 6-hour, 3-hour and 90-minute cycles. It was Kleitman (1972) who especially postulated that there is a more rapid rest/activity cycle with a phase of about 90 minutes, detected during polysomnographically recorded sleep as REM sleep, but occurring also in muted form throughout wakefulness. Such a rhythm in wakefulness, again a residue from our past but perhaps with continuing essential purpose, may nevertheless facilitate the episodic expression of what now reveal themselves as morbid sleep tendencies during wakefulness, such as narcolepsy.

More evident to everyone, is the usual 3–5-hour cycle of the infant, initially defiant of light and darkness and related to demand for food. Only with patience and skillful feeding, and sometimes overfeeding, can the developing infant be persuaded to forego an episode of what is presumably a hunger-related arousal in the middle of the night. What a myriad of opportunities there are for human diet and sleep to become influenced and distorted by human relationships! Normally, two (or more) 3–5-hour blocks of sleep become welded together but remain, or perhaps become, substantially different from each other. The first one has a preponderance of SWS, the second more light sleep and REM sleep. Starvation and reduced metabolism in later life can rupture the bond, or at least erode, the second block and thus selectively reduce REM sleep (Crisp 1967, Crisp et al 1970, Lacey et al 1975, Adam 1977).

There is still a widespread belief that human sleep is a time of near total inactivity rather like hibernation. This is the likely explanation of the fact that people, including doctors, talk about 'sleeping' pills when what they may be actually prescribing and consuming are central nervous system depressant drugs which produce semicoma. In fact, sleep is a time of important internal activity. The individual ceases to orientate himself to the outside world and becomes self-oriented. Sleep is almost certainly an important restorative process and Oswald (1970) and Adam & Oswald (1977, 1983) have been to the fore in presenting the case for this. SWS early in the night prompts the secretion of growth hormone. Corticosteroid levels are at their lowest and protein synthesis becomes optimal in the body. This process alternates with REM episodes when protein synthesis in the brain is probably at its highest. The predominance of complex mental content and autonomically based sexual activity during REM has led to the proposal that, at this time, the brain is updating itself by selectively mobilizing its personal and evolutionary data banks (and perhaps thereby permitting more ready access to them as Freud and Jung respectively proposed). Their reshaping proceeds, influenced by the previous day's experience, integrating social and sexual need in the process and thereby equipping the individual the best to deal with the various challenges of the next day. If there were to be some truth in such a view, then dreams would perhaps be our most prophetic moments as has been claimed. Furthermore, REM suppression would be damaging. Certainly, high alcohol consumption and accompanying malnutrition are associated with major REM suppression and can, as we know, lead eventually to a major failure of recent memory and apathy. Only then does the alcoholic stop drinking!

It has also been suggested that sleep plays a regulatory role not only in cognitive/emotional activity, but also in terms of nutritional activity and temperature control. The amount and quality of food we eat one day is influenced by, amongst other factors, the amount and kind of food we have eaten the previous day. Is this achieved solely by the moderating influence of the tightness of the belt or is there a more direct central mechanism? Recent work has shown a direct relationship between the amount of ingested carbohydrate and the amount of REM sleep during the subsequent night (Phillips et al 1975, Crisp et al 1986), whilst Seigel (1975) has shown, in small mammals at least, that there is a negative correlation between such REM sleep and carbohydrate intake during the next period of wakefulness and activity. It is therefore plausible and deserving of continued attention that there may be regulatory mechanisms within sleep, although not necessarily confined to its natural expression, and that these may exist so far as the above activities are concerned within what we can detect poly-somnographically as REM sleep.

Sleep, then, is intimately related to wakefulness in many ways. The impact of starvation and hunger have been referred to. Consummation within the sexual act is typically followed by sleep. Exercise promotes sleep, especially SWS (Oswald 1970, Shapiro et al 1981) and also raises the concurrent plasma level of growth hormone (Adamson et al 1974). Delaying sleep onset promotes sleep. Arousing moods are incompatible with sleep, not only anxiety but anger in particular (Crisp 1980, Crisp & Stonehill 1973, 1976). It is daunting to contemplate the complexity of possible sleep disturbances stemming from the interactions of such everyday variables as these which can become so distorted in modern man.

It might be argued then that complaints about sleep can be oblique or alternative ways of complaining about wakefulness: in particular, waking 'unrefreshed' to face the same problems as yesterday. Many depressed people, seeking sleep and therefore 'sleeping' tablets, are seeking oblivion — it is wakefulness about which they are really complaining, especially first thing in the morning.

Reference to this aspect of severe depression makes it timely to reflect on those morbid conditions with which we waken having gone to sleep relatively free from them. What has 'gone wrong' in sleep? The author's interest in this area was prompted by a study of people wakening with migraine having been free of it at sleep onset (Hsu et al 1977). During sleep preceding migraine, plasma catecholamine levels begin to rise around the time of the first REM episode instead of continuing to fall naturally. Waking, some hours later, is then often directly from a REM episode. This led to an hypothesis concerning the nature of migraine evoking the concept of its relationship to information processing and overload during sleep in this instance (Crisp 1979a, 1981).

Then again, the common complaint of morning stiffness was investigated by Acheson et al (1969) and Acheson & Ginsburg (1973) who found that one-third of the general population experienced it and that it was, of course, over-represented in those with frank arthritis, especially rheumatoid arthritis. Moldofsky and his colleagues in Toronto (Modolfsky et al 1975) have been exploring for many years the polysomnography and sleep chemistry of subjects with 'fibrositis'. Their initial finding, of persistent alpha rhythm within SWS in such subjects, has led them to explore aspects of the immune system, the processes within which they now conclude are dramatically related to SWS (Moldofsky et al 1986) and probably deranged in such syndromes. Here may be a regulatory mechanism gone wrong in non-REM sleep.

Finally, in the severe depressive syndrome, people are at their most inert and feel most helpless and hopeless on wakening. Crisp (1986) has suggested that this is the fundamental hallmark of such disorder and that the complaint of wakening too early is secondary to it and that it arises through the inability of the sleep process to prepare/programme the individual for an active solution to his problems on wakening.

Such studies indicate important links between sleep and physical wellbeing and serve to emphasise again the active nature of sleep and its indissoluble relationship with wakefulness. Furthermore, as the brain and its mind settles down within sleep to check and organise the inputs of the day as a preamble to their absorption, its first task is that of recognition. Failure to recognise and/or inability thereafter to handle such new substances/information concerned with body tissue repair and development other than in the brain, may result in the mobilisation of immunological responses within SWS and precipitate out such disorders as fibrositis or rheumatoid arthritis itself. Such failure in respect of information relevant to the mind, within processes operative in REM sleep, may express itself in such 'allergic' terms as migraine on waking, morning inertia, or failure to correlate to the outside world and rejection of it, characteristic of 'depression'.

SLEEP DISORDERS

The above disorders are not commonly amongst those that present in our sleep disorders clinic. Presentations there fall mainly and familiarly into a few categories such as the insomnias, the hypersomnias and the parasomnias. Whilst there are very few such clinics in the United Kingdom, there are many in the USA where considerable experience has now been gained.

In 1979 the Association of Sleep Disorders Centers and the Association for the Psychophysiological Study of Sleep produced a diagnostic classification of sleep and arousal disorders (Roffwarg 1979). They were broadly categorised into:

A. Disorders of initiating and maintaining sleep (DIMS) (the insomnias)

B. Disorders of excessive somnolence (DOES)

C. Disorders of the sleep/wake schedule

D. Dysfunctions associated with sleep, sleep stages or partial arousals (the parasomnias).

The authors had approached their task with circumspection, recognising that their effort was likely to prove no more than 'a provisional working construct'. They recognised both the overlap between syndromes and the interrelation between some of their broad categories of disorder. The insomnias (category A) were divided into seven subcategories:

1. Psychophysiological
2. Associated with psychiatric disorders:
   a. symptom and personality disorders
   b. affective disorders
3. Associated with use of drugs and alcohol
4. Associated with sleep-induced respiratory impairment (sleep apnoea)
5. Associated with sleep-related myoclonus and 'restless legs'
6. Associated with other medical, toxic and environmental conditions
7. Childhood onset insomnia.

These were followed by a collection of 'difficult to classify syndromes'. The disorders of excessive somnolence lent themselves to a rather similar subclassification, demonstrating in fact the possibility of relationships between these two major categories. Disorders of the sleep/wake schedule were simply divided into 1) transient, e.g. jet lag, work shift changes, and 2) persistent sleep/wake disorders. The category D) dysfunctions were broken down into 1) sleep walking, 2) sleep terror, 3) sleep-related enuresis, 4) a whole collection of other dysfunctions.

The rest of this chapter will be devoted to a report of the experience of the author and his colleagues and restricted to aspects of two categories of insomnias on the one hand, and excessive somnolence on the other, dubbed in the classification either 1) psychophysiological, or 2) associated with psychiatric disorders; also some reference to the subcategories of the parasomnias dubbed sleep walking and sleep terror respectively.

Insomnias and hypersomnias

Insomnia is a complaint about insufficient or inadequate sleep. People expect to waken refreshed and the complaint of insomnia may reflect the lack of this restorative experience. People also sometimes welcome loss of contact with the outside world and resent persistent or intermittent wakefulness during the night. The 1979 classification subdivided its psychophysiological insomnia into transient and situational on the one hand and persistent on the other, and breaks down insomnia associated with psychiatric disorders into those related to a) symptom and personality disorders, b) affective disorders, and c) other functional psychoses. The author will be looking at some of the relationships between these subcategories as well as touching briefly on one way in which an underlying nutritional diathesis links them with the hypersomnias, correspondingly subdivided into those identified as 'psychophysiological' and 'associated with psychiatric disorders' respectively.

The 1979 sleep disorders classification (Roffwarg 1979) proposes that 'transient physiological' insomnia is often situation-specific, e.g. bereavement, and usually obviously associated with general distress following an evident provocative life event. Sleeplessness may be pervasive or occur predominantly in the first or second halves of the night. In contrast, the 'persistent psychophysiological insomnias' are recognised as probably also being importantly related to stress, though unrecognised by the sufferer. The expression of the strain is channelled exclusively through the complaint of insomnia as the 'chosen path' of chronic somatised tension. Furthermore, it may have become self-perpetuating through conditioning and fearful expectation. Again, sleep may be shortened and disrupted throughout the night. During the day such people feel fatigued rather than sleepy. Typically, such patients have a total sleep time of 5–6 hours and, polysomnographically, show many sleep interruptions, much light sleep and very little slow wave sleep.

In contrast, the 1979 classification outlines insomnias associated with psychiatric disorders comprising 'symptom and personality disorders' as mainly reflecting sleep onset difficulties. These disorders are identified as including general anxiety and anxiety phobic states, hypochondriasis, personality disorder and, interestingly (vide infra), dissociative disorders. Sleep difficulty and complaint about sleep in the second half of the night is more a feature of major depressive illness. This distinction between impaired sleep in the two halves of the night is the traditional way of classifying so-called secondary insomnias in the psychiatric clinic. However, it is also recognised that depressive illness can occasionally be associated with hypersomnia.

Some years ago Crisp & Stonehill (1973, 1976) studied a consecutive series of 375 psychiatric outpatients in respect of their specific diagnostic status, mood and their weight and sleep changes within the illness. This was a clinical study using standardized measures. The hypothesis being tested was that sleep changes during the second half of the night, as well as total sleep time and number of overall sleep interruptions, would be related to nutritional changes as reflected in weight change and irrespective of diagnosis. The postulate was that nutritional changes can sometimes be profound within psychiatric illness. Normally, weight loss in particular is difficult to achieve — the set point mechanisms regulating body weight and protecting against weight loss are powerful. Yet in depression in particular, individuals may lose 10 or more pounds easily consequent on anorexia. They had previously shown that such weight loss in patients with anorexia nervosa and obesity was associated with erosion of sleep in the second half of the night, whilst restoration of body weight in these patients led to reconstitution of normal sleep independent of mood change.

Amongst the psychiatric population these associations were also found to hold (Fig. 7.1, Table 7.1), although it was inevitably the depressed patients who complained most about not sleeping sufficiently. In fact, the authors did not find the sleep of depressed people to be greatly reduced. Amongst other things they went to bed and thence to sleep earlier than their counterparts. The authors speculated as to whether this reflected a primary change in rhythms or whether it simply reflected the depressed person's tendency to withdraw. In contrast, there was no doubt that erosion of sleep in the first half of the night was much more likely to be associated with degree of disturbance of mood. Of all the moods reported anger was the most disruptive, a finding that is plausible enough. The findings in respect of sleep in the second half of the night were viewed in terms of energy balance (Fig. 7.2). Reduced calorie consumption associated with anorexia, leading to a negative energy balance, evoked arousal/foraging behaviour after a few hours of (unnourished) sleep. Increased calorie consumption, as characterised by some patients with depression, and associated with weight gain and positive energy balance, was also associated with increase in total sleep and later wakening. This hypersomnia, which was usually welcomed by the depressed patient, might further reinforce increased food intake in the search for escape from the outside world. Such food intake,

Table 7.1 Mean total sleep times of patient groups defined in Figure 7.1. Note those related to weight gain and weight loss greater than 10 lb

Total psychiatric population		Hours	Minutes
Premorbid	(n = 375)	7	16
Morbid	(n = 375)	6	52
Morbid — wt ↑ >10 lbs	(n = 46)	7	22
Morbid — wt ↓ >10 lbs	(n = 63)	6	14
Diagnostic categories			
Endogenous depression	(n = 43)	7	08
Neurotic depression	(n = 106)	6	18
Anxiety state	(n = 106)	7	07
Mood states			
Angry	(n = 27)	6	09
Anxious	(n = 100)	6	58
Sad	(n = 131)	6	39
Tense	(n = 109)	6	52
Less disturbed	—	7	01
Very disturbed	—	6	28

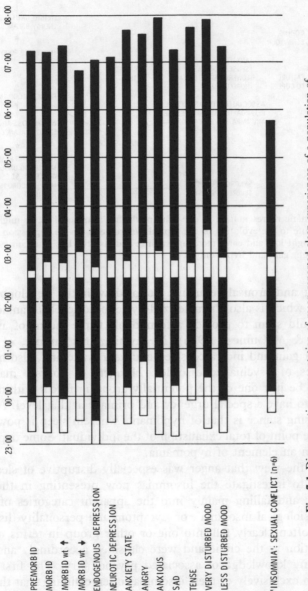
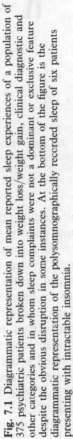

Fig. 7.1 Diagrammatic representation of mean reported sleep experiences of a population of 375 psychiatric patients broken down into weight loss/weight gain, clinical diagnostic and other categories and in whom sleep complaints were not a dominant or exclusive feature despite the obvious disruption in some instances. At the bottom of the figure is the diagrammatic representation of the polysomnographically recorded sleep of six patients presenting with intractable insomnia.

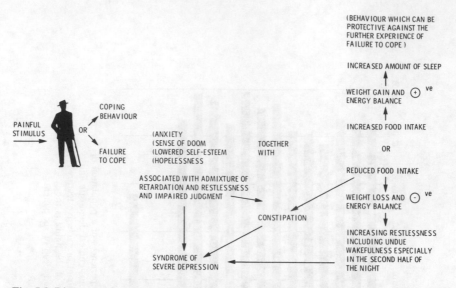

Fig. 7.2 Diagrammatic representation of one way in which a nutritional factor might sometimes contribute to the evolution of the typical syndrome of severe depression associated with weight loss and early morning waking, and also the less common syndrome of depression, weight gain and hypersomnia.

itself gratifying and arousal reducing, coupled with the development of formal obesity, which is also characterized by reduced levels of anxiety and depression, would seem to provide a formidable triple means of avoiding anxiety (Crisp & McGuiness, 1976). Meanwhile, this finding, of a link between weight gain and increased sleep and later wakening, also held for other categories of psychiatric disorder. Hunger, of course, may at a biological level be just one of the potentially arousing forces within sleep, but it is likely to have a special urgency and primacy at that level. Another obviously arousing stance is that of hypomania wherein sleep is powerfully disrupted to the point of total exhaustion of the individual. Some depressive illnesses contain an element of hypomania.

Armed with the view that anger was especially disruptive of sleep, the authors began to investigate the insomnias now presenting in the sleep disorders clinic and falling mainly into the apparent categories of either 'persistent physiological insomnia', or 'symptom and personality disorder'. Patients quite often clearly fell into one or other group in terms of their initial presentation at the clinic and were classified accordingly and independently of any knowledge of associated psychometry. The first group would complain exclusively of their insomnia, often claiming that they had not slept for several years (a complaint to take at its face value even though one can usually demonstrate fitful polysomnographic sleep, because we have very little knowledge of the chemistry of sleep which is presumably essential to its proper restorative function and which may be severely deranged in such patients). Personal distress of a broader kind was not acknowledged in the first instance. By contrast, the second group, although primarily complaining of chronic insomnia, also reported a wide mix of neurotic symptomatology, usually clearly anxiety based. All patients attending the clinic are expected to bring one or more family members, parents, spouse, etc., as the case may be. The consultation, lasting about two hours, is preceded by the completion of a number of self-report questionnaires, including the direction of hostility questionnaire (Caine et al 1967) and the Crown-Crisp Experiential Index (CCEI, a brief scale providing scores in six psychoneurotic categories, namely anxiety, anxiety phobia, obsessive compulsive, depression, functional somatic and hysteria). Scores range 0–16 (Crown & Crisp 1979).

Early on in the life of the clinic the author had become impressed by the history, in those presenting with persistent psychophysiological insomnia, of profound decompensations in personal relationships occurring in association with the onset of sleep symptoms and expressing themselves especially in sexual unfulfilment which would often come to symbolize the rift. Helpless anger was often another facet of such complex psychopathology and the combination appeared to comprise one reasonable basis of severely disrupted sleep in many patients (Crisp 1979b, 1980). Clinical assessments, involving family members, therefore include exploration of these aspects and, overall, the association has continued to hold. At the end of the consultations the aim is always to have sown the seed of greater insight by the patient (and family) into this underlying psychopathology. In recent times we have run an outpatient group-therapy programme for patients with such apparently intractable insomnia. In 12 sessions of therapy, with expert group leadership, these patients often do remarkably well (Matthews & Crisp 1986). The majority are able to gain insight into the basis of their own difficulties through learning about and sharing the problems of other group members. Sleep complaints diminish and the patients become less desperate and defiant and more depressed. Depression is the potential gateway to change, especially if further psychotherapeutic help is then provided, for instance together with a partner. However, some of our patients have remained much changed and/or improved without further intervention of this kind. We would suggest that many such patients have either an initial predilection to monosymptomatic complaint (about sleep in this case), or else have come to present themselves in this way over the years of their distress. It is perhaps the latter who can most likely be helped to unravel their difficulties.

The initial CCEI profiles of the two groups of patients show striking similarities (Fig. 7.3 A–E), indicating that they can actually impart their more general symptomatology by self-report questionnaire, even though they are inclined to deny it in the consultation. Thus the groups of insomniacs designated 'psychophysiological' and 'symptom and personality disorder' are very similar in profile, and both are similar on the first five subscales

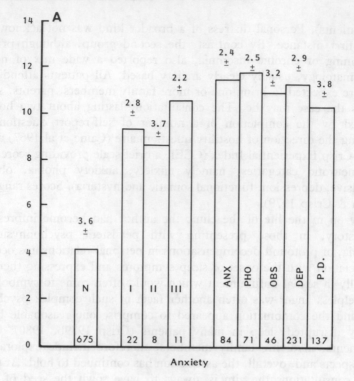

Anxiety

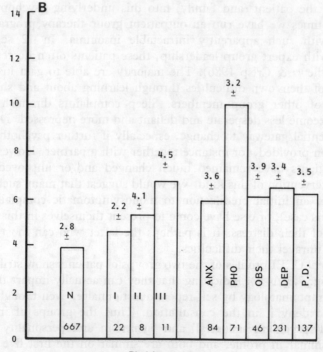

Phobic avoidance

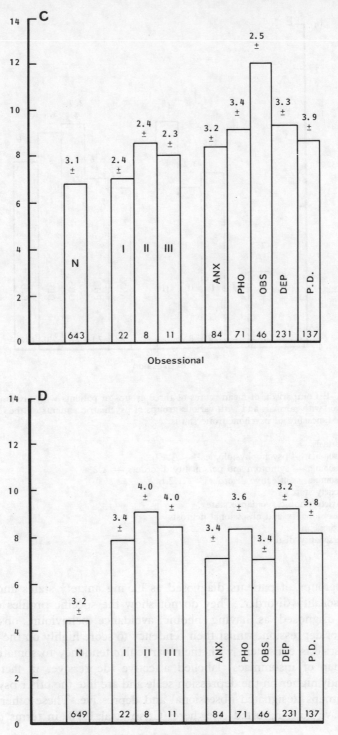

Obsessional

Somatic complaint

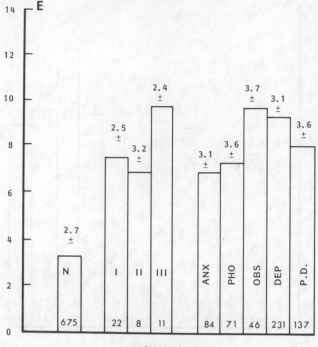

Fig. 7.3 A–E Comparison of mean scores of three groups of patients with insomnia (DIMS classification) with normals and with various groups of psychiatric patients on the CCEI — a standardised measure of psychoneurotic status.
Key:
N   = normals
I   = insomnia — psychophysiological — A.1.b.
II   = insomnia — symptom and personality disorders — A.2.a.
III   = insomnia — affective disorders — A.2.b.
Anx = anxiety state
Pho = anxiety/phobic avoidance state
Obs = obsessionality and obsessional neurosis
Dep = depression
PD   = personality disorder

to other groups of patients diagnosed as having anxiety states and others with personality disorder. They do not show the specific profiles of other patients diagnosed as having phobic avoidance behaviour, obsessional neurosis or depression, whilst their tendency to score highly on the psychosomatic scale is consistent with their particular tendency to somatise. The third group of insomniacs, labelled affective (depressive, in fact), score significantly higher on the depression scale and are like the other psychiatric patient groups designated obsessional and depressive. These other patient groups have been reported elsewhere (Crisp et al 1978) in terms of CCEI profiles. Such an instrument may therefore be helpful in the task of exploration of cases of insomnia.

Parasomnias

Sleep walking and night terrors are closely related polysomnographically and also clinically, perhaps in the same way as classical and common migraine. Sleep walking, arising out of a sudden arousal from slow wave sleep, needs to be differentiated from psychomotor epilepsy, fugue state (see Stengel 1943) and sleep drunkenness. Oswald (see Oswald & Evans 1985) has especially insisted that sleep walking is not an hysterical disorder. There is clearly substance to this view and it is based on the fact that the episode arises out of deep sleep and also the view that 'the sleeping mind is not in touch with reality and amnesia for events during sleep is usual'.

However, because of artefact caused by the activity following arousal from deep sleep, it has proved very difficult to identify the polysomnographic features of the sleep walking episode itself. Not all individuals experiencing such sudden and urgent arousals embark on sleep walking. Moreover, it could equally be argued that the cerebral prodromata to hysterical conversion behaviours and fugues are similar to those quoted above in relation to sleep walking. For this, of course, one needs also to postulate that the waking mind can be totally consumed by fantasy and that psychological mechanisms producing amnesia exist; moreover, that the process may be automatic and outside awareness. The issue has become prominent because of medicolegal implications. In the law, wakeful/conscious man, devoid of mental illness, is usually held responsible for his actions. In recent times there have been several murders committed during sleep-walking episodes (e.g. see again Oswald & Evans 1985), when a successful defence has been mounted on the grounds that the episode was occurring from within sleep and that the individual was not therefore responsible for his (the cases are nearly all male) actions. Clearly, under such circumstances it would be important to convince the court that the behaviour had not occurred outside sleep in either a fugue or dissociative state as a commonly recognised feature of hysteria, or else even in a simulated fugue state or a state retrospectively claimed to have been either a fugue state or sleep walking. The more elaborate and co-ordinated the activity during the state, the more likely it is to have occurred in full consciousness.

However, from a clinical standpoint it is interesting to consider whether such abrupt changes in the level of consciousness as occur in night terrors and sleep walking have any parallels with the hysterical mechanism. Hysterical conversion states and fugues are also often borne of intense anxiety and arousal and the mechanism of dissociation is invoked. Another perspective is allowed by finding that the patients we have seen with night terrors and sleep walking score very highly on the hysteria scale of the CCEI.

The eight items in this scale comprise the following:
1. Are your opinions easily influenced? Yes No
2. Have you, at any time in your life, enjoyed acting? Yes No
3. Are you normally an excessively emotional person? Yes No
4. Do you enjoy being the centre of attention? Yes No
5. Do you find that you take advantage of circumstances for your own ends? Never Sometimes Often
6. Do you often spend a lot of money on clothes? Yes No
7. Do you enjoy dramatic situations? Yes No
8. Do you sometimes find yourself posing or pretending? Yes No

Such patients may therefore either have a highly developed cerebral dissociative mechanism, involving the need/capacity to switch from one level of consciousness to another mutually exclusive one, or, alternatively or perhaps in complementary fashion, it may be those with such traits who elaborate their behaviour on waking, finding it possible to express themselves more freely than usual within such a context. Night terrors might characterise those who internalise conflict, sleep walking those who act it out.

CONCLUSION

The descriptive and polysomnographic approach to classification of sleep disorders has great advantage. It is the main way to make progress in the field at present. However, there are evident overlaps between the disorders so classified. The search therefore for common underlying diatheses and for links with the waking mind and its mechanisms can hopefully continue at the same time. Sufficient is already known about this complementary approach, in the author's view, for this to be of advantage in optimising our present capacity to understand and help our patients.

REFERENCES

Acheson R M, Yick Kwong Chan, Payne M 1969 New Haven survey of joint diseases. Journal of Chronic Disorders 21: 533–542

Acheson R M, Ginsburg G N 1973 New Haven survey of joint diseases XVI. Impairment, disability and arthritis. British Journal of Preventive and Social Medicine 27: 168–176

Adam K 1977 Body weight correlates with REM sleep. British Medical Journal 1: 813–814

Adam K, Oswald I 1983 Protein synthesis, bodily renewal and the sleep/wake cycle. Clinical Science 65: 561–567

Adamson L, Hunter W M, Ogunremi O O, Oswald I, Percy-Robb I W 1974 Growth hormone increase during sleep after daytime exercise. Journal of Endocrinology 62: 473–478

American Psychiatric Association 1980 Diagnostic and statistical manual Volume III (DSM III). American Psychiatric Press, Washington DC

Caine T M, Foulds G A, Hope K 1967 Manual of the hostility and direction of hostility questionnaire (HDHQ). University of London Press, London

Crisp A H 1967 The possible significance of some behavioural correlates of weight and carbohydrate intake. Journal of Psychosomatic Research 11: 117–131

Crisp A H 1979a Holistic speculations concerning the origin of migraine. Trends in Neurosciences 2: 116–118

Crisp A H 1979b Sexual psychopathology in the psychiatric clinic. British Journal of Clinical Practice 5 (supplement 4): 3–11

Crisp A H 1980 Sleep, activity nutrition and mood. British Journal of Psychiatry 137: 1–7

Crisp A H 1981 The relevance of an hypothesis concerning the laterality of migraine. Journal of Affective Disorders 3: 71–75

Crisp A H 1986 'Biological' depression; because sleep fails? Postgraduate Medical Journal 62: 179–185

Crisp A H, McGuiness B 1976 Jolly fat: the relation between obesity and psychoneurosis in the general population. British Medical Journal 1: 7–9

Crisp A H, Stonehill E 1973 Aspects of the relationship between sleep and nutrition: a study of 375 psychiatric outpatients. British Journal of Psychiatry 122: 379–394

Crisp A H, Stonehill E 1976 Sleep, nutrition and mood. Wiley, London

Crisp A H, Douglas J W B, Ross J M, Stonehill E 1970 Some developmental aspects of disorders of weight. Journal of Psychosomatic Research 14: 313–320

Crisp A H, Jones G M, Slater P 1978 The Middlesex Hospital questionnaire: a validity study. British Journal of Medical Psychology 51: 293–301

Crisp A H, Hartmann M K, Crutchfield M, Matthews B, Bhat A V 1986 Sleep, activity, nutrition and mood. In: Lacey J H (ed) Proceedings of the 15th European conference on psychosomatic research. John Libbey, London

Crown S, Crisp A H 1979 Manual of the Crown-Crisp experiential index. Hodder & Stoughton, London

Gagnon P, De Koninck J, Broughton R 1985 Reappearance of electroencephalograph slow waves in extended sleep with delayed bedtime. Sleep 8: 118–128

Hsu L K G, Crisp A H, Kalucy R S et al 1977 Early morning migraine. Nocturnal plasma levels of catecholamines, tryptophan, glucose and free fatty acids and sleep encephalographs. Lancet i: 447–451

Kleitman N 1972 Implications of the rest-activity cycle. In: Hartmann E (ed) Sleeping and dreaming. International Psychiatric Clinics 7: 13–14. Little, Brown, Boston

Lacey J H, Crisp A H, Kalucy R S, Hartmann M K, Chen C N 1975 Weight gain and the sleeping EEG, study of ten patients with anorexia nervosa. British Medical Journal iv: 556–559

Matthews B J, Crisp A H 1986 Some clinical and disposal characteristics of patients attending a sleep disorders clinic. Paper presented at 8th European congress on sleep research, Szeged, Hungary, September 1986

Merskey H 1975 Psychological aspects of pain. In: Weisenberg M (ed) Pain: clinical and experimental perspectives. C V Mosby, St Louis, p 24–35

Moldofsky H, Scarisbrick P, England R, Smythe H 1975 Muscularskeletal symptoms and non-REM sleep disturbance in patients with 'fibrositis syndrome' and healthy subjects. Psychosomatic Medicine 37: 341–351

Moldofsky H, Lue F A, Keystone E, Gorczynski R 1986 The relationship of interleukin 1 and immune functions to sleep in humans Psychosomatic Medicine 48: 309–318

Oswald I 1970 Sleep, the great restorer. New Scientist 46: 170–172

Oswald I, Evans J 1985 Serious violence during sleepwalking. British Journal of Psychiatry 147: 668–691.

Phillips F, Chen C N, Crisp A H et al 1975 Isocaloric diet changes and EEG sleep. Lancet ii: 723–725

Roffwarg H P 1979 Diagnostic classification of sleep and arousal disorders, 1st edn. Prepared by the Sleep Disorders Classification Committee, H P Roffwarg chairman, Association of Sleep Disorders Centers. Sleep 2: 1–137

Seigel J M 1975 REM sleep predicts subsequent food intake. Physiology and Behaviour 15: 399–403

Shapiro C M, Bortz R, Mitchell D 1981 Slow wave sleep: a recovery period after exercise. Science 214: 1253–1254

Stengel E 1943 Further studies on pathological wandering. Journal of Mental Science 89: 224–241

Disorders of verbal expression in neuropsychiatry

Sir Denis Hill was a superb clinical diagnostician with a knowledge of brain disorders involving many approaches. His interviewing skill stimulated the author to study the verbal output characteristics of neuropsychiatric disorders, an effort that Sir Denis strongly encouraged. Unfortunately, a printed tabulation can convey only a portion of the diagnostic information to be gleaned from a neuropsychiatric patient's communication efforts. The magic that was Sir Denis' interview of a mentally disordered patient cannot be reproduced. It can only be hoped that this information may prove useful to neuropsychiatrists developing their own diagnostic skills.

INTRODUCTION

Most psychiatrists are adept at analysing verbal output because, of all branches of medicine, the verbal output of a patient is most crucial to psychiatry. While all medical specialties utilise patient history to direct their examination, the psychiatrist often uses almost no other information for diagnosis. The patient's verbal expressions have long been accepted as the major building block of psychiatric diagnosis and almost all psychiatrists are skilled at noting disorders presented verbally. The psychiatrist, however, routinely utilises only a portion of the information available from the patient's verbalisations. In contrast, the neurologist often analyses totally different aspects of verbal output. Both approaches offer information of value for neuropsychiatric evaluation.

The content is the aspect of verbal output most closely analysed by psychiatrists. The content not only relates disordered beliefs or perceptions but also reflects the environmental background of the patient, the immediate social stresses and the familial, interpersonal and educational background against which these stresses are playing. The material is presented to the psychiatrist verbally and the interpretation of the content is accepted as diagnostically valid.

The neurologist, on the other hand, often concentrates on the physical characteristics of disordered verbal expression. The alterations of speech and language that accompany disease states involving the brain are pertinent. Aphasia, mutism, hypophonia, apraxia, the many types of dysarthria, and other disorders of verbal output often supply important diagnostic clues to the neurologist.

Verbal output is crucial to the understanding of many neuropsychiatric disorders and both verbal content and output mechanisms must be monitored. Characteristic alterations of verbal expression exist and the abnormalities of verbal output offer many clues needed to define a disorder. An outline of verbal characteristics, both positive and negative, for a number of neuropsychiatric entities will be presented.

METHODS

The material to be discussed here is an accumulation of observations, not the result of a formal investigation. The initial information stemmed from experience gained evaluating patients with structural brain damage at the Aphasia Research Center of the Boston Veterans Administration Hospital. Additional experience was obtained at the Maudsley Hospital in London with a considerably different experiential background. The psychiatric experience was general but the prior experience in language evaluation favoured concentration on the verbal variables of a variety of psychiatric patients. These experiences were later augmented by opportunities to perform both formal and informal speech and language studies on a variety of disease entitites (Alzheimer's disease, Huntington's disease, schizophrenia, frontal brain injury, posterior aphasia, limbic epilepsy, depression) at the Neuropsychiatric Institute of UCLA and the Brentwood (Cal.) Veterans Administration Medical Center.

The information in this chapter does not represent a single test battery administered to a variety of individuals with known disease states. Some of the information comes from formal investigations, but much more represents accumulated observations of patients in the clinic. Nine disorders will be discussed — psychotic depression, mania, schizophrenia (particularly catatonic or 'loose'), posterior aphasia, Huntington's disease, progressive supranuclear palsy (PSP), Parkinson's disease, Alzheimer's disease and temporal lobe epilepsy; distinctive characteristics of the verbal output of each disorder will be described.

DEFINITIONS

Crucial to this presentation is differentiation of *speech* from *language* and of both from *thought*. Common sense notes differences in the three but definitions that are simultaneously accurate and inclusive are almost impossible. It is common, in fact almost a rule, that individuals with a disturbance in one area will have problems in another. Separation of the three aspects of verbal output is pertinent, however, when attempting to understand the disease processes and/or diagnose the disease state.

It has long been acknowledged that speech and thought are distinct and separable (Pick 1931/1973). Similarly, a difference between speech and language is now accepted, although the differences are less distinct and often the two are not separated. Differentiation of language and thought is the least specific; in fact, a number of authorities deny that they should be separated (Arendt 1978, Mueller 1887). Others (Critchley 1970, Vygotsky 1962) demand that separation of thought from language is essential for the understanding of many mental functions.

Speech

Speech disorders can be defined as disturbances in verbal output based on abnormal function of the neuromuscular components necessary for production of the communication signal. Included among disturbances to oral speech would be various types of articulatory, phonatory and respiratory disturbances that produce a motor dysarthria (Darley et al 1975, Metter 1985). Prosody (the melody, rhythm, inflection and timbre of speech) is a major constituent. Speech problems are mechanical, not cognitive. The individual with a speech disorder not only knows exactly what he wants to express but has the necessary lexical and grammatical competency; only a mechanical disturbance interferes with the output. In pure speech disorder a linguistically and cognitively adequate verbal output is distorted by neuromuscular disturbance. In this context 'speech' would include oral, written and gestural communication. Current concepts of dysgraphia (Benson & Cummings 1985) note the presence of purely mechanical disturbances that account for some types of disordered written language that can be separated from dysgraphia due to abnormal language. Similarly, gestural disturbances caused by paralysis can be separated from those due to apraxia (abnormal ideation).

Language

The definition of a language disorder is less exact. Patients with language disorders have difficulty utilising the symbols of communication. Language disorders represent a breakdown in the ability to use the symbolic and grammatical structures needed to express ideas. A disturbance in speech may or may not accompany the language disorder; similarly, there may or may not be distortion of the ideation that underlies the language output. Aphasia may be a pure language defect but is often mixed with either speech or thought disorder or both.

Thought

The third entity, thought, is the most difficult to define and is often accepted without definition. Thought disorders indicate abnormalities in ideation; this is inadequate as a definition but the concept helps separate thought from speech and language. A major problem is that thought disorders are most often noted through verbal expression and are frequently but erroneously called language disturbances.

While the definitions appear ambiguous, relatively clean clinical examples are immediately available. Pure speech disorders occur with primary motor problems such as a lacerated tongue, laryngitis, bulbar paralysis, severe dystonia or rigidity (e.g. Parkinson's disease). Many disorders that seriously affect the mechanical aspects of verbal output produce no recognisable disturbance in either thought or language.

Disorders of language are, by definition, called aphasia and all true aphasic syndromes feature language disturbances. The aphasic patient has lost some ability to utilise the symbols and rules of communication. Both spoken and written output are usually involved. Separation of the articulatory, phonatory and mechanical aspects of verbal output from an inability to handle the constituents of language is relatively straightforward once the problem is demarcated. Separation from disordered thought is far more difficult, but many aphasic patients appear to have normal thinking capability (Basso et al 1975, Benson 1979).

Clear examples of thought disorder with little or no disturbance of language or speech are also well known. The classic example is, of course, the psychotic verbal production of a schizophrenic (Faber et al 1983); the output is often voluminous, is both grammatically and lexically complex and appears to express with accuracy the disturbed, bizarre thought processes of the individual (Gerson et al 1977). Other disorders of thought, expressed with more or less adequate speech and language, include mania, depression, and some types of dementia. While the verbal content in these disorders is obviously abnormal, sufficient idiosyncracies of expression may be present to suggest concurrent language or even speech disorder. Careful consideration of the characteristics of speech, language and thought, however, easily demonstrates the primary problem as thought disorder. Major differentiating points in the verbal output that characterises the nine disease processes under consideration are presented in Tables 8.1–8.4, subdivided into speech, language, thought performance and thought constituent categories.

VERBAL OUTPUT DISORDERS IN DISEASE STATES

Depression

Anhedonic affective disorder ranks as one of the most common neuropsychiatric disturbances. Depression is not a single disease state or even a unitary clinical syndrome; variations produce differences in symptomatology reflected in the verbal output. Nonetheless, some verbal characteristics strongly suggest depression and are routinely monitored by the clinician.

Table 8.1 Speech qualities

	Rate	Initiation of verbalization	Clarity of pronunciation	Prosodic qualities
Depression	slow	slow, hesitant	indistinct, hypophonic	monotonous, long inter-word pause duration
Parkinson's disease	slow	slow	indistinct, hypophonic	monotonous
PSP	slow	slow	indistinct, hypophonic	monotonous, altered rhythm
Posterior aphasia	rapid	normal	normal	normal
Schizophrenia	moderately fast	variable	clear	normal
Epilepsy	rapid	normal	normal	normal
Mania	fast	rapid	clear	normal or exaggerated
Huntington's disease	slow	variable, usually slowed	indistinct, dysarthic	poorly controlled
Alzheimer's disease	moderately fast	rapid	clear	normal

In depression the rate of verbal output is consistently slow, but may vary from only mildly sparse to a near total absence. Speech pause time (the interval between phonations) is increased (Greden & Carroll 1981). The verbal output is often indistinct, lacks crisp articulation and shows a flat melodic line and decreased inflection and rhythm qualities. Pauses between words, and particularly between phrases, are elongated (Szabodi et al 1976). Language capability appears intact but the output tends to be simplified and is often presented in incomplete phrases. Decrescendo, a decreasing vocal volume as the phrase is uttered, significantly decreases comprehensibility; the phrase may not even be completed. There is some limitation of lexicon and, if monitored carefully, a proportional increase in the number of words with negative or morbid connotation (Hinchcliffe et al 1971). A matching slowness and impoverishment of non-verbal expression is present; the patient looks as flat as he sounds.

Thinking appears slowed in depression and there is a ponderousness to the stream of thought, but a tight maintenance of thought control can usually be demonstrated. The depressed individual often shows an over-whelming, almost always morbid, ideation; this may be a single, strongly fixed belief that can properly be called a delusion. When asked to manipulate thought, not only slowing but inadequacy is noted; cognitive competency is decreased in depression. Testing of the constituents of thought demonstrates that learning ability is preserved, although not at a normal level; retrieval of learned material is adequate but often requires prompting. The mood is morose and abnormal beliefs often represent a significant portion of the seriously depressed individual's verbal output.

Table 8.2 Language Qualities

	Syntax	Semantics	Non-verbal expression
Depression	simplified, incomplete	limited, morbid lexicon	impoverished
Parkinson's disease	simplified, economical	normal, full lexicon	markedly decreased
PSP	simplified, economical	normal, economical use of lexicon	markedly decreased
Posterior aphasia	normal	anomic, paraphasic	normal, tendency to stereotypy
Schizophrenia	normal but simplified	normal, full but bizarre	decreased
Epilepsy	normal	normal	normal
Mania	normal, incomplete sentences	repetitive, clang, rhyming, use of words	exuberant
Huntington's disease	normal	normal	erratic, reduced
Alzheimer's disease	normal	word-finding problems, paraphasia	normal

In advanced cases the verbal output of depression is striking and diagnostic. With less advanced disease a considerable potential for cross-diagnosis exists, particularly with other disorders featuring psychomotor
retardation and slow, hypophonic, poorly articulated verbal output.
Parkinson's disease and progressive supranuclear palsy have many similar
features. Table 8.5 shows findings differentiating these three entities.

Parkinson's disease

Parkinson's disease is a common neurological problem with such striking
clinical features that the diagnosis is usually obvious. Among many features
that distinguish the disorder are a number of alterations in verbal
expression. Parkinsonian patients usually speak slowly with at least some
degree of indistinct articulation. Output can range from severe hypophonia
(a barely discernible whisper) with a slurred, poorly articulated output to
a soft monotone and mild loss of clarity of enunciation. Initiation of speech
is often slow (latency) and the prosodic quality is altered; pause duration,
pitch change and loudness are strikingly muted (Darkins et al 1988). While
the Parkinsonian may produce a simplified verbal output, it is grammatically correct and contains an adequate lexicon. The simplification probably
represents economy of effort, the difficulty of verbal output being sufficiently great that the patient strives for simplicity. Parkinsonian patients
also show a notable decrease in non-verbal language; gestures, facial
expressions and bodily movements are distinctly decreased but not absent.

The rate of thinking is also slow, reflecting (and augmenting) the slowing of movement and speech with an apparent slowing of the stream of thought. Parkinsonian patients maintain control of their line of thought, but the ability to manipulate information may be hindered by mental slowing. They often are forgetful, having difficulty retrieving information already learned. Many investigators report dementia in Parkinson's disease (Celesia & Wanamaker 1972, Mayeux et al 1981, Pollock & Hornabrook 1966). Some suggest this represents an Alzheimer dementia superimposed on the Parkinsonism (Boller et al 1980), others postulate a clinically distinct 'subcortical' dementia (Albert 1979), and still others accept that both may occur during the course of the disease (Benson 1984).

Parkinson's disease patients frequently appear depressed (Brown & Wilson 1972, Mindham 1970); whether the depression is the same as the psychiatric depression just described, or a separate entity unique to Parkinson's disease is debated (Horn 1974, Marsh & Markham 1973). Psychomotor retardation is notable in both disorders and many other features of major depression, both vegetative and psychological, occur in Parkinsonian patients; differentiation of Parkinson's disease from major depressive disorder can be difficult. Table 8.5 shows some characteristics that help differentiate Parkinson's disease from depression and progressive supranuclear palsy.

Progressive supranuclear palsy (PSP)

A relatively rare degenerative disorder of the elderly first demonstrated by Steele et al (1964) may produce cross-diagnostic problems. Four cardinal findings of progressive supranuclear palsy (PSP) include axial dystonia (a rigidity that is far more pronounced in axial than appendicular musculature), pseudobulbar palsy, disturbance of extraocular movements (particularly of vertical gaze) and dementia. The course is slow, persistent and insidious; many years often pass between the onset (as noted by the victim) and a sufficiently clear clinical picture to allow diagnosis. In this dilemma careful attention to speech, language and thought may be of help.

The verbal output in PSP is slow, poorly articulated and hypophonic and, as the disease progresses, eventually disappears completely (mutism). Initiation of speech is slow; the output is flat with decreased prosodic qualities. In contrast, basic language remains normal. While some simplification of syntactical structure is apparent, this is obviously based on output difficulties, a compensatory economy. The semantic content appears normal. There is also marked limitation of non-verbal gesture so that communication by either voice or gesture is limited.

In PSP, thinking appears slow and long latencies before initiation of a response are common (Albert et al 1974). The stream of thought is also slow but PSP patients tenaciously maintain control of their own thought processes. There appears to be no loss of cognitive function until the end

Table 8.3 Thought performance

	Rate	Stream of thought	Control (possession)	Manipulation (cognition)
Depression	slow	ponderous	maintained	slowed
Parkinson's disease	slow	slow	maintained	dilapidated
PSP	slow	slow	maintained	dilapidated
Posterior aphasia	normal	normal	occasionally lost	deficient
Schizophrenia	normal	irregular (difficult to judge)	interrupted (internal cues)	bizarre
Epilepsy	normal to fast	normal	excellent, tenacious	normal
Mania	rapid	rapid changes	interrupted (internal and external cues)	adequate
Huntington's disease	slow	slow	maintained	dilapidated
Alzheimer's disease	slow	irregular	interrupted	deficient

stages, but the ability to demonstrate cognitive capability is severely compromised by the output disturbance. The dementia of PSP is more apparent than real. The ability to learn new material remains normal until deep into the course and, except for the tremendous latency, retrieval of learned information remains good. Depression is common and the appearance may be exaggerated by the physical features of the disease; nonetheless, true and significant depressions do occur. Rarely does a PSP patient tell of either hallucinatory or delusional intrusions.

PSP is difficult to diagnose until fairly advanced, most often misdiagnosed as either Parkinson's disease or depression. Table 8.5 demonstrates verbal output features that help raise suspicions until the pathognomonic physical features appear.

Posterior (fluent) aphasia

A number of aphasic syndromes are characterized by a fluent verbal output that appears confused or nonsensical (Benson 1979) and are easily misinterpreted as psychiatric disturbances. Almost without exception, a fluent aphasic output indicates pathology located posteriorly in the dominant (usually left) hemisphere. Many individuals with posterior aphasia show no evidence of basic neurological defect, such as paresis or sensory loss. The aetiology may be stroke, tumour or brain trauma and so obvious that the condition presents no diagnostic problem. Not infrequently, however, the diagnosis is not obvious and the strikingly abnormal verbal output may lead to misdiagnosis as schizophrenia or mania.

A number of characteristics of posterior aphasia clearly differentiate the disorder. The verbal output is rapid and the quantity of words produced per minute is normal (from 100 to 200). Initiation, articulation and prosodic qualities of speech remain normal and the use of relational (syntactic) language structures is normal. On the other hand, the verbal content is notably lacking in specific, substantive words; pauses, circumlocutions and/or substitutions are frequent. Paraphasia is common and may be literal (substitution of a phoneme), verbal (substitution of a word) or neologistic (substitution of a group of phonemes to produce an unreal word). With a rapid rate and frequent paraphasias, the verbal output becomes an incomprehensible gibberish, a true jargon, and must be differentiated from glossolalia, schizophrenic word salad (Bleuler 1912/1950) and manic hyperverbosity.

Both schizophrenia and mania can be cross-diagnosed with posterior aphasia. The rate and quantity of verbal output is increased in all three disorders but word-finding difficulty is far more prevalent in posterior

Table 8.4 Thought constituents

	Memory (learning)	Memory (retrieval)	Mood/ affect	Abnormal perception (hallucinations)	Abnormal beliefs (delusions)
Depression	preserved (but limited)	often need prompting	morose	not uncommon	common, fixed
Parkinson's disease	normal	slow, need cues	often depressed	rare	rare
PSP	normal	slow but good	often depressed	rare	rare
Posterior aphasia	variable, normal to poor	poor	often unconcerned	not uncommon	not uncommon
Schizophrenia	preserved	good	blunted, inappropriate	common, auditory > visual	common, often systematised
Epilepsy	variable, normal to limited	good	intense feelings	not uncommon	common
Mania	preserved (limited by poor attention)	good	euphoric	not uncommon	uncommon, simple
Huntington's disease	normal until late	poor, need cues	may be depressed	common	common
Alzheimer's disease	lost	poor	unconcerned	confabulatory	confabulatory

aphasia, with less tendency to use a consistent, idiosyncratic word (a characteristic of some schizophrenic and manic outputs). Most important, the posterior aphasic is more concerned than either of the psychotic types that the listener understand. Table 8.6 presents a number of features differentiating schizophrenia, mania, Huntington's disease, epilepsy and posterior aphasia. With careful attention, misinterpretation of posterior aphasia as a psychotic output is less likely.

Schizophrenia

Even more than other psychiatric disorders, schizophrenia presents with a multitude of different features including fascinating abnormalities of verbal expression. Unfortunately, in some countries, schizophrenia has been overdiagnosed and, once the label is applied, it persists. Many individuals have been called schizophrenic, and some of their symptoms accepted as schizophrenic, even though different disease processes are known to be present. With effective treatments now available for schizophrenia, accurate diagnosis has become important. Evaluation of speech, language and thought often offers crucial clues in the differential diagnosis.

The verbal output in schizophrenia may be moderately fast, not to the degree of mania but may equal hypomanic outputs. Articulation is usually normal but the initiation of speech may be delayed with long pauses preceding vocalization. Prosodic qualities are normal and the language of the schizophrenic is also normal, although slight simplification of sentence structure may be seen. The lexicon is usually full, but during psychotic phases may feature bizarre words and phrases. Amongst the bizarre vocabulary is a tendency toward idiosyncratic word usage, neologisms made up of normal phonemes (often parts of normal words) consistently used to represent the same symbolisation in the psychotic thought process. In rare instances the psychotic schizophrenic may substitute individual phonemes (literal paraphasia) in substantive words to produce a jargon known as schizophrenic word salad (Bleuler 1912/1950); in the current practice of psychiatry this is a rare occurrence. Gesture is almost invariably decreased in the schizophrenic, at times producing a notable difference between the rapid and loquacious verbal output and a decreased quantity of gesture. The movement disorders of antipsychotic medication or true catatonia may produce an increase in motion, but not in gesture.

It is in thinking that the diagnostic abnormalities are most notable. The schizophrenic's rate of thinking appears normal, but the stream of thought is often difficult to follow. Control of thought appears interrupted and is surmised as responses to internal cues. The patient appears to respond to hallucinated voices, intruding thoughts, misrepresented external stimuli, etc., most of which are unavailable to the examiner. While most schizophrenics can perform cognitive tasks adequately the results may suffer from interruptions to the stream of thought. The schizophrenic can learn new

Table 8.5 Differential features of slow output disorders

Characteristic	Depression	Parkinson's disease	Progressive supranuclear palsy
Verbal output	soft, decrescendo	soft, poorly articulated	soft, monotonous, poorly articulated
Lexicon	morbid	full	economical
Syntax	simple — often incomplete	simplified for economy	simplified for economy
Swallowing	normal	dysphagic, drooling	dysphagic, drooling
Posture	stooped	stooped	hypererect
Gait	slow	abnormal, short steps, shuffling, en bloc turns, retropulsion	unstable, falls are frequent
Motor tone	normal	rigidity, limb > axial	rigidity, axial > limb
Tremor	none	common, resting, pillrolling	uncommon

material, even during the psychotic phase (unless too heavily drugged) and the ability to retrieve old information, if it can be tested, remains adequate. A blunted, inappropriate affect, often described as shallow, is common. Both hallucinations and delusions are common with the latter sufficiently pervasive and systematised that everyday activities are misinterpreted into a delusional system.

Similar findings, particularly the psychotic features, are often accepted as proof of schizophrenia even though they appear in the course of other recognized disorders. Thus, depression, mania and Huntington's disease all produce delusions and/or hallucinations, disordered thought and inappropriate affect. Careful attention to verbal output differences may avert some misdiagnoses. Table 8.6 outlines important verbal differentiating characteristics.

Epileptic personality

While the topic remains controversial, there is growing agreement that some of those individuals with complex-partial seizure disorder develop a striking personality disorder. Geschwind (1979) called the behavioural complex of temporal lobe seizures the most characteristic of all psychiatric syndromes and many now refer to this complex as the Geschwind syndrome. While the disorder includes alterations of sexuality and an intensification of both cognitive and emotional thought, the most characteristic feature involves verbal expression (Blumer & Benson 1982). The verbal output has been called circumstantial output, but it is imperative not to confuse epileptic circumstantiality with schizophrenic circumstantiality; these are distinctly different disorders of expression. In the affected epileptic (most epileptics do not show the disorder) the verbal output is both excessive and over-inclusive. The epileptic wants to be certain that the listener understands, totally and exactly, what is meant by the response. This produces a tenaciousness in communication, reflected in both verbal output and interpersonal relationships, a status often called clinging or viscous. The verbal output is overlong, hyperdetailed and contains many side explanations. Loose association can be suspected, but if allowed sufficient time, the epileptic returns to the original topic, the side discussions and overly detailed explanations proving pertinent to the idea expressed. If the patient is literate, circumstantiality is often expanded into hypergraphia (Waxman & Geschwind 1974), a tendency to express ideas in voluminous writings. Some turn to poetry, others write novels, essays or books. Many keep extensive logs or diaries detailing the mundane activities of their life. Letters to politicians, newspaper editors and their physicians are frequent, hyperdetailed and often difficult to understand.

Through all this output grammar is intact, the lexicon is adequate and there are no speech abnormalities. Only the control of thought is disordered, as demonstrated by the verbal expression (Bear 1979, Blumer 1975, Blumer & Benson 1982). Typically the epileptic personality disorder occurs in patients who are seizure free and need little or no anticonvulsant medication; the behavioural problem is easily misinterpreted as a primary psychiatric disorder but proves remarkably resistant to routine psychotherapy measures. Differential diagnosis includes schizophrenia and posterior aphasia and diagnostic points are presented in Table 8.6.

Mania

Fullblown mania is usually not a diagnostic problem, but lesser degrees may be misinterpreted as either schizophrenia or posterior aphasia. Characteristics of verbal output worthy of attention include a fast accelerating, clearly articulated output that is rapidly initiated but with normal prosodic quality. Except for the rapid rate, speech quality is normal. Language shows little abnormality. Grammar is normal, except that the patient almost invariably speaks in phrases rather than sentences. There is a tendency for repetitiveness in the lexicon, sometimes with changing meaning for a single word. Verbal output may be incessant, apparently triggered by clang sounds, puns and both external and internal associations. An exuberance of both verbal output and non-verbal gestures is prominent.

Thought, as monitored by verbal output, is rapidly processed with characteristically abrupt changes in the stream of thought, interrupted by either internal or external cues (the flight of ideas). Control of thought processes is poor. If controlled sufficiently for testing, the manic patient will show an adequate but inefficient ability to manipulate knowledge. The ability to learn new material is preserved as is a relatively good ability to

Table 8.6 Differential features of rapid output disorders

Characteristic	Mania	Schizophrenia	Huntington's	Epilepsy	Posterior aphasia
Movements	hyperkinetic	normal or reduced	bizarre, choreiform	normal	normal
Articulatory clarity	slight impairment, rushed	normal	indistinct, variable, articulatory errors	normal	normal
Prosody	normal	normal	poorly controlled, variable	normal	normal
Semantic quality	normal, tend to be repetitive	normal, tendency to bizarre word selection	normal	normal	anomic, paraphasic
Non-verbal communication	exuberant, excessive	decreased	unpredictable	normal	normal or decreased
Rate of thought performance	rapid	normal	slow	normal to fast	normal to fast
Control of thought	interrupted (internal and external cues)	interrupted (internal cues)	maintained	excellent, tenacious, excessive	fairly good
Mood/affect	euphoric	blunted, inappropriate	depressed	intense	unconcerned
Delusions	uncommon, simple	common, systematised	common, non-systematised	common, intense, may be systematised	occasional
Concern about listener's reaction	mild	limited	moderate	strong	strong

retrieve old learned information. Mood is obviously, often overwhelmingly, euphoric and abnormal perceptions (hallucinations) are not infrequent. Simple delusions are not uncommon but persistence of a delusion is unusual.

Mania is to be differentiated from other disorders featuring rapid verbal output, including the fluent output of a posterior aphasic or the circumstantial output of a temporal lobe epileptic, but is most often cross-diagnosed with schizophrenia. Table 8.6 presents features useful for these differentiations.

Huntington's disease

The verbal output in the genetically determined degenerative process, Huntington's disease, varies with the progression of the disorder. In general, while appearing rapid because of the uneven, explosive output, word counts demonstrate that verbal output is decreased. With progression, clarity of articulation is lost and disturbed prosody (abnormal melody, rhythm, timbre and inflection) is evident. Initiation of speech is often delayed. Language remains intact except for a decrease in lexicon in late stages. Control of non-verbal expression becomes erratic; inappropriate grimaces and bodily movements are frequent. Thought performance is slow. Mental control is often disturbed; paranoid and/or hallucinatory disturbances occur, particularly as the disorder progresses. The ability to manipulate knowledge decreases and is totally lost in the late stage. Evaluation of memory in Huntington's patients demonstrates only a retrieval problem until late in the disease course, when learning ability becomes affected (Caine et al 1977). Depression is common (Trimble 1981) and often occurs early, not infrequently preceding the onset of chorea (McHugh & Folstein 1979). There may be no pathognomonic motor or verbal expression abnormalities to differentiate the depression of the early Huntingtonian from other forms of depression and, indeed, they respond to physical treatments for depression (McHugh & Folstein 1979). Severe depression may also occur during the course of the disorder; suicide is common (McHugh & Folstein 1979). Hallucinations and paranoid ideation are not uncommon and delusions may be noted. Thus, the patient with Huntington's disease at times presents a depressive, at others a schizophrenia-like, picture; usually some degree of subcortical dementia is present. Most often the movement disorder, dementia and family history will identify the disorder but speech characteristics may help.

Alzheimer's disease

Although long recognized (Alzheimer 1907), only recently has this degenerative dementing disorder become a major public health threat. Inevitably, the massive publicity given to Alzheimer's disease in the past decade has lead to overdiagnosis and misdiagnosis, a serious error as the incorrect label may conceal a treatable dementing disorder (Benson 1982). Dementia may pose a diagnostic problem and among the most valuable of differentiating features are those of verbal output (Cummings et al 1985). It must be recognized, however, that Alzheimer's disease is progressive and all features change with time. No static description remains correct. The verbal output in the early stages may be moderately fast (not as rapid as mania or schizophrenia) and the articulation distinct and clear with normal prosodic quality. A language problem, anomia, is the first verbal output abnormality noted and rapidly worsens. Syntax remains normal until late in the course, a valuable diagnostic feature when contrasted to the early and progressive decrease in the availability of words. Problems with comprehension are eventually noted and, finally, verbal and/or neologistic paraphasias intrude. Repetition of spoken language remains relatively intact until late; a transcortical sensory aphasia syndrome eventually becomes prominent (Cummings et al 1985). Non-verbal gesture also decreases but is difficult to quantify.

There is a slowing and irregularity of the stream of thought and the control of thought appears interrupted, based on word-finding and memory problems. The ability to manipulate old knowledge (cognition) deteriorates early and becomes a major defect. The ability to learn new material is also impaired early, usually the first problem noted by family or physician. The ability to retrieve old information decreases more slowly but eventually almost all old memories are lost. The patient with Alzheimer's disease shows progressively less concern about the mental deficits, a state of unawareness and unconcern bordering on euphoria. Crude disorders in both perception and belief may be noted but are clearly confabulatory, attempts to substitute for information that is not available.

Alzheimer's disease may begin at age 50 or 60 but more often involves the older individual; most have no history of prior psychiatric disorder. This, plus the slow progression and characteristic mental features, is suggestive but not diagnostic in the early stages. Verbal expression in Alzheimer's disease is strikingly different from that of depression (see Tables 8.1–8.4) and yet these are often considered the two forms of mental impairment most difficult to differentiate in the elderly. Study of the differences in verbal output make this differential problem relatively easy.

DISCUSSION

Tables 8.1–8.4 outline findings useful for differentiating nine neuropsychiatric disorders with characteristic abnormalities of verbal expression. As with any abbreviated description or tabular outline, the tables are inadequate and only highlight a few features. Four aspects — speech, language, thought performance and thought constituents — can be monitored. Each can provide significant information, either characteristic abnormalities or, often just as valuable, retention of normal function. Familiarity with each avenue of verbal expression provides the clinician with a diagnostic tool of potential value. All psychiatrists and neurologists use some of the features presented in Tables 8.1–8.4 but too few are knowledgeable in all. The neurologist may overlook the depression in a patient with Parkinson's disease while the psychiatrist may miss the Parkinsonian features in a depressed patient. Similarly, the psychiatrist may use a label of schizophrenia for an epileptic behavioural disturbance while the neurologist does the opposite. Analysis of verbal output can provide diagnostic aid in these and many other neuropsychiatric problems.

Several clusters of neuropsychiatric features are prone to cross-diagnosis, particularly those featuring either slow or relatively rapid output. Tables 8.5 and 8.6 present a number of verbal and non-verbal characteristics for the clinical entities most likely to present with these altered rates of output. While the disorders are often easily separated, on occasion distinctive features are not clear and attention to the verbal features separating the disorders may prove valuable for the clinician.

Even though most of the entities discussed are well known, diagnostic errors are not uncommon. Now that effective specific treatment is available for many neuropsychiatric problems, correct diagnosis becomes imperative. Mere treatment of a symptom can prove fruitless or even detrimental. For instance, the use of neuroleptics in the treatment of hallucinations due to covert complex partial epilepsy may dangerously exacerbate the seizure problem. Diagnostic information from all sources may be needed and the disorders of verbal output often provide the clues needed for proper diagnosis. Most accomplished clinicians do monitor several aspects of verbal output, often without consciously noting individual features, and use this information to gain an overall diagnostic impression. The individual practicing neuropsychiatry needs this information for evaluating his patients.

REFERENCES

Albert M L 1979 Subcortical dementia. In: Katzman R, Terry R D, Bick K L (eds)
   Alzheimer's disease: senile dementia and related disorders. Raven, New York, p 173–180
Albert M L, Feldman R G, Willis A L 1974 The subcortical dementia of progressive
   supranuclear palsy. Journal of Neurology, Neurosurgery and Psychiatry 37: 121–130
Alzheimer A 1907 Über eigenartige Erkrankung der Hirnrinde. Allegemeine
   Zeitschrift für Psychiatrie 64: 146–148
Arendt H 1978 The life of the mind. Harcourt, New York
Basso A, Faglioni P, Vignolo L A 1975 Etude contrôlee de la reéducation du langage dans
   l'aphasie: Comparison entre aphasiques traités et non-traités. Revue Neurologique
   131: 607–614
Bear D M 1979 The temporal lobes: An approach to the study of organic behavioral
   changes. In: Gazzaniga M S (ed) Handbook of behavioral neurobiology. Vol 2:
   Neuropsychology. Plenum Press, New York, p 75–95
Benson D F 1979 Aphasia, alexia and agraphia. Churchill Livingstone, New York

Benson D F 1982 The treatable dementias. In: Benson D F, Blumer D (eds) Psychiatric aspects of neurologic disease, vol 2. Grune & Stratton, New York, p 123–148

Benson D F 1984 Parkinsonian dementia: cortical or subcortical? In: Hassler R G, Christ J F (eds) Advances in neurology. Vol 40: Parkinsonian-specific motor and mental disorders. Raven Press, New York, p 235–240

Benson D F, Cummings J L 1985 Agraphia. In: Vinken P J, Bruyn G W, Frederiks J A M (eds) Handbook of clinical neurology, 2nd edn. Vol 45: Clinical neuropsychology. Elsevier Press, Amsterdam, p 457–472

Bleuler E (trans. Zinkin J) 1912/1950 Dementia praecox. International University Press, New York

Blumer D 1975 Temporal lobe epilepsy and its psychiatric significance. In: Benson D F, Blumer D (eds) Psychiatric aspects of neurologic disease. Grune & Stratton, New York, p 171–197

Blumer D, Benson D F 1982 Psychiatric manifestations of epilepsy. In: Benson D F, Blumer D (eds) Psychiatric aspects of neurologic disease, vol 2. Grune & Stratton, New York, p 25–47

Boller F, Mizutani T, Roessmann V, Gambetti P 1980 Parkinson disease, dementia and Alzheimer disease: clinicopathological correlations. Annals of Neurology 7: 329–335

Brown G L V, Wilson W P 1972 Parkinsonism and depression. Southern Medical Journal 65: 540–545

Caine E D, Ebert M A, Weingartner H 1977 An outline for the analysis of dementia. Neurology 27: 1087–1092

Celesia G G, Wanamaker W M 1972 Psychiatric disturbances in Parkinson's disease. Diseases of the Nervous System 33: 577–583

Critchley M 1970 Thinking and speaking: verbal symbols in thought. In: Critchley M Aphasiology. Edward Arnold, London, ch 13, 159–173

Cummings J L, Benson D F, Hill M A, Read S 1985 Aphasia in dementia of the Alzheimer type. Neurology 35: 394–397

Darkins A W, Fromkin V A, Benson D F 1988 A characterization of the prosodic loss in Parkinson's disease. Brain and Language 34: 315–327

Darley F L, Aronson A E, Brown J R 1975 Motor speech disorders. Saunders, Philadelphia

Faber R, Abrams R, Taylor M A, Kasprison A, Morris C, Weisz R 1983 Comparison of schizophrenic patients with formal thought disorder and neurologically impaired patients with aphasia. American Journal of Psychiatry 140: 1348–1351

Gerson S N, Benson D F, Frazier S H 1977 Diagnosis: schizophrenia versus posterior aphasia. American Journal of Psychiatry 134: 966–969

Geschwind N 1979 Behavioural changes in temporal lobe epilepsy (Editorial). Psychological Medicine 9: 217–219

Greden J F, Carroll B J 1981 Psychomotor function in affective disorders: an overview of new monitoring techniques. American Journal of Psychiatry 138: 1441–1448

Hinchcliffe M K, Lancashire M, Roberts F J 1971 Depression: Defense mechanism in speech. British Journal of Psychiatry 118: 471–472

Horn S 1974 Some psychological factors in Parkinsonism. Journal of Neurology, Neurosurgery, and Psychiatry 37: 27–31

McHugh P R, Folstein M F 1979 Psychopathology of dementia: implications for neuropathology. In: Katzman R (ed) Congenital and acquired cognitive disorders. Raven Press, New York, p 17–30

Marsh G G, Markham C H 1973 Does levodopa alter depression and psychopathology in parkinsonism patients? Journal of Neurology, Neurosurgery, and Psychiatry 36: 925–935

Mayeux R, Stern Y, Rosen J, Leventhal J 1981 Depression, intellectual impairment and Parkinson disease. Neurology 31: 645–650

Metter E J 1985 Speech disorders. Spectrum Publications, New York

Mindham, R H S 1970 Psychiatric symptoms in Parkinsonism. Journal of Neurology, Neurosurgery and Psychiatry 33: 188–191

Mueller M 1887 The science of thought. Scribner, New York

Pick A 1931/1973 Aphasia. Charles C Thomas, Springfield, Illinois

Pollock M, Hornabrook R W 1966 The prevalence, natural history and dementia of Parkinson's disease. Brain 89: 429–488

Steele J C, Richardson J C, Olszewski J 1964 Progressive supranuclear palsy. Archives of Neurology 10: 333–359

Szabodi E, Bradshaw C M, Besson J A O 1976 Elongation of pause time in speech: A single, objective measure of motor retardation in depression. British Journal of Psychiatry 129: 592–597

Trimble M 1981 Neuropsychiatry. Wiley, New York

Vygotsky L S 1962 Thought and language. (Trans. Hanfmann and Vakar) MIT Press, Cambridge, Mass.

Waxman S G, Geschwind N 1974 Hypergraphia in temporal lobe epilepsy. Neurology 24: 629–638

9

D. J. Cutting

Body image disturbances in neuropsychiatry

INTRODUCTION

The body image is a relatively stable collection of beliefs, memories and sensory and motor representations concerning the body. It may evoke a particular set of emotions when some part enters consciousness, and subconsciously plays a major role in determining personality and reactions to events in the environment. It is largely non-verbal in its development and structure, but contains a linguistic representation of body parts to allow one, for example, to point immediately to any of these on command. Overall, the most striking feature about the body image, compared with the image of things and events in the outside world, is the relative unimportance of language and sound in its composition, and the powerful influence and interplay of kinaesthetic, tactile, and, to a lesser extent, visual sensations.

In the definition of body image given above, I have included motor as well as cognitive elements, and beliefs and memories as well as sensory representations. This is a wider concept than has at times been recommended, but can be justified for the following reasons. First, information concerning the body does not only provide knowledge about *what* is happening, but also affects *how* we do things. It contributes to both *declarative* and *procedural* knowledge. Secondly, a powerful belief about the size or shape of one's body can have quite dramatic repercussions in all spheres of life, more so, in some ways, than a complete loss of sensation on one side of the body. For these reasons the concept of body image should, in my view, be a broad one, so long as it is appreciated that the representations of ideas, sensations and movements are each different in the factors involved in their structure and in the rules governing their function.

An examination of the history of the concept should clarify the issues involved in definition.

The notion of a body image is relatively new in the history of ideas. Few psychiatrists, psychologists or neurologists during the 19th century referred to anything like it, and the first real discussion was initiated by a French neurologist, Bonnier, in 1905 and by two British neurologists, Head and Holmes, in 1911. Its interest at this epoch can partly be attributed to what

Foucault (1966), the French historian of ideas, called the contemporary 'preoccupation with man's subjectivity' and partly to the discovery of the cortical localisation of functions, which occurred at that time.

The originators of the concept — Bonnier, Head and Holmes — were interested in the cortical representation of sensation, and the first notion of a body image was in essence a physiological explanation of how tactile (Bonnier) or postural (Head and Holmes) sensation was represented in the brain. These authors used the term 'schema' for this. Head and Holmes defined their 'schema' as a 'standard resulting from previous postures and movements to which immediate reference is made when a fresh position is recognised . . . for this combined standard against which all subsequent changes in posture are measured before they enter consciousness we propose the word schema'.

Schilder, an Austrian neuropsychiatrist, then enlarged the concept in his book *The Image and Appearance of the Human Body* published in 1935. Like Freud he had trained as a neurologist, but then turned to psychoanalysis. He was influenced by several factors. First, by this time a number of patients with body image disorders had been reported, some of whom had intact peripheral sensation. Secondly, a handful of intriguing optical experiments had been carried out, in which a subject wore inverting lenses continuously for up to eight days. Visually, the world was seen as completely inverted, but the most surprising finding was the marked distortion of the experience of movement and tactile localisation which resulted. It was clear from this that the body schema could not be an isolated representation of postural and tactile sensation, but must have a prominent visual component as well. Thirdly, Gestalt psychology was at its height at the time, the central tenet being that the whole is greater than the sum of the constituent parts. Applied to the concept of body image, this meant that even if the physiological representations of all the sensory modalities took part in a complex cerebral interaction, this would still not explain the *psychological* entity of a body image. A psychological Gestalt such as the body image could not even be reduced to its perceptual elements, according to this theoretical school, and certainly not to a physiological level. Finally, Schilder was much influenced by Freud and went as far as claiming that the body image was essentially an *emotional* complex, underpinned by sexual energy.

Schilder's body image as a libidinous psychological entity and Head's body schema as a physiological representation of postural sensation are clearly worlds apart. And in subsequent decades most writers on the subject took up a position somewhere between these two extremes. French neurologists, in particular Lhermitte (1939) and Hecaen (Hecaen and Ajuriaguerra 1952), wrote extensively on the subject, defending the Gestalt position about the irreducibility of the body image into physiological elements, but eschewing any fundamental emotional basis to it. The most significant advance in recent years has come from the new discipline of neuropsychology, with the realisation that the right hemisphere subserves specific higher functions, and is not merely a reserve for the left hemisphere. This has confirmed the earlier suspicions of some neurologists that the body image is largely represented in the right hemisphere and that most body image disorders both result from right hemisphere dysfunction and involve the left side of the body. The most contentious development in this period has been the extension of the concept into areas such as personality typology and neurosis.

In the rest of this chapter I shall review the range of body image disorders which have been described, and consider the particular types which occur in specific neurological and psychiatric disorders. One of the problems in the literature is the abundance of terms, often synonymous or with only subtle differences in meaning. Many of these are neologisms, with a dubious etymological basis in Greek. I shall try to group the terms into broad categories, each with some common feature. Another problem is the difficulty, more so than in other psychopathological enquiries, in establishing the precise phenomenological basis for many of the disorders. For example, if a subject reports that they have a 'double', is this a belief or a perceptual experience? If the latter, does it have visual, tactile, or even auditory components? A further problem concerns the link between disorders of self-awareness (e.g. depersonalisation, multiple personality) and disordered bodily awareness. Some might argue that one should exclude the former, because the condition affects the way a subject views the entire world, external surrounding as well as body. I have included them, however, because the body image is usually markedly altered, albeit secondarily, and because such disorders often occur at the same time as, for example, visual hallucinations of the body, and appear to be closely linked in terms of the shared mechanism.

The broad categories which I shall deal with are altered awareness of one side of the body, denial of bodily disability, the experience of a phantom, impaired identification of bodily parts, altered awareness of pain, abnormal awareness of movement, abnormal visual experiences of the self, abnormal tactile experiences, abnormal consciousness of the self, abnormal beliefs about the body, and abnormal preoccupations with the body.

ALTERED AWARENESS OF ONE SIDE OF THE BODY

(Includes neglect, hemiasomatognosia, alloesthesia, and forms the basis for some instances of anosognosia, abnormal tactile experiences and a particular abnormal belief about the body, known as somatoparaphrenia)

Definition

The essential feature of this group of disorders is an altered awareness of one side of the body. It is impossible to be more specific because the two main conditions which are included within the category — conscious (or active) neglect (or hemiasomatognosia), and unconscious (or passive) neglect (or hemiasomatognosia) — have very different features.

The terms neglect and hemiasomatognosia (literally lack of knowledge of one side of the body) are used interchangeably in the literature. Of the four main writers on the subject, Critchley (1953) and Heilman (Heilman et al, 1985) favour neglect, while Hecaen (Hecaen & Albert, 1978) and Frederiks (1985) favour hemiasomatognosia. This disputed terminology is understandable, but it is curious that the writers who favour the term neglect are not aware of the contradiction implied in the division into conscious and unconscious varieties. One cannot be actively conscious of something which one neglects; one would take steps to remedy the situation. For this reason, I would recommend the use of the term 'altered awareness of one side of the body', and call the two main subgroups subjective alienation of limb and unawareness of limb.

In what has been known as passive or unconscious neglect, a subject has *no experience* at all of the limb and behaves as if it were not there. He may fail to put on a slipper on that side, fail to shave on that side and leave his arm hanging over the bed as if it did not exist.

In the active or conscious variety, a subject has a definite *positive experience* that the limb is strange or does not belong to him. Subjects vary in the way they describe this experience, and may report complex perceptual experiences, such as shrinking, enlargement and qualitative distortions (see case 3).

It is probable that the varieties of altered awareness of one side of the body, known as active or passive neglect, share the same physiological mechanism of a central blocking of stimuli from the periphery, but it is clear that the psychological consequences of this can be quite different. (The contradictions inherent in the usual terminology can probably be attributed to the false assumption that psychological phenomena have a simple point-to-point correspondence with physiological abnormalities.)

Illustrative cases

Case 1: A 70-year-old right-handed woman was admitted to hospital complaining that she had 'had another stroke', and that she could not hold anything in her left hand. She had suffered a left hemiplegia three months previously but had made a full and rapid recovery from this. On examination on this admission she had virtually no weakness apart from a slight falling away of the outstretched left arm. She did, however, have a left field defect, left visuospatial neglect, and left-sided sensory loss to touch and joint position. She said: 'My hand doesn't belong to me; when I was in before it was just like a plastic hand; it used to come flop on me; it was stone cold; I used to feel that someone else was touching me; I used to say, 'Who's touching me'; now it feels more filled out'.

(Subjective alienation — personal series)

Case 2: A man of 75 developed weakness in his left arm three days before being examined. He had undergone an amputation of his left leg 11 years before, and of his right leg two years ago, for peripheral vascular disease. There was no field defect and no gross impairment of tactile sensation, but he had left-sided tactile inattention and impaired joint position sense. On request he could raise his left arm above his head, but usually he just let it hang down over the edge of the bed and seemed unaware of it.

(Unawareness — personal series)

Case 3: A woman of 72 developed an acute left hemiplegia four days before being examined. At this time she had total weakness, total sensory loss and a field defect on the left. She said: 'My arm feels like a child's rubber doll; I felt it had actually left my body; all my fingers seemed to have shrunk to short fat fingers'.

(Illusory distortion with alienation — personal series)

Case 4: A man of 30 developed left-sided focal motor seizures. At the age of 37 a right parietal meningioma was diagnosed and removed, which left him with a mild left hemiparesis and slight left-sided astereognosis and tactile inattention. At the age of 46 he developed the belief that the left side of his body was evil and controlled by the devil, that the left side had slipped behind the right side making the latter more prominent, and that there was another person, possibly his father, to the left of him. He also had visual hallucinations of his father in the left field of vision.

(Somatoparaphrenia — Nightingale 1982)

Varieties and associated phenomena

Subjective alienation of limb (conscious neglect, active neglect, conscious hemiasomatognosia, active hemiasomatognosia) In these cases, a subject experiences the limb as not belonging to them (case 1). There may or may not be associated weakness, but tactile sensation is nearly always impaired. In my series of 100 hemiplegics (Cutting 1978) 16 patients reported the experience, 13 with sensory loss. The left arm was the focus of the experience in 13, and 2 of those with a right-sided experience had global cognitive impairment.

Unawareness of limb (passive neglect, unconscious neglect, passive hemiasomatognosia, unconscious hemiasomatognosia)

Here the subject simply ignores the limb, even to the extent of letting it hang over the side of the bed (case 2). When asked to touch the limb their intact hand will approach the affected limb and then waver above it. There is usually associated weakness and impaired joint position sense, but tactile sensation may be surprisingly good. It was confined to left hemiplegics in my series.

Sensory displacement (alloesthesia, exosomesthesia)

Some subjects experience a stimulus in another part of the body from that actually touched, or even claim to experience it outside the body altogether (Shapiro et al 1952), on a chair, for example.

Illusory distortions (microsomatognosia, macrosomatognosia)

The subjective experience of alienation may be complicated by illusory distortions of the affected limb. I have called these 'illusory' because there is an underlying sensory impairment, whereas the same experience of distortion may also occur in other conditions, organic or functional, with intact sensation, and must then be regarded as an hallucination. The condition is illustrated by case 3. (Frederiks 1963 reported three epileptics who had transient experiences that their limbs were 'inflated', 'shortened' or 'extremely small'. He called these microsomatognosia and macrosomatognosia, though it is possible that these were hallucinations rather than illusions.)

Delusional elaboration of alienation (somatoparaphrenia)

Some subjects develop quite elaborate and bizarre beliefs about their affected limb. Nightingale's (1982) patient (case 4) illustrates this well. Another patient reported by von Angyal & Frick (1941) believed that he had a paralysed brother beside him; when asked to lift his left arm, he replied, 'He doesn't hear. He won't answer. He has mental paralysis'.

Denial of paralysis (anosognosia for hemiplegia)

Although some examples of this condition probably originate with unawareness of the limb, this was not true of all cases in my series (Cutting 1978) and I shall treat denial of disability as a separate set of conditions.

Altered awareness of entire body (total body asomatognosia)

The early French writers on the subject of body image (Bonnier 1905, Deny & Camus 1905) reported cases of total body asomatognosia. However, there are no subsequent reports of any convincing examples of this in subjects with definite brain damage, and the phenomenon they described is more suggestive of psychotic depersonalisation. (Deny and Camus' patient, for example, was a young woman, greatly distressed by her lack of bodily feeling, who threw herself naked into the snow in an attempt to experience some powerful sensation. Such dramatic attempts to experience the body as they remember it before their illness is not uncommon in schizophrenia — see case 18).

Cause

Almost invariably it is the left side of the body which is ignored or the focus of abnormal experiences, and the right side of the brain which contains the lesion. Exceptions to this rule have either been left-handed subjects or have had an associated global cognitive disturbance as in delirium or dementia.

Within the right hemisphere the most pathogenic site is the parietal lobe, although frontal lobe, cingulate gyrus and thalamus have all been cited (Heilman et al 1985). Frederiks (1985) regards the experience of alienation as an effect of cortical dysfunction and unawareness as arising from subcortical damage.

The commonest pathology is a cerebrovascular accident; more rarely a cerebral tumour, a postictal state and right-sided ECT may produce the phenomenon.

It is assumed that the physiological mechanism is insufficient integration and synthesis of somatosensory sensation, a situation Denny-Brown et al (1952) referred to as 'amorphosynthesis'. Other writers (e.g. Schilder 1935, Lhermitte 1939) have been reluctant to attribute the disorder to physiological dysfunction, maintaining the Gestalt principle that perceptual 'wholes' cannot be reduced to physiological elements. In my view, of all the body image disorders, altered awareness of one side of the body is the one most plausibly explained using physiological principles. The varieties and elaborations, such as somatoparaphrenia, can be accounted for by the additional influence of associated psychological dysfunction such as clouding of consciousness or thought disorder.

DENIAL OF BODILY DISABILITY

(Includes anosognosia, anosodiaphoria, personification, overestimation of strength and misoplegia)

Definition

Denial or minimisation of physical disability is one of a range of psychological reactions to illness. Most of this is a normal adaptation to illness and cannot be regarded as a disorder of body image. Beyond a certain level, however, it must be regarded as pathological. Lloyd (personal communication) encountered a man who had suffered a serious heart attack and who was being monitored in the intensive care unit, and yet steadfastly denied that there was anything wrong with him. When pressed to explain his current situation he would only admit to being 'in for a rest', all this despite having been told about the true state of his health.

The form of pathological denial about which most has been written is denial of a hemiplegia. Babinski (1914) was the first to draw attention to it. He called it anosognosia (literally lack of knowledge of disease). Since then the term anosognosia has also been applied to unawareness of cortical blindness (Anton's syndrome) and unawareness of aphasia (always of the Wernicke type), but these are not body image disorders.

A number of other abnormal attitudes towards a paralysed limb may occur, and are usually grouped with denial: minimisation and inappropriate joviality — anosodiaphoria, giving the limb a nickname — personification, overestimation of the strength of the limb — overestimation, and anger towards limb — misoplegia.

Illustrative cases

Case 5: A right-handed man of 58 was admitted to hospital with a coronary thombosis six days before I saw him, and then developed left-sided weakness one day before I saw him. On examination by me he had a left visual field defect, left-sided sensory loss for joint position and fine touch, and a left hemiparesis, affecting the arm and face more than the leg. Although he admitted he had suffered a heart attack he denied that his left arm was in any way weak. He accepted that it felt different — 'heavy', 'swollen' — but even when I showed him that he could not hold his left arm to the same height as the right, he still denied any idea of a stroke or weakness. He had no neglect: he could point accurately to his left middle finger, his left ear and his left thumb. He was correctly orientated in time and place, and had no attention or memory defect. The only associated neuropsychological deficits were mild left visuospatial neglect and a marked visual agnosia for pictures.

(Anosognosia — personal series)

Case 6: A right-handed woman of 65 was examined seven days after admission. She had a left hemiplegia, sensory loss, field defect and was disorientated in time and place, but had no neglect. She said: 'I've no use down the left side. I must have lost an arm and they've stuck another one on. The leg's the same'. On being asked if it were a nuisance, she replied, 'Not much', and when asked if she had had a stroke said, 'We'll have to see about that'.

(Anosodiaphoria — personal series)

Case 7: A left-handed woman of 68 was examined seven days after an acute stroke. She had total weakness on the left side, a left-sided sensory loss and a visual field defect. She admitted her condition but went on to say, 'The nurse called my leg Fred and I called my arm little Fred. I'm one-handed pandy'.

(Personification — personal series)

Case 8: A right-handed man of 66 was examined six days after the onset of a stroke. He had mild left-sided weakness and a field defect, but no detectable sensory loss. He denied any weakness, even when watching the left arm fall away much lower than the right. When pressed to give an explanation he said that he was a football coach and had always had a strong right hand.

(Overestimation — personal series)

Case 9: A right-handed man of 61 was seen two days after the onset of a right hemiplegia. He was weepy and depressed and had total weakness, but only minimal sensory loss. He stated: 'I do feel angry. I'm buggered because I'm right handed. I feel like cutting the bloody thing off.'

(Misoplegia — personal series)

Varieties and associated phenomena

Denial of hemiplegia (anosognosia)

This is the main variety, and the commonest. It was present in 25 of 48 left hemiplegics in the first week and 2 of 52 right hemiplegics in my study, and similar figures have been reported in other large surveys (Nathanson et al 1952, Gross & Kaltenbäck 1955). It is not certain if there are subgroups of denial or not. Based on the degree of insight, I identified three groups: those with complete denial of any illness or disability, those who fluctuated in the course of the interview, denying weakness, one minute, admitting it the next, and those who readily admitted to a stroke, but denied weakness. There was a tendency for the first group to have more profound weakness, sensory loss and unawareness of the limb itself than the others, and I suggested that, following Lissauer's (1890) classic distinction between apperceptive (lower level) and associational (higher level) types of visual agnosia, anosognosia might also be so divided.

Anosodiaphoria

This was also first described by Babinski in his paper on anosognosia in 1914, and later reviewed by Critchley (1957). It was rather rare for minimisation and joviality to be associated in my series (4%), it could occur with a right or a left hemiplegia and appeared to be more in the nature of an understandable reaction than a pathological response (see case 6).

Overestimation

Anastasopoulos (1961) reported five patients with weakness of the right arm who overestimated the strength of this abnormal limb. His original paper has been misunderstood by subsequent authors who have taken the term 'overestimation' to mean overestimating the strength of a normal right limb in compensation for a paralysed left limb. Either variety is rare, only two of the latter and none of the former being observed in my series (case 8).

Personification

Juba (1949) and Critchley (1955) drew attention to this phenomenon, in which the paralysed limb is given a nickname by the subject. Only one subject in my series did this (case 7), despite all subjects being specifically asked about the matter. It is probably, like anosodiaphoria, more an adaptation response than a specific body image disorder.

Hatred towards the limb (misoplegia)

The occasional presence of a morbid fear or dislike of the limb was first noted by Critchley (1962). It was relatively common in my series (9%) and was the only phenomenon which was more common with a right than a left hemiplegia. It was usually associated with depressed mood (case 8) and was almost certainly an adaptation reaction and not a body image disorder.

Cause

The cause of anosognosia for a hemiplegia has been the subject of much discussion.

Like altered awareness of a limb, almost all cases have involved denial of a left hemiplegia, and have had a right hemisphere pathology. In my series the only patients who denied a right hemiplegia were markedly disorientated in time and place, implying generalised cerebral dysfunction.

The necessary site of damage within the right hemisphere is disputed. Some authorities maintain that it is parietal, others that is is thalamic, yet others that both these areas have to be involved. It is possible that subcortical damage might be responsible for the apperceptional variety, and cortical for the associational type.

The precise physiological or psychological cause has been formulated in a variety of ways since Babinski's original description. Babinski himself appears to have favoured a psychodynamic explanation, as he noticed that the relatives of his two patients had colluded with the nurses and doctors to conceal the true nature of the condition from the patient. This approach was emphasised by Ullman (1962), who took the view that anosognosia was merely a severe tendency to deny or minimise any unpleasant incident in one's life. Most writers on the topic, however, have acknowledged that anosognosia for a hemiplegia belongs to a different class of things and have tried to explain it in terms of disordered physiological or neuropsychological functioning or disordered body image.

Waldenström (1939) and Frederiks (1985) believed it was due to kinaesthetic hallucinations, which made the subject believe that the limb was moving when it was still. Purdon Martin (1949) regarded it as a disorder of consciousness, in which awareness of the body, but not the outside world, was selectively affected. Weinstein & Kahn (1955) considered it to be due to a disorder of language — metaphorical language — which they claimed the right hemisphere had a monopoly of. If the right hemisphere were damaged, they argued, the correct idiom for referring to a paralysis would be lost. Roth (1949) regarded it as a primary perceptual deficit, a true agnosia for the body, a view I would support from the results of my study, where visual agnosia for the outside world was the most consistent neuropsychological association. (Disorientation, inattention, unawareness of limb, visuospatial neglect, language disorder and sensory loss were all present in the majority of cases, but were less closely associated with denial.) Pötzl (1924) and Gerstmann (1958) favoured some disintegration of the body image itself, but Potzl's precise suggestion of an incongruence between visual and kinaesthetic components is almost certainly incorrect, because patients maintain their denial, even when asked to look at the paralysed limb.

EXPERIENCE OF A PHANTOM

Definition

According to Weinstein (1969), a phantom is the 'report of the awareness of a non-existent or deafferent bodily part in a mentally competent individual'. It is experienced by virtually all amputees and may persist for years, but eventually the phantom becomes smaller and less 'real', a phenomenon known as 'telescoping'. Pain is the most distressing aspect.

Varieties

Phantom limb, following amputation of a limb, is the commonest variety. Breast removal and tooth extraction are rarer causes of a phantom. Some patients with a left hemiplegia experience what is known as a supernumerary phantom (Ehrenwald 1931). They sense the presence of another limb or even a nest of limbs in a different position from their real limb. (This variety is probably rare as none of my 100 acute hemiplegics reported it.)

Cause

The experience is generally thought to originate centrally, because modification of peripheral sensation at the stump gives, at best, only temporary relief, and the phantom has been known to disappear after a cerebrovascular accident (Head & Holmes 1911) and parietal lobe surgery (Frederiks 1985).

IMPAIRED IDENTIFICATION OF BODILY PARTS

(Includes autotopagnosia, finger agnosia, right-left disorientation and Gerstmann's syndrome)

Definition and varieties

There are a number of related disorders in which a subject has difficulty in identifying parts of their body. Autotopagnosia is an inability to localise and name body parts. Finger agnosia is a selective variety of this, affecting only finger identification. Right-left disorientation is an impairment in pointing to and naming the correct side of the body when requested to. Gerstmann, who first described finger agnosia in 1924, noted that it was often associated with right-left disorientation, agraphia without alexia, and acalculia, and this tetrad is referred to as the Gerstmann syndrome. In fact, the presence of all four in any one patient is extremely rare.

Subjects with any of these disorders have additional problems in identifying body parts in pictures and on the bodies of others, and their drawings of bodies are usually inadequate.

Cause

Some authorities regard all these conditions as disorders of a 'verbal body image', the linguistic representation of the body. It is not clear from the literature, however, whether this is correct. Some investigators (e.g. De Renzi & Scotti 1970) have found that the difficulty in identification extends to parts of a machine (e.g. bicycle), and it may be that finger agnosia and autotopognosia are merely examples of a more fundamental problem in dealing with parts of a whole. Others (e.g. Selecki & Herron 1965) consider them a form of aphasia, in which the expression or comprehension of words for body parts is more affected than for other words.

Whatever the link with other functional deficits, however, all authorities accept that some brain-damaged patients do have particular difficulty in this sphere, out of proportion to their performance on other language tasks. There is also good agreement that a lesion in the angular gyrus of the left parietal lobe is the usual pathological basis for them.

ALTERED AWARENESS OF PAIN

(Includes asymbolia for pain and preoccupation with painful body areas in the thalamic syndrome)

Definition and varieties

Pain is a subjective experience, the intensity of which varies according to the strength of the provoking stimulus and a number of central factors (personality, current emotional state, current life situation, expectations, etc.). And most subjects whose reports of pain appear out of proportion to what one would expect in the light of all these factors cannot be said to have a body image disorder. Two types of pain disorder, are, however, usually included in any discussion of body image disorder. The first is asymbolia for pain (Schilder & Stengel 1931); the second is an elaborate type of the thalamic syndrome where pain is experienced without any provoking stimulus and the affected body part becomes a focus for powerful emotions. The justification for even regarding these as body image disorders is slender, in my view. They owe their inclusion to the original comment by Schilder and Stengel, when describing asymbolia for pain, that 'pain must be brought into connection with recognition of the model of the body in order to be appreciated fully'.

Asymbolia for pain

This is extremely rare. Only 20 cases had been reported in the world literature up to 1978, all with normal peripheral sensation, but with acquired
cerebral lesions, usually in the left supramarginal gyrus. The condition is
characterised by a diminished response (verbal and behavioural) to a
stimulus which would normally produce a marked response. Subjects have
been known to inflict 'pain' on themselves in astonishment at their lack of
response. It is claimed that the loss of meaning attached to painful stimuli
may extend to any danger signal.

Elaborate thalamic syndrome

It is well known that thalamic lesions may produce exacerbated pain
responses or even spontaneous pain. Rarely, this can give rise to preoccupation with the painful area. Van Bogaert (1934) reported a man in which
a left thalamic lesion produced spontaneous pain in the right arm, and a
feeling that the right arm was lying behind his head. During the day he
could overcome this feeling but at night he would call out to other patients
to alter the position of his arm. Vasilescu & Mares (1958) described three
patients with a left hemiparesis in whom pain in the weak limb, of thalamic
origin, was induced by emotion and certain odours and, like van Bogaert's
case, this gave rise to a preoccupation with the arm.

Other 'pain syndromes'

It is doubtful if any other pain syndrome can usefully be regarded as a body
image disorder, although the condition known as congenital indifference to
pain (Jewesbury 1970) is similar to asymbolia for pain, except that it is
present from birth, and subjects with neurotic conditions such as atypical
facial pain (Feinmann & Harris 1984) become preoccupied with the affected
area.

ABNORMAL AWARENESS OF MOVEMENT

(Includes motor impersistence, 'alien hand sign', experience of non-spontaneity and kinaesthetic hallucinations)

Definition

The body image not only provides a cognitive representation of a *static* body
(with respect to space, prevailing somatic stimuli, and the links between
the various body parts), but also supplies information about the body as
a *dynamic* entity. If one considers each movement or action to originate as
a motor programme with its particular pattern of neuronal circuits, then
there must be a second set of neuronal circuits which provides the sensory

representation of the movement or action. This second set allows one to monitor the movement and recognise a change in routine. Of course, the monitoring of well-learned routines, such as walking, is largely carried out subcortically, and cannot be said to form part of a body image, as it is doubtful if one can even be potentially conscious of every movement (although those who engage in yoga may improve in this). The relevance of such considerations to body image disorders is that the sensory representation of movement derives information from two sources: a central signal that the motor programmes is to take place or is completed, and peripheral stimuli informing of a change in body position. It is theoretically possible, therefore, that a cerebral lesion could interfere with one of these channels, and produce a distorted image of movement.

Most disorders of movement cannot be regarded as body image disorders because they involve a breakdown in performance with preserved awareness of the deficit. A Parkinsonian patient with bradykinesia, for example, is only too aware of their limitations. Apraxia is also primarily a disruption of the motor programme itself. But there are some movement disorders in which the abnormality either lies in an inefficient monitoring of performance or in a distorted awareness of movement which in itself is normal. It is justified, in my view, to call these body image disorders, because there is either neglect or an abnormal experience of the body in movement, which corresponds to unawareness (neglect) and alien experiences (hemiasomatognosia) of the static body, discussed earlier.

Examples of such disorders are motor impersistence (Fisher 1956) or intentional neglect (Heilman et al 1985) in right hemisphere lesions; the 'alien hand sign' (Brion & Jedynak 1972) or autocriticism (Bogen 1979) in callosal lesions; the subjective experience of non-automatic or non-spontaneous movement in schizophrenia (McGhie & Chapman 1961); and kinaesthetic hallucinations, regarded by Waldenström (1939) and Frederiks (1985) as the basis of anosognosia.

Illustrative cases

Case 10: A man of 41 was admitted to hospital complaining of poor memory. He was found to have a glioma invading the posterior half of the corpus callosum. He was noticed to have great trouble in dressing, one hand often becoming entangled in the other. At such times he would say, 'Let go of my hand, you're preventing me from dressing'.

(Callosal lesion — Brion & Jedynak 1972)

Case 11: A young schizophrenic described the early stages of his condition as follows: 'I am not sure of my own movements any more. It's very hard to describe this but at times I'm not sure about even simple actions like sitting down. It's not so much thinking out what to do, it's the doing of it that sticks me. People just do things but I have to watch first to see how you do things. I have to do everything step by step, nothing is automatic now. Everything has to be considered.'

(Schizophrenia — McGhie & Chapman, 1961)

Varieties

Motor impersistence (intentional neglect)

Fisher (1956) drew attention to patients with a left hemiplegia who had great difficulty in maintaining a simple posture or persisting in a simple act. Heilman et al (1985) widened the concept to include any 'inability to initiate movement which could not be attributed to a defect in the motor unit or pyramidal system'. They called this 'intentional neglect or akinesia'. Typical manifestations of these are difficulty in keeping the eyes closed or the tongue protruded. According to Carmon (1970), the essential feature is a failure of kinaesthetic feedback, in my terms an unawareness of bodily movement and posture.

'Alien hand sign' (autocriticism)

It was first noticed in the celebrated callosal section operations conducted by Bogen and Sperry, that in the immediate postoperative period some patients would have 'antagonistic movements'. With one hand they would attempt to put on their trousers, with the other they would pull them off. Brion & Jedynak (1972) then reported three patients with a tumour of the corpus callosum who experienced the movement of one of the hands involved in such antagonistic movements as alien. One of these (case 10) said, 'Let hold of my hand, you stop me dressing'. Another said, 'My hand doesn't belong to me'. The latter remark is identical to the remarks made by patients with hemiasomatognosia, but in the present case it originates with an altered experience of movement and not tactile awareness. Bogen (1979) called the same phenomenon autocriticism, the expression of astonishment that the left hand was behaving independently of the 'self'. He regarded it as one of the diagnostic signs of callosal dysfunction.

Experience of non-spontaneity

McGhie & Chapman (1961) analysed the subjective experiences of schizophrenics in the early stage of the condition. Several, including case 11 above, noticed that they were more aware of their movements than before, sometimes to a degree that spontaneous action became impossible, because every step had to be considered separately. Such experiences may provide a clue to the occurrence of catatonic phenomena, particularly catalepsy, in schizophrenia. I have argued (Cutting 1985) that 'frozen actions' such as waxy flexibility could arise if the experience of non-spontaneity were exaggerated to the point of total immobility.

Kinaesthetic hallucinations

Waldenström (1939) and Frederiks (1985) suggested that anosognosia for a hemiplegia could result from kinaesthetic hallucinations which incorrectly informed a paralysed subject that movement was occurring. If, they argued, the central efferent signal from the motor programme, that movement was under way, was still intact, and signals from the periphery, that the body position had not changed, were ignored, then the subject would continue to experience movement. This intriguing explanation is weakened by my study of hemiplegics, where only two subjects reported kinaesthetic hallucinations, neither of whom had anosognosia, and by the fact that most anosognosic subjects maintained their denial even when forced to look at the arm (faced with visual evidence of weakness).

ABNORMAL VISUAL EXPERIENCES OF THE SELF

(Includes autoscopy, Doppelgänger, out-of-body experience, near-death experience)

Definition and varieties

As discussed in the introduction most body image disorders are difficult to categorise phenomenologically. This is particularly true of abnormal experiences which occur in subjects free of focal brain damage. It is probable that a phenomenon such as seeing one's self, autoscopy or heautoscopy, which can occur in a variety of anomalous situations and pathological disorders, has different combinations of perceptual and ideational elements in these different conditions. However, the phenomenon is so transient and so difficult to describe subjectively that the difference between an epileptic's experience and that of a lone mountaineer is unclear. In Maack & Mullen's (1983) report of a Doppelgänger in a psychotic, it was partly a belief and partly a perceptual experience involving three modalities — sight, sound and touch. In Gabbard et al's (1981) study of 'near-death' experiences and Twemlow et al's (1982) of 'out-of-body' experiences, what subjects remembered most vividly was their emotional state at the time, which in some cases had been so powerful that it produced a lasting spiritual change. Despite these differences in phenomenological interpretation, the common element in autoscopy, Dopplegänger, the double, 'out-of-body' and 'near-death' experiences is the visual experience of seeing oneself.

Illustrative cases

Case 12: 'I knew that he would come that night, so close that I would be able to touch him . . . So I pretended to be reading . . . and suddenly I sensed something and I was certain that he was standing behind me, over my shoulder, that he was there, touching my ear . . . I looked in the mirror in front of me; it was clear, empty; my reflection wasn't there at all and yet I was directly in front of it; the entire mirror was free of any reflection from top to bottom . . . how I was frightened; and I felt that although he was there, he was escaping me yet again, he whose invisible body had swallowed up my reflection; then suddenly I began to see myself as if in a mist at the back of the mirror . . . . . the fog clearing slowly making my face clearer, second by second.'

(Autoscopy — *Le Horla*, Maupassant)

Case 13: A man in his early 50s was admitted to a psychiatric hospital with the complaint that wherever he went he had a double. He and his double would travel by bus together, in different seats, but would reunite as they left the bus. It was, he said, 'not unlike looking at and being in the mirror at the same time'. When separated, the two beings knew and felt each other's presence. He had depressed mood and bizarre bodily delusions and it was not clear whether the diagnosis was schizophrenia or depressive psychosis.

(Doppelgänger in functional psychosis — Maack & Mullen 1983)

Case 14: This subject was involved in a serious car accident and nearly died as a result of his injuries. He remembered later: 'As the two vehicles collided I suddenly found that I was watching the scene from several yards up in the air, as if I were suspended above the road. I saw our own Land-Rover colliding with a large lorry. I watched as I was thrown from the Land-Rover . . . . . I remember thinking that I looked a terrible mess lying there on the road . . . The whole experience, even after all these years, has left me completely unafraid of death'.

(Out-of-body/near-death experience — Dawson 1980)

Cause

The phenomenon has been reported in a variety of conditions, some of which, as Maack & Mullen (1983) noted, have been accepted uncritically from reviewer to reviewer. It is reliably reported in temporal lobe epilepsy (Lukianowicz 1958, Williams 1968) (and Maupassant himself was said to suffer from epilepsy), encephalitis (Mize 1980), depressive illness (Lukianowicz 1958), hypnagogic states (Lhermitte 1941), delirium (Lhermitte & Hecaen 1942), and anomalous physiological states such as occur at the limits of human endurance, e.g. near death (Gabbard et al, 1981). It is rare in schizophrenia, if, in fact, it ever occurs. Maack & Mullen's (1983) case, although diagnosed as schizophrenia, did not fit conventional criteria and in my careful records of over 200 schizophrenics it was not mentioned once.

The psychological mechanism is unclear. Williams (1968) believed that autoscopy was characteristic of temporal lobe lesions, because this part of the brain, he believed, was a superordinate association area linking all modalities of sensation with emotion and a representation of the 'self'. Todd & Dewhurst (1955) suggested a combination of several factors — narcissistic personality, exceptional visual imagery and primitive thinking. None of these is very convincing, in my view, and the best approach to uncover aetiology is to consider the conditions in which it is most frequent and to identify common features.

The common psychological deficit of all the reliably reported conditions in which autoscopy occurs is altered consciousness or a deficit in attention. There are dreamy states in temporal lobe epilepsy (Jackson 1888) and the temporal lobe is usually involved in encephalitis, attention is particularly affected in depression; and extreme physiological and psychological distress, in which autoscopy often occurs, is marked by a disturbance in attention and consciousness. For these reasons, and because of the common experience of seeing oneself in dreams, I favour an explanation of autoscopy in terms of altered consciousness and dream-like thinking.

ABNORMAL TACTILE EXPERIENCES

(Includes tactile, body and somatic hallucinations)

Definition and varieties

Subjects with a variety of neurological and psychiatric conditions may experience abnormal tactile experiences in various body parts. Sometimes these have a basis in sensory impairment or altered awareness of a limb (e.g. case 3), in which case they must be correctly regarded as illusions. Other subjects report abnormal tactile experiences in the absence of any discernible physiological dysfunction, and their experience must be regarded as an hallucination.

Limbs may be changed in shape (e.g. 'hands like cat paws' — Lukianowicz 1967), position (e.g. 'arm twisted round and round' — Lunn 1965), size (e.g. 'my legs are so long that there is no room for them in the bed' — Lunn, 1965) or mass (e.g. 'my legs feel heavy' — Lunn, 1965). Other parts of the body or the whole body may be the focus of abnormal experiences: e.g. ballooning of the head (Lippman 1952), disintegration of the body (personally observed schizophrenic) or sexual experiences — intercourse, burning (personally observed schizophrenics).

Illustrative cases

Case 15: A woman of 48, with no family history of schizophrenia or antecedent brain damage, developed a series of abnormal experiences in her body. Her bed felt particularly hot at night, the earth occasionally shook, she felt her heart pounding and whenever she made love with her husband she experienced intense and strange feelings such as she had never had before. These experiences were associated with other perceptual experiences and beliefs which fulfilled diagnostic criteria for schizophrenia.

(Tactile hallucinations in schizophrenia — personal series)

Case 16: A woman of 48 was well until 10 days after a laminectomy operation for a prolapsed disc. She then developed a delirious illness in which she believed frightening events were going on around her. She had visual, auditory and tactile hallucinations. She felt the bed moving beneath her, her body felt wet and she had the experience that her husband and a friend were underneath her bed turning it round.

(Tactile hallucinations in delirium — personal series)

Cause

Reported causes include epilepsy (Arseni et al, 1966), migraine (Lippman 1952), delirium from a variety of causes (Cutting 1987), schizophrenia (Lunn 1965), cocaine intoxication (Siegel 1978) and hypnagogic states (Oswald 1962).

The mechanism in cases where there is no sensory impairment is best regarded as a projection on to the body of physiological dysfunctions in those parts of the brain which subserve tactile sensation.

ABNORMAL CONSCIOUSNESS OF SELF

(Includes depersonalisation, multiple personality, false identity, transexualism, altered generic image, alien influences on self and ecstasy)

Definition

There are a number of disorders in which the common element is not a change in the way the body is experienced or thought about, but a change in the way the self experiences or thinks about everything, body and outside world. One might not regard them as body image disorders at all, in that they do not selectively affect the image of the body, but they all involve a marked change in the way the self experiences or thinks about all matters, and in that sense one's image of self is affected and, secondarily, one's body image. Habitual perceptual, emotional and thought patterns are experienced as radically different from before, and this colours all areas of one's life.

Illustrative cases

> Case 17: A man of 26 had experienced attacks of feeling strange for five years. In these attacks things looked dull, flat and lifeless. The experience of bladder and rectal fullness was diminished and the other sensations, such as taste, tickle and pain, were reduced. His hands and feet felt detached, as if they did not belong to him, and sometimes seemed to disappear altogether. He felt clumsy in his movements and unsteady. His mouth seemed like 'an empty cavern'.
>
> (Neurotic depersonalisation — Ackner 1954)

> Case 18: A man of 24 complained of no zest for life. He had been diagnosed as schizophrenic three years previously on the basis of several discrete episodes of florid psychosis. Now he was on neuroleptics, neither deluded nor hallucinated, but complained bitterly about his mental state. The world around looked 'eerie', he felt no appetite and no interest in anything. He wished he could feel some emotion when he watched a film or made love to his girlfriend, but had none. He had thought of suicide, if only to experience some feelings again.
>
> (Psychotic depersonalisation — personal series)

Case 19: A girl of 19 was admitted for a second opinion, as she had been behaving oddly for several years (withdrawn, angry, frightened for no apparent reason). Several admissions to another hospital had revealed no overtly psychotic behaviour or ideas. On this admission she denied that she was called Susan X, and wished to be referred to as Mary Y. She said that her parents were not her parents at all, and that her sister was not related. During the admission she changed names several times, and presented these changes with no emotion. She resisted attempts to uncover her reasons for this behaviour and refused abreaction. Occasionally she mentioned paranoid ideas and talked about voices.

(Psychotic false identity — personal series)

Varieties

Depersonalisation

This is the commonest of these disorders of altered self-consciousness. Schilder (1935) defined it as a state in which 'the individual feels himself changed throughout in comparison with his former state . . . . this change extends to both the self and the outer world and leads to the individual not acknowledging himself as a personality . . . his actions seem automatic and he observes his actions like a spectator'. Ackner (1954) stressed the highly distressing quality of the experience.

Depersonalisation, with accompanying derealisation of the outside world, can be a neurotic condition in itself, a state which Roth (1959) termed the phobic anxiety-depersonalisation syndrome. It may occur during a depressive illness. It may be a feature of schizophrenia, when it is particularly intense and distressing (case 18). It may be induced by hallucinogenic drugs, in the phase of intoxication, by LSD for instance (Katz et al 1968), or as a sequel, particularly of psilocybin ingestion (Benjamin 1979). It is a prominent feature of all anomalous physiological and psychological states, however produced (e.g. sensory deprivation, sleep deprivation, mystical states), and is closely linked with autoscopic experiences.

Multiple personality

A rare, but dramatic condition is that in which a subject, usually a woman, develops two, three or four separate personalities. These alternate and have a curious inter-relationship, in that there is often a primary personality, not always the premorbid one, which is acquainted with the others, and subsidiary personalities whose existence is entirely unknown to one another.

The most celebrated case was described by Prince (1905), where the dissociation had occurred following a bang on a window by a man during a thunderstorm. One personality was prude, one mischievous, one stupid, and one briefly appeared in the course of hypnosis. Larmore et al (1977) showed that, in their case, each personality had its own MMPI profile and unique psychophysiological responses. The cause is almost always a form of hysterical dissociation, although, rarely, temporal lobe lesions may predispose (Mesulam 1981), and occasionally it is seen in the course of schizophrenia (Cutting 1985).

False identity

Loss of personal identity or adoption of false identity is a rare condition which can be neurotic or psychotic. The neurotic form is seen in hysterical or psychogenic amnesia, induced by some insoluble personal situation aggravated by depressive mood and secondary gain (e.g. release from intolerable situation, excuse for criminal behaviour). The psychotic form is seen in mania (Koehler & Jacoby 1978), when the adopted identity is of a celebrity, or schizophrenia (Yarden & Raps 1981) when it may be quite bizarre (case 19).

Transexualism

Sexual identity may be selectively altered. This may occur transiently during a psychotic illness. A male schizophrenic patient of mine experienced his body as '10% feminine' and 'half Chinese', and changed his name from Colin McSweeny (incorrect to preserve confidentiality, but similar) to Colina Sweeny-Cheng. Most transexuals (Pauly 1965) are not formally psychotic, but hold a strong belief that they should be the opposite sex, and may go to extreme lengths, even self-mutilation, to achieve this end.

Altered generic image

A curious 'freezing' of self-consciousness occurs in Korsakoff's syndrome. Because of their retrograde amnesia, Korsakoff patients still regard themselves as they were in bygone times. Zangwill (1950) referred to this as an altered generic image. Asked to draw transport and fashion as they thought it was, they depict it as it was several decades ago, and if asked to describe their body or give their age, they refer to themselves as several decades younger than they really are.

Alien influences on self

A central feature of schizophrenia is the belief that will, emotions, thinking and movement are no longer under the control of self. There is a sense that some alien force has taken over, and that they are an automaton or zombie, vulnerable to outside influences. Indeed this phenomenon has become one of the most widely used diagnostic criteria for the condition, and is the common denominator for many of the 'first-rank symptoms' used to diagnose the condition. Such passivity experiences, delusions of influences, or disorders of 'ego consistency' (Scharfetter 1981) cannot be excluded from any discussion of body image disorders, because they represent the core psychopathology of one of the commonest psychiatric disorders and intimately affect the way a subject with such a condition must regard their body. Nasrallah (1982) made the intriguing suggestion that they were the psychological manifestation of a physiological deficit in corpus callosal transfer. The left hemisphere, according to Nasrallah, with a monopoly of expressive language and 'consciousness', becomes unduly aware of the workings of the right hemisphere, through increased callosal transfer. The left hemisphere's 'conscious' response is to assume that something or someone has taken control of it, because it has no idea that its fellow hemisphere has any mental activity: hence delusions of control, passivity experiences and thought interference.

Ecstasy

A final category of altered consciousness of the self are those experiences in which the individual feels that the boundary between themselves and the outside world has been broken down, and that their mind and body are intermingled with those of other individuals and nature as a whole. Such ecstatic experiences can occur in mania (Anderson 1938), cycloid psychosis (Perris 1974), LSD intoxication (Katz et al 1968), temporal lobe epilepsy (Bear 1979) and as a mystical experience in normals (Buckley 1981). It has links with depersonalisation and mania, but is qualitatively different from either, and is best regarded as the consequence of the intense emotion that accompanies the most fulfilling experiences that humans are capable of — love, religious devotion, altruism.

Cause

The cause in each of these is different. It may be an intense (ecstasy) or displaced emotion (multiple personality, neurotic false identity); it may be amnesia (altered generic image); it may be subtle disturbances of consciousness itself (depersonalisation, alien influence on self); it may be a psychotic perception (psychotic transexualism); or it may be a powerful belief (neurotic transexualism). The heterogeneous nature of these disorders illustrates, however, the variety of influences which play on the body and self-image, and underlines the mutual interdependence of body and self.

ABNORMAL BELIEFS ABOUT THE BODY

(Includes hypochondriacal and bizarre bodily delusions, monosymptomatic hypochondriacal psychosis and Cotard's syndrome)

Definition and varieties

Abnormal beliefs about the external form or internal workings of the body occur in all psychoses, functional and organic.

Depressive bodily delusions

These are the most well-known variety. Lewis (1934), in his classic survey of depressive states, obtained the following examples: 'bones alive with worms', 'sexual parts swollen up and noticeable to passers-by', 'something inside the chest gnawing', 'inability to walk' and 'hands no longer human hands but canary's claws'. Cotard (1882) had earlier described 'délire des négations' (nihilistic delusions, later termed Cotard's syndrome). Patients would maintain for example, that they had no head, no bowels or no brain.

Schizophrenic bodily delusions

Such delusions tend to be particularly bizarre and incongruent with mood. They are remarkably common, probably exceeded, amongst delusions, only by delusions of influence, thought interference and paranoid delusions. Of 74 acute schizophrenics, interviewed with particular reference to their delusions (Cutting 1987) 16 had bodily delusions: pregnancy, brain rotating, blood sucked out, turned into a dog, turned into a different person, back broken, body will wash away if he has a shower, vagina burnt, half Chinese and 10% woman, right side of body empty, throat cut, head blown up, testicles to be cut off, bleeding to death, throat diseased and died in past.

Isolated bodily delusional disorder (monosymptomatic hypochondriacal psychosis)

Some subjects entertain isolated delusions about their body, in the absence of any other diagnostic criteria for one of the major psychoses. A variety of terms have been proposed for this condition — the best, in my view, being 'delusional disorder' (Winokur 1977), which links them with other isolated delusional states such as erotomania and paranoia, which they closely resemble in terms of premorbid personality, course and response to treatment. Munro (1980) suggested the term monosymptomatic hypochondriacal psychosis.

Organic bodily delusions

Delirium, dementia and specific neurological disorders, such as anosognosia, may give rise to elaborate bodily delusions. The last-named has been given a particular name — somatoparaphrenia (case 4). In my series of 74 cases of delirium (Cutting 1987) 5 had bodily delusions: something in head turned to dust, contracted venereal disease, carrot in windpipe, decomposed matter being transmitted into neck and doctors injecting blood into neck.

Illustrative cases

Case 20: A woman of 69 was admitted to hospital in a third discrete psychotic episode. She was convinced that if she sat down her body would split in two and that there was nothing inside her. She was attentive to her surroundings, denied depressed mood on questioning, and spent all day standing up to prevent what she believed would be her disintegration.

(Cotard's syndrome — personal series)

Case 21: A man of 32 had been an inpatient in the back wards of a mental hospital for 10 years. When interviewed, he believed that he had '20 000 bones' in his body, that he was stunted, and that this was because his bones were growing wrongly. He was preoccupied with his height and weight (which were in fact normal) and kept drawing diagrams to illustrate what he saw as his abnormal body.

(Chronic schizophrenia — personal series)

Cause

Lewis (1934) believed the mechanism in depressive bodily delusions was a 'changed feeling of self, affecting to a greater or lesser extent the somatic or psychic aspect of personality'. In other psychoses the mechanism is undoubtedly different, and a discussion of this would involve all the theories of delusional formation in general (Cutting 1985).

ABNORMAL PREOCCUPATION WITH THE BODY

(Includes anorexia nervosa, dysmorphophobia and hypochondriasis)

Definition

The last major category of body image disorders is an amalgam of various neurotic conditions which share a preoccupation with bodily size or shape, without delusional intensity, without abnormal bodily perceptions and without any general alteration in consciousness about the self. It is an area of psychiatry and psychology about which there is most doubt as to whether the term body image disorder is appropriate.

The conditions usually included are anorexia nervosa, hypochondriasis and dysmorphophobia. If one widens the concept even further then one enters the area of personality typology based on attitude to body (e.g. the notion of field dependent and field independent individuals, differing according to whether they use the body as a fixation point for estimating changes in the world around them, or vice versa — Witkin 1965). One also enters into a discussion of how normal people react to loss or disfigurement of body parts, e.g. breast removal, facial injuries. It is not my intention to cover these issues as they are not the focus for body image disorders, but the cause of a spectrum of reactions ranging from preoccupation at one end to denial at the other.

Three neurotic conditions — anorexia nervosa, dysmorphophobia and some forms of hypochondriasis — do, however, merit inclusion, because there is a marked concern with the body, there is a distortion of memories and ideas (though probably not perceptions) about the body, and they cause the subject considerable distress and even lead to death, all through bodily preoccupation.

Illustrative case

Case 22: A boy of 18 was admitted to hospital complaining that the left side of his face was flatter than the right, and that his cheek bone on the left was damaged. The conviction fluctuated from day to day and he attributed the disability to a singing lesson he had had six months before when the teacher had made him, in his view, overstretch his facial and vocal muscles. There was no visible abnormality and his condition allowed him to postpone indefinitely an audition he had planned for entry to drama school.

(Dysmorphophobia — personal series)

Varieties

Anorexia nervosa

A central diagnostic feature of anorexia nervosa is the idea, almost a conviction in some cases, that their body is too fat, when relative to others it may be too thin and even cachexic. Loss of weight, amenorrhoea and determined attempts to lose weight, the other criteria, are common to other conditions, whereas the alteration in body image is unique. There is some experimental evidence (Slade & Russell 1973) that anorexics do overestimate their body size at the height of their condition, a finding which reverts to normal after weight gain. As pointed out by the philosopher Bain, action is the measure of belief, and someone who dies weighing five stones, still convinced she is fat, is clearly suffering from grossly abnormal beliefs about her body image. In fact, it is always a surprise to me that the condition is not included with paranoia, erotomania and other delusional disorders (see above), as the condition is in many ways more psychotic than neurotic.

Dysmorphophobia

This is the neurotic version of monosymptomatic hypochondriacal psychosis, although the distinction between the two is often difficult to make. Cases where the belief appears largely understandable in terms of personality and life situation, where the conviction is less than total, and where there is some gain to the individual in maintaining their belief are usually given the present label (Hay 1970). Common preoccupations are shape of nose, quantity of hair, breast size or shape and size of penis. They are often remarkably difficult to treat, whether by drugs, psychotherapy or behaviour therapy, and patients often manage to obtain surgical operations which are then usually disappointing.

Hypochondriasis

Hypochondriasis is a broad term for a condition in which the complaint of physical disability or illness exceeds the cultural norm for the actual physical illness they are suffering from. Sometimes there is no pathology at all. Kenyon (1976) argued cogently that it was a symptom or phenomenon and even when one excluded definite cases of depressive illness and schizophrenia, the remaining patients still formed a heterogenous group. In some it is a life-long tendency to somatise emotional problems, in others learned behaviour that a medical solution for personal disappointment exists. There may be a subgroup, however, who do fall within the definition of a body image disorder. Macdonald & Bouchier (1980), for example, noted that constant attenders at a gastrointestinal clinic, with no organic explanation for their symptoms, tended to be obsessional, ruminative types, who were preoccupied with the physiological workings of their body. Another feature, which suggests that a body image disorder is an appropriate explanation for some cases, is the finding (Kenyon 1964) that lateralised hypochondriacal complaints (pain in the arm, headache, etc.) are more likely to be left sided, a finding which corresponds to the distribution of the more definitive body image disorders in neurological practice.

CONCLUSIONS

The body image is a useful notion to both neurologists and psychiatrists as it explains many otherwise inexplicable conditions. The physiological and psychological components, the interplay between tactile and visual elements, the balance between perceptual and ideational aspects, and links with language, movement and emotion all make for a complex but versatile concept.

Body image disorders are then neurological and psychiatric conditions in which perception, belief or consciousness concerning the body are abnormal. The boundary of what should be regarded as a body image disorder is still hazy, but it is probable that the concept will continue to be discussed and refined, and may prove one of the major influences in reuniting neurology and psychiatry.

REFERENCES

Ackner B 1954 Depersonalisation. Journal of Mental Science 100: 838–872
Anastasopoulos G K 1961 Die nosoagnostische Uberschätzung. Psychiatria, Neurologia (Basel) 141: 214–228
Anderson E W 1938 A clinical study of states of ecstasy occurring in affective disorders. Journal of Neurology and Psychiatry 1: 80–99
Arseni C, Botez M I, Maretsis M 1966 Paroxysmal disorders of the body image. Psychiatria, Neurologia (Basel) 151: 1–14

Babinski M J 1914 Contribution à l'étude des troubles mentaux dans l'hémiplégie organique cérebrale. Revue Neurologique i: 845–848

Bear D M 1979 The temporal lobes. In: Gazzaniga M S (ed) Handbook of behavioural neurobiology, vol 2. Plenum, New York

Benjamin C 1979 Persistent psychiatric symptoms after eating psilocybin mushrooms. British Medical Journal i: 1319–1320

Bogen J E 1979 The callosal syndrome. In: Heilman K M, Valenstein E (eds) Clinical neuropsychology. Oxford University Press, New York

Bonnier P 1905 L'aschématie. Revue Neurologique 13: 605–609

Brion S, Jedynak C-P 1972 Troubles du transfert interhémisphérique: à propos de trois observations de tumeurs du corps calleux. Le signe de la main étrangère. Revue Neurologique 126: 257–266

Buckley P 1981 Mystical experience and schizophrenia. Schizophrenia Bulletin 7: 516–521

Carmon A 1970 Impaired utilization of kinaesthetic feedback in right hemispheric lesions. Neurology 20: 1033–1037

Cotard J 1882 Du délire des négations. In: Hirsch S R, Shepherd M (eds) Themes and variations in European psychiatry. J Wright, Bristol

Critchley M 1953 The parietal lobes. Hafner, New York

Critchley M 1955 Personification of paralysed limbs in hemiplegics. British Medical Journal ii: 284–286

Critchley M 1957 Observations on anosodiaphoria. Encéphale 46: 540–546

Critchley M 1962 Clinical investigation of disease of the parietal lobes of the brain. Medical Clinics of North America 46: 837–857

Cutting J 1978 Study of anosognosia. Journal of Neurology, Neurosurgery and Psychiatry 41: 548–555

Cutting J 1985 The psychology of schizophrenia. Churchill Livingstone, London

Cutting J 1987 The phenomenology of acute organic psychosis: comparison with schizophrenia. British Journal of Psychiatry 151: 324–332

Dawson J 1980 The disembodied self. In: The unexplained, vol 1. Orbis, London, p 101–103

Denny-Brown D, Meyer J S, Horenstein S 1952 The significance of perceptual rivalry resulting from parietal lobe lesions. Brain 75: 433–471

Deny G, Camus P 1905 Sur une forme d'hypocondrie aberrante due à la perte de la conscience du corps. Revue Neurologique 13: 461–467

De Renzi E, Scotti G 1970 Autotopognosia: fiction or reality? Archives of Neurology 23: 221–227

Ehrenwald H 1931 Anosognosie und Depersonalisation. Nervenarzt 4: 681–688

Feinmann C, Harris M 1984 The diagnosis and management of psychogenic facial pain disorders. Clinical Otolaryngology 9: 199–201

Fisher M 1956 Left hemiplegia and motor impersistence. Journal of Nervous and Mental Diseases 123: 201–218

Foucault M 1966 The order of things: an archaeology of the human sciences. Tr 1970, Pantheon, New York

Frederiks J A M 1963 Macrosomatognosia and microsomatognosia. Psychiatria, Neurologia, Neurochirurgia 66: 531–536

Frederiks J A M 1985 Disorders of the body schema. In: Frederiks J A M (ed) Handbook of clinical neurology, vol 45. Elsevier, Amsterdam, ch 25, p 373–393

Gabbard G O, Twemlow S W, Jones F C 1981 Do 'near-death experiences' occur only near death? Journal of Nervous and Mental Disorders 169: 374–377

Gerstmann J 1924 Fingeragnosie: eine umschriebene Störung der Orientierung am eigenen Körper. Wiener klinische Wochenschrift 37: 1010–1012

Gerstmann J 1958 Psychological and phenomenological aspects of disorders of the body image. Journal of Nervous and Mental Diseases 126: 499–512

Gross H, Kaltenbäck E 1955 Die Anosognosie. Wiener Zeitschrift für Nervenheilkunde 11: 374–418

Hay G G 1970 Dysmorphophobia. British Journal of Psychiatry 116: 399–406

Head H, Holmes G 1911 Sensory disturbances from cerebral lesions. Brain 34: 102–254

Hecaen H, Ajuriaguerra J 1952 Méconnaissances et hallucinations corporelles. Masson, Paris

Hecaen H, Albert M L 1978 Human neuropsychology. J Wiley, New York

Heilman K M, Valenstein E, Watson R T 1985 The neglect syndrome. In: Frederiks
    J A M (ed) Handbook of clinical neurology, vol 45. Elsevier, Amsterdam, ch 12,
    p 153–183
Jackson J H 1888 On a particular variety of epilepsy ('intellectual aura'). In: Selected
    writings of John Hughlings Jackson, vol 1 1931. Hodder and Stoughton, London
Jewesbury E C O 1970 Congenital indifference to pain. In: Vinken P J, Bruyn G W (eds)
    Handbook of clinical neurology, vol 8. N Holland Pub Co, Amsterdam, ch 15,
    p 187–204
Juba A 1949 Beitrag zur Struktur der ein — und doppelseitigen Körperschemastörungen.
    Monatsschrift fur Psychiatrie und Neurologie 118: 11–29
Katz M M, Waskow I E, Olsson J 1968 Characterizing the psychological state produced by
    LSD. Journal of Abnormal Psychology 73: 1–14
Kenyon F E 1964 Hypochondriasis: a clinical study. British Journal of Psychiatry
    110: 478–488
Kenyon F E 1976 Hypochondriacal states. British Journal of Psychiatry 129: 1–14
Koehler K, Jacoby C 1978 Acute confabulatory psychosis: a rare form of unipolar mania.
    Acta Psychiatrica Scandinavica 57: 415–425
Larmore K, Ludwig A M, Cain R L 1977 Multiple personality — an objective case study.
    British Journal of Psychiatry 131: 35–40
Lewis A 1934 Melancholia: a clinical survey of depressive states. Journal of Mental Science
    80: 277–378
Lhermitte J 1939 L'image de notre corps. Nouvelle Revue Critique, Paris.
Lhermitte J 1941 Sur un syndrome catoplectique accompagné d'alteration de la
    personnalité. Revue Neurologique 73: 590–591
Lhermitte J, Hecaen H 1942 L'héautoscopie onirique. Revue Neurologique 74: 226
Lippman C W 1952 Certain hallucinations peculiar to migraine. Journal of Nervous and
    Mental Diseases 116: 346–351
Lissauer H 1890 Ein fall von seelenblindheit nebst einen beitrag zur theorie derselben.
    Archiv für Psychiatrie 21: 222–270
Lukianowicz N 1958 Autoscopic phenomena. Archives of Neurology and Psychiatry
    80: 199–220
Lukianowicz N 1967 Body image disturbances in psychiatric disorders. British Journal of
    Psychiatry 113: 31–47
Lunn V 1965 On body hallucinations. Acta Psychiatrica Scandinavica 41: 387–399
Maack L H, Mullen P E 1983 The Doppelgänger, disintegration and death — a case
    report. Psychological Medicine 13: 651–654
Macdonald A J, Bouchier I A D 1980 Non-organic gastrointestinal illness: a medical and
    psychiatric study. British Journal of Psychiatry 136: 276–283
Maupassant G Le Horla. Le Livre de Poche, Paris
McGhie A, Chapman J 1961 Disorders of attention and perception in early schizophrenia.
    British Journal of Medical Psychology 34: 103–115
Mesulam M-M 1981 Dissociative states with abnormal temporal EEG: multiple personality
    and the illusion of possession. Archives of Neurology 38: 176–181
Mize K 1980 Visual hallucinations following viral encephalitis: a self report.
    Neuropsychologia 18: 193–202
Munro A 1980 Monosymptomatic hypochondriacal psychosis. British Journal of Hospital
    Medicine 24: 34–38
Nasrallah H A 1982 Laterality and hemispheric dysfunction in schizophrenia. In: Henn
    F A, Nasrallah H A (eds) Schizophrenia as a brain disease. OUP, New York
Nathanson M, Bergman P S, Gordon G C 1952 Denial of illness. Its occurrence in 100
    consecutive cases of hemiplegia. Archives of Neurology and Psychiatry 68: 380–387
Nightingale S 1982 Somatoparaphrenia: a case report. Cortex 18: 463–467
Oswald I 1962 Sleeping and waking. Elsevier, Amsterdam
Pauly I B 1965 Male psychosexual inversion — transexualism. Archives of General
    Psychiatry 13: 172–181
Perris C 1974 A study of cycloid psychosis. Acta Psychiatrica Scandinavica
    supplement 253
Pötzl O 1924 Über störungen der selbstwahrnehmung bei linksseitigen hemiplegie.
    Zeitschrift für die gesamte Neurologie und Psychiatric 93: 117–168
Prince M 1905 The dissociation of a personality. Reprinted 1957. Meridian, New York

Purdon Martin J 1949 Consciousness and its disturbances. Lancet i: 48
Roth M 1949 Disorders of the body image caused by lesions of the right parietal lobe. Brain 72: 89–111
Roth M 1959 The phobic anxiety-depersonalisation syndrome. Proceedings of the Royal Society of Medicine 52: 587–595
Scharfetter C 1981 Ego-psychopathology: the concept and its empirical evaluation. Psychological Medicine 11: 273–280
Schilder P 1935 The image and appearance of the human body. Kegan Paul, Trench, Trubner, London
Schilder P, Stengel E 1931 Asymbolia for pain. Archives of Neurology and Psychiatry 25: 598–600
Selecki B R, Herron J T 1965 Disturbance of the verbal body image: a particular syndrome of sensory aphasia. Journal of Nervous and Mental Diseases 141: 42–52
Shapiro M F, Fink M, Bender M B 1952 Exosmesthesia or displacement of cutaneous sensation into extrapersonal space. Archives of Neurology and Psychiatry 68: 481–490
Siegel R K 1978 Cocaine hallucinations. American Journal of Psychiatry 135: 309–314
Slade P D, Russell G F M, 1973 Experimental investigations of body perception in anorexia nervosa and obesity. Psychotherapy and Psychosomatics 22: 359–363
Todd J, Dewhurst K 1955 The double: its psycho-pathology and psycho-physiology. Journal of Nervous and Mental Diseases 122: 47–55
Twemlow S W, Gabbard G O, Jones F C 1982 The out-of-body experience: a phenomenological typology based on questionnaire responses. American Journal of Psychiatry 139: 450–455
Ullman M 1962 Behavioural changes in patients following strokes. Charles C Thomas, USA
Van Bogaert L 1934 Sur la pathologie de l'image de soi. Annales médicopsychologiques 92: 519–555
Vasilescu N, Mares A 1958 Alterations of body picture during the thalamic syndrome. Rumanian Medical Review 2: 53–55
Von Angyal L, Frick F 1941 Beiträge zur Anosognosie und zu der Regression des Phantomgliedes. Zeitschrift für die gesamte Neurologie und Psychiatrie 173: 440–447
Waldenström J 1939 On anosognosia. Acta Psychiatrica Scandinavica 14: 215–220
Weinstein E A, Kahn R L 1955 Denial of illness. Charles C Thomas, Springfield
Weinstein S 1969 Neuropsychological studies of the phantom. In: Benton A L (ed) Contributions to clinical neuropsychology. Aldine, Chicago
Williams D 1968 Man's temporal lobe. Brain 91: 639–654
Winokur G 1977 Delusional disorder. Comprehensive Psychiatry 18: 511–521
Witkin H A 1965 Development of the body concept and psychological differentiation. In: Wapner S, Werner H (eds) The body percept. Random House, New York.
Yarden P E, Raps C S 1981 Identity alterations and prognosis in schizophrenia. British Journal of Psychiatry 138: 495–497
Zangwill O L 1950 Amnesia and the generic image. Quarterly Journal of Experimental Psychology 2: 7–13

Neuropsychology: memory and hippocampal pathology*

Memory disorder is a symptom of the utmost importance in psychiatric practice, in that it is often the decisive clinical feature which indicates the presence of underlying cerebral disease.

Lishman 1987

Neuropsychology is a particular area of neurology of common interest to neurologists, psychiatrists, psychologists and neurophysiologists.

Jeeves 1987, quoting from *Neuropsychologia* editorial, 1963

Just as clinical memory disorders constitute a meeting point for neurology and psychiatry, likewise attempts to establish the neural basis of memory have formed a major ground for contact between neuropsychologists and other neuroscientists — to those enumerated by Jeeves and the first editor of *Neuropsychologia* should surely be added neurosurgeons and neuropathologists. As so often in brain research, much of the endeavour has originated from studying epilepsy and its treatment and, like memory, epilepsy is a major point of contact between neurology and psychiatry. It is appropriate therefore to recognise here that the first reports from the United Kingdom of the outcome of temporal lobectomy as a treatment for a series of patients with drug-resistant epilepsy were by Sir Denis Hill and Mr Murray Falconer from the Maudsley Hospital in papers which appeared consecutively in the *Proceedings of the Royal Society of Medicine* for 1953 (Hill 1953, Falconer 1953). Both authors considered the same 14 patients, of whom 12 had been inpatients at the Maudsley Hospital. Hill recorded that his role was 'to discuss first the identification and selection of patients for whom this operation would appear to offer a hope of amelioration, and secondly to describe some of the results obtained'. These have remained the role of the physician ever since. Hill mentioned that previous reports from North America, describing the effects of temporal lobe surgery in the treatment

* This chapter develops an idea originally presented at the Beaune (France) meeting of the International Neuropsychology Symposium in June 1984, and at the Manchester (England) meeting of the Association of British Neurologists in April 1985 (Oxbury J, Oxbury S 1986 Memory impairment following hippocampal damage in early childhood. Journal of Neurology, Neurosurgery and Psychiatry 49: 729).

of epilepsy, had not recorded any 'particular memory loss'. Clearly this situation was soon to change. Falconer described his technique of en bloc resection mentioning that:

> . . . at first we did not have electrocorticography available to delineate the irritable area, and so at the outset we adopted the policy of removing as much of the affected temporal lobe as possible without crippling the patient. In this way we hoped not only to remove the epileptogenic area but also to secure the affected tissue for histological study.

A similar technique of en bloc excision is still practised by some epilepsy surgeons, including Mr Christopher Adams in Oxford, and has been extremely fruitful not only to the patients but also to the advancement of knowledge. The anterior 5–6 cm of temporal lobe is removed, including the anterior 2–3 cm of hippocampus, producing a specimen with fixed weight of around 45 grams.

Hill mentioned that the operation did not produce any significant change of 'formal intelligence' or 'Rorschach responses', but he did not comment on any change of memory function. However, two years later Meyer & Yates (1955) described the findings from pre- and postoperative psychological testing of 18 patients who underwent temporal lobectomy at the Maudsley Hospital. They reported a verbal memory and learning deficit after left-sided operations in patients who were left hemisphere dominant. They showed that such patients have a marked impairment on the paired associate learning test from the Wechsler Memory Scale, and a similar deficit on a new word learning task. No deficit was found in patients who had undergone right temporal lobectomy.

At much the same time Scoville (1954) and Scoville & Milner (1957) reported on the effects of bilateral temporal lobe excisions as a treatment for schizophrenia and/or epilepsy. Excisions which encroached upon both hippocampi, but not those restricted to uncus and amygdala, produced amnesia whose severity depended upon the extent of the hippocampal removal. One of these patients, HM, developed a very severe amnesic syndrome which has persisted. He has been extensively studied since his operation and he has probably been the subject of more case reports than any other person immortalised by the neurosciences literature. It was these reports from Scoville and Milner which gave rise to the view that the hippocampus has a major importance in memory function. Previously, there had been isolated reports of severe persistent amnesia associated with bilateral temporal lobe pathology (see Brierley 1966). Subsequently, such amnesia has been described in a wide range of pathological conditions affecting the medial parts of the temporal lobes including herpes simplex virus encephalitis (Oxbury & MacCallum 1973), degeneration of the type associated with malignant disease (Corsellis et al 1968), posterior cerebral artery territory infarction (Benson et al 1974; De Renzi et al 1987), hypoxia/ischaemia (Cummings et al 1984), and of course in the early stages of Alzheimer's disease (Kemper 1984).

EFFECTS OF UNILATERAL TEMPORAL LOBECTOMY ON
MEMORY

The observations of Meyer & Yates (1955) were considerably extended by
Milner (1958, 1962, 1967). She used both the paired associate learning test
and the paragraph recall subtests of the Wechsler Memory Scale. Scores for
the initial learning of the paired associates and for the immediate recall of
the paragraphs were combined together to give a 'combined immediate
score'. Similarly, scores for recall of the paired associates and for recall of
the paragraphs after a delay of $1-1\frac{1}{2}$ hours were combined to give a
'combined delayed recall score'. The combined scores were considerably
depressed for at least 10 years after left temporal lobectomy. No deficits
seemed to follow right temporal lobectomy, or non-temporal excisions from
either hemisphere.

Milner's findings of a left temporal verbal memory and learning deficit
have been repeatedly confirmed. A deficit on immediate paragraph recall
was found by Rausch & Crandall (1982), Novelly et al (1984), Ojemann
& Dodrill (1985), and Powell et al (1985). Novelly et al (1984) also found
a deficit on delayed paragraph recall. A deficit on the initial learning of the
paired associates was reported by Blakemore & Falconer (1967) and by
Rausch & Crandall (1982).

The relationship between the postoperative deficit and particular structures within the temporal lobe is not so clear. Milner, using the combined
delayed recall measure, found that the severity of the deficit varied both
with the extent of the hippocampal excision and with the extent of the
neocortical excision. Inspection of her data (see Table 12 in Milner 1967)
suggests that the hippocampus might be the more important structure. In
contrast, Ojemann & Dodrill (1985) found that the severity of the
immediate paragraph recall deficit depended more on the extent of the
neocortical removal than on the amount of the hippocampus removed.
Further investigations in Professor Milner's laboratory indicated that
whether or not the extent of the hippocampal removal is a major factor may
depend on the type of testing technique that is used (Milner 1970, & 1971,
Jones-Gotman & Milner 1978, Jones-Gotman 1987).

In contrast to the situation after left temporal lobectomy, there have been
only occasional reports of impaired performance on verbal memory tasks
after right temporal excisions. Samuels et al (1972), using an auditory
version of the Peterson task, did find that patients with right temporal
excisions including a 'large' hippocampal removal were impaired relative to
normal controls, and they performed at the same level as patients with left
temporal lobectomies which had included only a small part of the hippocampus. Likewise, Jones-Gotman & Milner (1978) found that right
temporal excisions including a large portion of the hippocampus caused
more difficulty with a word-pair memory task in which the use of a visual
imagery mnemonic was required than did those including only a small part

of the hippocampus, although both caused less difficulty than did left temporal excisions and the basis of the right temporal defect may have been other than purely verbal. Memory impairment after right temporal excisions has tended to be elusive. It has been found especially when using test material which is difficult to code verbally, such as when required to remember relative spatial location (Smith & Milner 1981). As with verbal memory tasks after left temporal lobectomy, some tests seem sensitive to the extent of the hippocampal removal whereas others do not (Jones-Gotman 1987).

The conclusion which has been drawn from memory testing after unilateral temporal lobectomy has been that there is a dichotomy such that left-sided operations produce a specifically verbal memory deficit and right-sided operations produce a non-verbal memory deficit. There has been some suggestion that the extent of these deficits is related to the extent of the hippocampal removal, but this certainly is not a consistent effect. For reasons that have not been elucidated, the importance of the hippocampal factor seems to vary according to the task used. Indeed some investigators have considered that with verbal memory tasks the left temporal neocortex is of at least as much importance as the hippocampus (Ojemann & Dodrill 1985, Ojemann & Engel 1987). There are a number of reasons why it is difficult to use the postoperative data to throw light on the relationship between memory and individual brain structures, especially the hippocampus. One is that a number of different structures, are inevitably involved in, or damaged by, the excision. These include not only the hippocampal-amygdala system, but also the temporal stem (Horel 1978) and neocortex. It is possible that the neocortical component of any deficit could be evaluated by comparing the effects of standard excisions with those of amygdalohippocampectomy (Yasargil & Weiser 1987), but as yet sufficient data are not available. However, the opportunity to assess the effects of hippocampal neurone depletion is already available because many, but not all, patients who are to undergo temporal lobectomy have this pathology. Consequently, a time-honoured method for establishing a relationship between a particular disorder of behaviour and an anatomical locus of cerebral pathology can be applied — that is, to select a group of patients on the basis of a known locus of pathology and to ascertain whether they show a behaviour disorder not present in those without pathology at that site.

HIPPOCAMPAL NEURONE LOSS IN TEMPORAL LOBE EPILEPSY

For well over a century it has been recognised that there is a depletion of hippocampal neurones in some patients with severe and long-standing epilepsy (Babb & Brown 1987, Armstrong & Bruton 1987). The studies of Margerison & Corsellis (1966) on autopsy material demonstrated that a

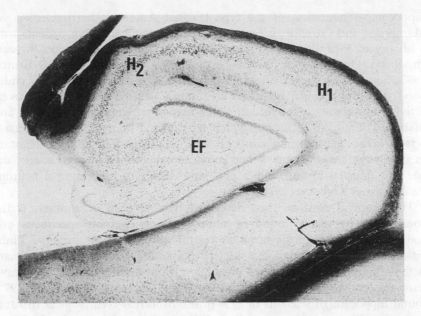

Fig. 10.1 To show the hippocampal zones.

depletion of hippocampal neurones was found especially in those whose seizures had conformed to the pattern of temporal lobe epilepsy and whose electroencephalograms had shown a temporal lobe focus. They noted that the most severe form of neuronal depletion, which they labelled Ammon's horn sclerosis as a subvariety of hippocampal sclerosis, was associated with onset of the epilepsy at a particularly young age. The neuronal depletion of Ammon's horn sclerosis affected the H_1 zone, especially in the region of the border with H_2, the end-folium and the dentate gyrus (Fig. 10.1). Amongst those with any degree of hippocampal neurone depletion, 50% had unilateral Ammon's horn sclerosis, approximately half of them with a lesser degree of hippocampal neurone loss in the opposite hippocampus, and 11% had bilateral Ammon's horn sclerosis. Stated another way, 82% of those with the Ammon's horn sclerosis lesion had it on one side only. It is important to appreciate that a neuronal loss in other parts of the brain almost invariably accompanies the Ammon's horn sclerosis. In the Margerison and Corsellis series all but 1 of the 22 cases with Ammon's horn sclerosis had neuronal loss in the amygdala and/or cerebellum and/or thalamus. Only one case had a loss of neurones in the amygdala without an associated Ammon's horn sclerosis, which was nearly always ipselateral.

The fact that the neuronal loss is characteristically multifocal led to the introduction of the term mesial temporal sclerosis, by Falconer, Serafetinides & Corsellis (1964), to describe the findings in temporal lobe excision specimens. There is much evidence that the most profound depletion of hippocampal neurones, of the type labelled Ammon's horn sclerosis by Margerison and Corsellis, is found in excision specimens from patients with a history of a prolonged, or otherwise 'complicated', convulsion in early childhood (Ounsted et al 1966, Babb & Brown 1987, Armstrong & Bruton 1987, Sagar & Oxbury 1987). It seems that, at a stage during early childhood, the hippocampal neurones are unduly sensitive to metabolic overactivity during such a convulsion which may cause irreparable damage; and that somehow a hippocampus which is sclerosed because of such damage acts as a focus, producing temporal lobe seizures which may be resistant to antiepileptic medication. When convulsions have commenced at an older age it is unusual to find such a profound degree of hippocampal neurone loss (Sagar & Oxbury 1987).

Hippocampal neurone loss, described by one term or another, is the commonest pathology found in temporal lobe excision specimens and confers a good prognosis for a successful outcome from surgery. Thus, Falconer (1971a) reported that mesial temporal sclerosis was the primary pathology in 47% of his series of temporal lobectomies and 92% of those with this pathology had a good postoperative outcome. Mathieson (1975) found hippocampal sclerosis in 27% of the Montreal Neurological Institute series in whom a definite pathological diagnosis could be made. Ammon's horn sclerosis was the underlying pathology in 33% of the Oxford series of temporal lobectomies, with lesser degrees of hippocampal neurone loss in a further 13% (Adams et al 1987), making the total with hippocampal neurone loss virtually identical to the 47% with mesial temporal sclerosis reported by Falconer from the Maudsley. Seventy-one per cent of the Oxford Ammon's horn sclerosis group remained completely seizure free at the end of the first postoperative year, compared to only 36% of those with lesser degrees of neurone loss. So, Ammon's horn sclerosis is not only common but also rewarding to treat.

PREOPERATIVE MEMORY ASSESSMENT

It is probable that several thousand people worldwide have now undergone excision of temporal cortex as a treatment for epilepsy. A large proportion of them will have suffered their epilepsy on the basis of hippocampal sclerosis. The diagnosis of this condition is largely dependent upon clinical acumen, electroencephalography and neuropsychology (Adams et al 1987). It is surprising therefore that, despite the large number of *postoperative* studies designed to investigate hippocampal function (Jones-Gotman 1987), preoperative studies are very sparse (Rausch 1987). A preoperative deficit on verbal memory/learning tasks has been elusive. Meyer & Yates (1955) did observe that patients who were to have a left temporal lobectomy performed poorly on a new-word learning test prior to operation. Milner (1958, 1962, 1967) also noted that delayed recall scores were lower preoperatively amongst those who were to have a left temporal excision than amongst those who were to have right temporal or extratemporal excisions. However, a number of other authors have failed to find any preoperative laterality difference amongst those destined for temporal excisions (Blakemore & Falconer 1967, Rausch & Crandall 1982, Novelly et al 1984, Powell et al 1985).

The difficulty in finding preoperative effects may have been because most studies have taken into account only the laterality of the intended operation and not the locus or nature of the underlying pathology. In this way, the patient population has been considered as homogeneous within each laterality group which may not be justifiable. Blakemore et al (1966) did attempt to relate preoperative IQ scores to whether or not mesial temporal sclerosis was found in the specimen excised by Falconer, but memory attempt to correlate preoperative neuropsychological data with the preoperative pathology requires a detailed histopathological examination which is virtually impossible unless the surgery utilises some form of en bloc excision technique of the Falconer type. It would be a difficult study to carry out in conjunction with surgical techniques relying on tissue removal by subpial suction.

CORRELATION OF PREOPERATIVE VERBAL MEMORY AND HIPPOCAMPAL NEURONE DENSITY

During the last 15 years approximately 100 people have undergone temporal lobectomy in Oxford — 60% of them during the last 6 years — as a treatment for drug-resistant temporal lobe epilepsy. The operations have all been carried out by Mr Christopher Adams who uses a modification of the technique described by Falconer (1953, 1971b). The anterior 5.5–6.5 cm of temporal lobe, including the anterior 2–3 cm of hippocampus, is excised in a single piece usually weighing 35–45 g when fixed. Most of the patients have been examined pre- and postoperatively by one or both of us. The excision specimens have all been examined by Dr J T Hughes, who has kindly provided the hippocampal neurone counts (Table 10.1). We have explored the relationship between performance on preoperative verbal memory tests and the density of the hippocampal neurones found in the excision specimens by comparing the performances of patients whose subsequently excised hippocampi were shown to be severely depleted of neurones with those of patients whose hippocampi showed little if any neuronal depletion. Only 30 patients were considered suitable for inclusion in the analysis. They were the total number who satisfied the following criteria:

1. They had all undergone full neuropsychological assessment preoperatively.

2. They were at least 12 years old at the time of the preoperative neuropsychological assessment.

Table 10.1 Age, IQ, and hippocampal neurone counts in the 30 patients divided according to pathology and laterality

Pathology groups	Ammon's horn sclerosis (AHS)		Hippocampus intact (HI)	
Side of operation	LEFT	RIGHT	LEFT	RIGHT
Number of patients	7	10	4	9
Age at operation				
mean (years)	20.4	16.4	24.8	27.7
range (years)	15–29	12–20	15–34	14–43
IQ (WAIS, WISC, or WISC-R)				
verbal	94.6	100.5	104.8	100.1
performance	104.6	105.0	109.8	106.8
Hippocampal Neurones* (per sq mm)				
(H_1 at H_1–H_2 border)	1.1		23.5	
EF	5.2		17.1	
dentate	35.6		93.7	

* Our gratitude is due to Dr J T Hughes (Department of Neuropathology, Radcliffe Infirmary) for providing us with these counts

3. They were either right handed without evidence of atypical language dominance, or if left handed they had been shown to be left hemisphere language dominant by intracarotid amytal examinations (Oxbury & Oxbury 1984).

4 Neuropathological examination of their excision specimens showed *either* :

a. Severe depletion of hippocampal neurones in the H_1 zone bordering on H_2, in the end folium and in the dentate gyrus conforming to the pattern of Ammon's horn sclerosis (see Sagar & Oxbury 1987) without other significant pathology; and in addition they had a history of a convulsion prior to their fourth birthday of the sort known to be very strongly associated with severe hippocampal neurone loss (see Berti et al 1988). *Seventeen patients in this category constituted the AHS group.*

or b. No marked degree of hippocampal neurone loss; and these were only included if they had *not* suffered a convulsion, or indeed any other epileptic seizure, prior to their fourth birthday. *Thirteen patients in this category constituted the hippocampus intact (HI) group.* Four of them did have some other form of pathology (traumatic scar 2, cortical malformation 1 and calcified cavernous angioma 1), but all those with indolent gliomas were excluded.

Some basic data for the groups are shown in Tables 10.1 and 10.2. The AHS group were significantly younger at the time of operation ($p < .002$, Mann-Whitney). Patients with this pathology often have severe temporal lobe epilepsy during late childhood and adolescence, and their response to surgery is good. So, our policy in Oxford when this pathology is suspected

Table 10.2 The relief from seizures following temporal lobectomy

Pathology group	Ammon's horn sclerosis (AHS)	Hippocampus intact (HI)
Duration of follow up (mean years)	3.8	5.8
Seizure free		
off medication	9	4
on medication	5	3
Occasional seizures (on medication)	3	6
Total Number	17	13

has been to recommend surgery if possible at age 12–15 years. For a large proportion operated at this age the epilepsy is abolished before leaving school. This is in contrast to a usual preoperative seizure frequency of around 200–250 per year. Also, it will be seen that all groups have a performance IQ (WAIS, WISC or WISC-R) higher than their verbal IQ, irrespective of pathology or laterality, but it is only the left AHS group which has a particularly depressed verbal IQ. The hippocampal neurone counts amongst the AHS group were considerably lower than amongst the HI group in all three hippocampal zones (H_1 at the H_1–H_2 border, end folium, and dentate gyrus) — the difference was significant well beyond the $p < .002$ level (Mann-Whitney) in each zone.

During the routine preoperative assessment, which was always carried out within 6 months of surgery, verbal memory was measured using the logical memory passages and the paired associate learning test from the Wechsler Memory Scale. Recall of the logical memory passages (or equivalent forms), or of short stories of similar length and equivalent difficulty for those younger than 15 years, was tested immediately after presentation and again without warning after a 1-hour delay; a maximum score of 22 was obtainable on each occasion. The paired associate learning test was administered in the standard fashion, giving a maximum score of 21; and a delayed recall trial was administered after 1 hour, again without warning, giving a maximum score of 10. The immediate combined score (C_i) is derived by adding the immediate paragraph recall (logical memory) score to the score for learning the paired associates, thus the maximum C_i is 43; and the combined delayed recall score (C_d) is derived by adding the delayed paragraph recall score to the score for delayed recall of the paired associates, giving a maximum of 32.

The mean preoperative verbal memory test scores for each group are shown in Table 10.3. The C_i scores were treated by a two-factor analysis of variance for pathology × laterality. Similar analyses were made of the following scores: C_d, immediate paragraph recall, initial learning of the paired associates. In each of the four analyses the pathology effect was significant (see Table 10.4), but there was no significant laterality effect nor any interaction. A separate two-factor analysis of variance was carried out within the AHS group comparing laterality and paragraph recall scores (immediate and delayed). This showed a significant immediate v delayed

Table 10.3 Preoperative verbal memory test scores, means for each pathology × laterality group

Pathology groups	Ammon's horn sclerosis (AHS)		Hippocampus intact (HI)	
Side of operation	LEFT	RIGHT	LEFT	RIGHT
Combined immediate (C_i) — max = 43	20.4	24.9	28.8	29.4
Combined Delayed (C_d) — max = 32	12.4	16.3	19.8	19.8
Paragraph Recall immediate — max = 22	7.9	10.1	12.8	12.2
Paragraph recall delayed — max = 22	5.1	7.7	11.3	10.8
Paired associate initial learning max = 21	12.5	14.9	16.0	17.2
Paired associate delayed recall max = 10	7.4	8.6	8.5	9.5

Table 10.4 Summary of analyses of variance on data from Table 10.3

Scores	F (ratios (df 1, 26) A-laterality (right, left)	B-pathology (AHS, HI)	A × B
Combined immediate (C_i)	1.07	9.64**	0.87
Combined delayed (C_d)	1.90	14.82**	1.89
Paragraph recall immediate	0.46	8.84**	1.40
Paired associates, initial learning	1.39	4.32**	1.06

** $p < 0.01$

difference ($p < .01$), which would be expected, but there was no laterality effect nor any interaction.

The implication of these findings is that severe hippocampal neurone depletion is associated with a verbal memory defect irrespective of which side is primarily affected. Inspection of the results suggests that primary involvement of the left hippocampus was associated with the greater memory impairment but on statistical analysis the laterality difference did not approach significance. This may be partly attributable to considerable variance within each laterality group. Thus, some patients with severe left hippocampal neurone depletion have surprisingly good verbal memory scores and may obtain a C_i score in the range of 25–30, although it is very unusual for a C_d to reach 20. Conversely, some patients with severe right hippocampal neurone depletion obtain C_i scores as low as 15 and C_d scores as low as 10.

We do not have any definite explanation for the phenomenon of high verbal memory scores in occasional patients in whom intracarotid amytal examination firmly indicates left hemisphere language dominance and in whom there is severe left hippocampal neuronal depletion indistinguishable from that of other patients with poor verbal memory scores. However, it is possible that they are patients in whom the ipselateral amygdala is intact despite the hippocampal damage (although Mr Adams removes the amygdala, this part is usually by suction and rarely appears in the block for histopathological examination). This explanation involves the idea of dual circuits underlying memory function, as suggested by Mishkin (1982), one involving the hippocampus and the other the amygdala. ·

Low scores in patients with severe right hippocampal neurone loss could be attributed to concomitant neuronal loss in the opposite (left) hippocampus, or to an involvement of the right hippocampus in verbal memory. The former suggestion seems unlikely. The selection process prior to surgery is rigorous in an attempt to pick only those with severe neuronal loss in one hippocampus and the high proportion who become seizure-free postoperatively (Table 10.2) suggests that this is successful. The right AHS group may have a minor degree of neurone loss in the contralateral (left) hippocampus, but such minor loss also exists in the left 'hippocampus intact' group whose performance is superior. Involvement of the right hippocampus in verbal memory seems the more likely explanation. A

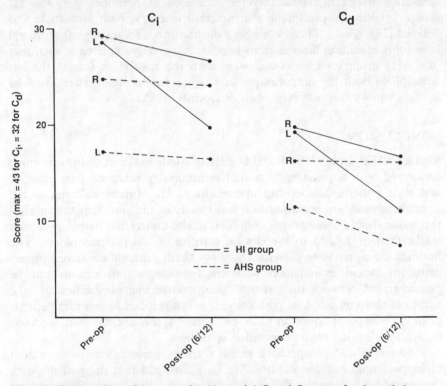

Fig. 10.2 Preoperative and postoperative (6 months) C_i and C_d scores for the pathology groups (AHS and HI) divided according to the side of temporal lobectomy. Note that the scores for the left AHS group are not as in Table 10.3. This is because two of the group who were available for examination before operation were not available at 6 months after operation because they had returned to their countries of origin (both spoke English as their first language).

further test of this view is that, if it is correct one would expect a post-operative decline in verbal memory following right temporal lobectomy including hippocampus, with no or only mild neuronal depletion. Inspection of the *postoperative* scores (Fig. 10.2) shows that this is what occurs.

Following right temporal lobectomy the C_i scores of the HI group decline, but this just fails to achieve statistical significance (Wilcoxon T = 6.5 with N = 9, T = 6 required for p =<. 05 figure 2-tailed). However, the drop in their C_d scores does achieve the $p < .01$ level of significance (Wilcoxon T = 2.5, N = 9). In contrast, there is virtually no change in the scores of the AHS group after right temporal lobectomy. Preoperatively, the two groups had differed pathologically only in the extent of their hippocampal neurone depletion (+ or - the amygdala which is probably abnormal preoperatively in many of the AHS group, but may not be in the HI group). The implication is that it is the hippocampus-amygdala system of the right hemisphere, rather than neocortical structures, which is involved in verbal memory function. As expected, left temporal lobectomy including hippocampus not severely depleted of neurones (i.e. the HI group) produced a precipitate fall in verbal memory, both immediate and delayed (Fig. 10.2). There was also a decline in C_d following left temporal lobectomy including hippocampus previously severely depleted of neurones (the AHS group), which is consistent with the suggestion that in the left hemisphere both the hippocampus and neocortical structures are involved in the memory function (Ojemann & Dodrill, 1985).

CONCLUSIONS

Sir Denis Hill, in his 1953 Royal Society of Medicine discussion, was much concerned with the matter of mental symptoms in temporal lobe epilepsy and their possible relationship to pathology. Mr Murray Falconer in the immediately subsequent discussion was clearly of the view that the surgical technique should allow proper definition of the underlying pathology which might then be related to the clinical features of the patients illness. The findings which we have presented support these contentions. Given proper histopathological examination of excised tissue, a relationship can be demonstrated between the patients' preoperative mental abilities and the nature of the temporal lobe pathology. It is not justified to consider patients prior to temporal lobectomy to be neuropsychologically homogeneous except for the side of their intended operation.

We have related preoperative verbal memory performance to the extent of hippocampal neurone density. We hasten to add that the patients with the lowest hippocampal neurone counts were also those most likely to have a significant depletion of neurones in the amygdala and the thalamus; likewise they may have had neuronal loss in temporal neocortex and white matter gliosis (Falconer et al 1964). Unfortunately we have not had the opportunity for a proper histopathological assessment of the amygdala and so it may be safest to associate the memory impairment with hippocampus-amygdala pathology, since the patients with severe hippocampal neurone depletion are likely to have concomitant neuronal loss from the ipsilateral amygdala (Margerison & Corsellis 1966). The extent of any neocortical or white matter involvement in our two groups seemed similar and the major anatomical difference seemed to be in the hippocampus. We have not as yet made any attempt to relate memory capacity to neuronal densities in specific hippocampal zones or particular parts along its antero-posterior dimension (Babb et al 1984). A loss of dentate gyrus granule cells may be particularly common after prolonged early childhood convulsions (Babb et al 1984, Sagar & Oxbury 1987). However, the case of severe amnesia following cardiopulmonary arrest reported by Cummings et al (1984) had well-preserved dentate granule cells, despite a severe loss of hippocampal pyramidal neurones. This may be a hint that the poor verbal memory associated with Ammon's horn sclerosis is likely to be related particularly to the loss of pyramidal neurones.

The findings suggest that both cerebral hemispheres, not just the left, have a role in verbal memory function and that this is differently organised on the two sides. On the right the hippocampus-amygdala system appears to be the only temporal lobe structure of importance, whereas on the left there seems to be involvement of both the hippocampus-amygdala system and temporal neocortex. Such a differential organisation would also explain the finding that left intracarotid amytal produces memory failure in the presence of right-sided severe hippocampal neurone loss, but right intra-carotid amytal does not necessarily do so in the presence of the same pathology on the left (Carpenter et al 1988, Oxbury et al 1988).

From the clinical point of view, it is important to appreciate that the neuropsychological data are difficult to interpret, especially when deciding whether or not to recommend surgery, unless it is possible to predict the pathology with reasonable accuracy. For instance, a low verbal memory score may not be a contraindication to right temporal lobectomy in a patient with suspected Ammon's horn sclerosis, but could be in a patient with other pathology because it might then imply that there was also pathology on the left. Similarly, the effects of temporal lobectomy on memory will depend at least partly on the pre-existing pathology and on the extent of any preoperative memory impairment, both of which may themselves be inter-related. In our experience, the most bitter complaints that operation has precipitated memory impairment come from patients whose preoperative memory was good and whose lobectomy has included left hippocampus (± amygdala) with only minor or no neuronal depletion. Also, patients who have had a normal or only mildly abnormal right hippocampus excised not uncommonly complain that their memory is not as good as preoperatively, citing failures of verbal memory as examples. In contrast, this complaint is relatively unusual from patients whose excised hippocampus showed severe neuronal depletion.

The study of the relationship between temporal lobe pathology and mental abilities is only in its infancy, despite the stage having been set by Mr Murray Falconer and Sir Denis Hill approximately 25 years ago. This paucity is in marked contrast to the very many and far-reaching studies of postoperative effects of temporal lobectomy pioneered by Professor Brenda Milner and her associates at the Montreal Neurological Institute. Since our first 1984 report suggesting that patients with right Ammon's horn sclerosis might have a verbal memory impairment, McMillan et al (1987) from the Guys Maudsley Neurosurgery Unit have also reported data to suggest that patients with 'hippocampal sclerosis', defined as neuronal loss and gliosis of any degree in the hippocampus without involvement of the amygdala, may have had some degree of preoperative verbal memory impairment irrespective of the side of the subsequent operation. It is to be hoped that there will now be an increasing number of such reports of clinicopathological correlations.

ACKNOWLEDGEMENTS

We would like to acknowledge our gratitude to our patients and many colleagues for the help given in the preparation of this chapter. Of our colleagues we would particularly like to mention Christopher Adams, Trevor Hughes, Peter Fenwick, Elizabeth Beardsworth, and Katherine Carpenter. We would also like to thank Sandra Horsburgh for her help and great patience in the preparation of the manuscript.

REFERENCES

Adams C B T, Anslow P, Molyneux A, Oxbury J 1987 Radiological detection of surgically treatable pathology. In: Engel J Jr (ed) Surgical treatment of the epilepsies. Raven Press, New York, p 213–233
Armstrong D D, Bruton C J 1987 Postscript: What terminology is appropriate for tissue pathology? How does it predict outcome? In: Engel J Jr (ed) Surgical treatment of the epilepsies. Raven Press, New York, p 541–552
Babb T L, Brown W J, Pretorius J, Davenport C, Lieb J P, Crandall P H, 1984, Temporal lobe volumetric cell densities in temporal lobe epilepsy. Epilepsia, 25: 729–740
Babb T L, Brown W J 1987 Pathological findings in epilepsy. In: Engel J Jr (ed) Surgical treatment of the epilepsies. Raven Press, New York, p 511–540
Benson D F, Marsden C D, Meadows J C 1974 The amnesic syndrome of posterior cerebral artery occlusion. Acta Neurologica Scandinavica. 50: 133–145
Berti A, Oxbury J M, Adams C B T, Oxbury S M, Hughes J T Jeffries M 1988 Drug-resistant epilepsy following early childhood convulsions treated by temporal lobectomy. Submitted for publication
Blakemore C B, Falconer M A 1967 Long-term efffects of anterior temporal lobectomy on certain cognitive functions. Journal of Neurology, Neurosurgery and Psychiatry 30: 364–367
Blakemore C B, Ettlinger G, Falconer M A 1966 Cognitive abilities in relation to frequency of seizures and neuropathology of the temporal lobes in man. Journal of Neurology, Neurosurgery and Psychiatry 29: 268–272

Brierly J B 1966 The neuropathology of amnesic states.In: Whitty C W M, Zangwill O L (ed) Amnesia. p 150–180

Carpenter K N, Oxbury S M, Oxbury J M, Anslow P, Hughes J T 1988 Intracarotid sodium amytal in the diagnosis of hippocampal pathology. In preparation

Corsellis J A N, Goldberg G J, Norton A R 1968 'Limbic encephalitis' and its association with carcinoma. Brain 91: 481–496

Cummings J L, Tomiyasu V, Read S, Benson D F 1984 Amnesia with hippocampal lesions after cardiopulmonary arrest. Neurology 34: 679–681

De Renzi E, Zambolin A, Crisi G 1987 The pattern of neuropsychological impairment associated with left posterior cerebral infarcts. Brain 110: 1099–1116

Falconer M A 1953 Discussion on the surgery of temporal lobe epilepsy: surgical and pathological aspects. Proceedings of the Royal Society of Medicine 46: 971–975

Falconer M A 1971a Genetic and related aetiological factors in temporal lobe epilepsy: a review. Epilepsia 12: 13–31

Falconer K A 1971b Anterior temporal lobectomy for epilepsy.In: Robb C, Smith R (eds) Operative surgery, vol 14: Neurosurgery. Butterworth, London, p 142–149

Falconer M A, Serafetinides E A, Corsellis J A 1964 Etiology and pathogenesis of temporal lobe epilepsy. Archives of Neurology 10: 233–248

Hill D 1953 Discussion on the surgery of temporal lobe epilepsy: the clinical study and selection of patients. Proceedings of the Royal Society of Medicine 46: 965–971

Horel J A 1978 The neuroanatomy of amnesia: a critique of the hippocampal memory hypothesis. Brain 101: 403–445

Jeeves M A 1987 Neuropsychology. In Gregory R L (ed) The Oxford companion to the mind. Oxford University Press, Oxford, p 545–549

Jones-Gotman M 1987 Testing hippocampal function. In: Engel J Jr (ed) Surgical treatment of the epilepsies. Raven Press, New York, p 203–211

Jones-Gotman M, Milner B 1978 Right temporal-lobe contribution to image-mediated verbal learning. Neuropsychologia 16: 61–71

Kemper T 1984 Neuroanatomical and neuropathological changes in normal aging and dementia. In Albert M L (ed) Clinical neurology of aging. Oxford University Press, Oxford, p 9–52

Lishman W A 1987 Organic psychiatry: the psychological consequences of cerebral disorder. Blackwell Scientific Publications, Oxford, p 24

McMillan T M, Powell G E, Janota I, Polkey C E 1987 Relationship between neuropathology and cognitive functioning in temporal lobectomy patients. Journal of Neurology, Neurosurgery and Psychiatry 50: 167–176

Margerison J H, Corsellis J A N 1966 Epilepsy and the temporal lobes. A clinical, electroencephalographic and neuropathological study of the brain in epilepsy with particular reference to the temporal lobes. Brain 89: 499–530

Mathieson G 1975 Pathology of temporal lobe foci. In: Penry J K, Daly D D (eds) Advances in neurology, vol 11. Raven Press, New York, p 163–185

Meyer V, Yates A J 1955 Intellectual changes following temporal lobectomy for psychomotor epilepsy: preliminary communication. Journal of Neurology, Neurosurgery and Psychiatry 18: 44–52

Milner B 1958 Psychological defects produced by temporal lobe excision. Proceedings of the Association for Research in Nervous and Mental Disease 35: 244–257

Milner B 1962 Laterality effects in audition. In: Mountcastle V B (ed) Interhemispheric relations and cerebral dominance. John Hopkins Press, Baltimore, p 177–195

Milner B 1967 Brain mechanisms suggested by studies of temporal lobes. In: Darley F C (ed) Brain mechanisms underlying speech and language. Grune and Stratton, New York, p 122–145

Milner B 1970 Memory and the medial temporal regions of the brain. In: Pribram K H, Broadbent D E (eds) Biology of memory. Academic Press, New York, p 29–50

Milner B 1971 Interhemispheric differences in the localisation of psychological processes in man. British Medical Bulletin 27: 272–277

Mishkin K 1982 A memory system in the monkey. Philosophical Transaction of the Royal Society of London B, 298: 85–95

Novelly P A, Augustine E A, Mattson R H et al 1984 Selective memory improvement and impairment in temporal lobectomy for epilepsy. Annals of Neurology 15: 64–67

Ojemann G A, Dodrill C B 1985 Verbal memory deficits after temporal lobectomy for epilepsy. Journal of Neurosurgery 62: 101–107

Ojemann G A, Engel J 1987 Acute and chronic intracranial recording and stimulation. In: Engel J Jr (ed) Surgical treatment of the epilepsies. Raven Press, New York, p 263–288

Ounsted C, Lindsay J, Norman R 1966 Biological factors in temporal lobe epilepsy. William Heinemann Medical Books, London

Oxbury J M, MacCallum F O 1973 Herpes simplex virus encephalitis: clinical features and residual damage. Postgraduate Medical Journal 49: 387–389

Oxbury S M, Oxbury J M 1984 Intracarotid amytal test in the assessment of language dominance. In: Rose F C (ed) Progress in aphasiology, advances in neurology, vol 42. Raven Press, New York, p 115–123

Oxbury S M, Carpenter K N, Oxbury J M 1988 Carotid amytal memory loss: a defect of retrieval associated with severe hippocampal neurone loss. Acta Neurologica Scandinavica 77: 348

Powell G E, Polkey C E, McMillan T 1985 The new Maudsley series of temporal lobectomy. I: short-term cognitive effects. British Journal of Clinical Psychology 24: 109–124

Rausch R 1987 Psychological evaluation, In: Engel J Jr (ed) Surgical treatment of the epilepsies. Raven Press, New York, p 181–195

Rausch R, Crandall P H 1982 Psychological status related to surgical control of temporal lobe seizures. Epilepsia 23: 191–202

Sagar H J, Oxbury J M 1987 Hippocampal neurone loss in temporal lobe epilepsy: correlation with early childhood convulsions. Annals of Neurology 22: 334–340

Samuels I, Butters N, Fedio P 1972 Short-term memory disorders following temporal lobe removals in humans. Cortex 8: 283–298

Scoville W B 1954 The limbic lobe in man. Journal of Neurosurgery 11: 64–66

Scoville W B, Milner B 1957 Loss of recent memory after bilateral hippocampal lesions. Journal of Neurology, Neurosurgery and Psychiatry 20: 11–21

Smith M L, Milner B 1981 The role of the right hippocampus in the recall of spatial location. Neuropsychologia 19: 781–793

Yasargil M G, Wieser H G 1987 Selective amygdalohippocampectomy at the University Hospital, Zurich. In: Engel J Jr (ed) Surgical treatment of the epilepsies. Raven Press, New York, p 653–658

11
C. D. Marsden

Movement disorders in neuropsychiatry

INTRODUCTION

Denis Hill had a lively interest in disorders of movement. No doubt he was influenced by Hughlings Jackson, who once commented 'these "mental centres" . . . they are motor too — they are the highest motor centres'. Denis Hill, like many of his contemporaries, had the hunch that the disorders of movement seen in patients with psychoses and neuroses held a clue to the functional (used in its proper sense) pathophysiology of mental illnesses. Denis Hill was sure that schizophrenia and depression disturbed movement and, like Kleist, he flirted with the notion that this was due to functional disturbance of the basal ganglia. Given my own interest in diseases of the basal ganglia, this lead to lively private discussion and argument between us, but with no resolution of the problem!

Nevertheless, movement is one of the robust bridges between neurology and psychiatry, built upon solid observations that tantalise those in both disciplines. What are these foundations, and how do they illuminate the shared ground between brain disease and mental illness?

Abnormal movement is a feature of untreated schizophrenia, depression, obsessive-compulsive disorders and hysteria. The schizophrenic displays a range of disturbances of movement, from catatonia to the bizarre eccentricities of stereotypies and mannerisms. The retarded depressed individual superficially resembles, and sometimes is confused with, the bradykinetic Parkinsonian. The motor behaviour of the obsessive-compulsive hints at basal ganglia dysfunction. One of the commonest expressions of hysteria is a movement disorder.

In each of these conditions, the diagnostic disturbances of the mind are accompanied by disorders of movement. Do the latter represent the results of an alteration of function in the motor areas of the brain similar to that in the regions of the brain responsible for thought, emotion and perception? If so, understanding the reasons for movement disorders in psychiatric illness may provide a window into comprehending the mental disorders.

MOVEMENT DISORDERS IN SCHIZOPHRENIA

Unfortunately, the modern interpretation of motor abnormalities in psychotic schizophrenic patients has been contaminated by the well-nigh universal administration of neuroleptic drugs. Since their introduction in the early 1950s, it has become exceedingly difficult to disentangle movement disorders associated with the untreated illness from those produced by neuroleptic drugs. Earlier, a similar problem arose during the epidemic of encephalitis lethargica in the 1920s and 1930s; this illness caused both mental and motor consequences. Nowadays it is difficult to find schizophrenic patients who have not received neuroleptics. Even those who would appear never to have taken such drugs, may have required medication during acute psychotic episodes which has gone unrecorded in their drug charts.

However, earlier classic descriptions of schizophrenia, such as those of Kraepelin and Bleuler, clearly documented movement disorders in schizophrenia in elaborate detail.

Stereotypies (pointless, repetitive, apparently voluntary normal movements) may occur in about a quarter of schizophrenics, especially early in the illness. They vary from simple tic-like events to highly complicated ritualistic gestures or actions. These repetitive behaviours may continue for years, becoming a motor characteristic of the individual patient which may dominate their life.

Mannerisms (bizarrely executed, unnatural exaggerations of normal voluntary movements) also feature in some schizophrenics. Mannerisms vary from minor quirks of performance to ludicrous antics which lay observers equate with the popular picture of the lunatic.

The abnormal spontaneous stereotypies and the abnormal manneristic execution of movement in schizophrenics may be accompanied by other interferences with normal motor behaviour. Thus, perservation (persistence of normal purposeful activity after the need for it has ceased) and motor blocking (sudden cessation of movement before it is completed) are not uncommon. Rarely, automatic obedience and echopraxia occur.

All these movement disorders may affect speech as well as bodily activity. They were most evident in catatonic schizophrenia, the incidence of which has declined. The catatonic syndrome, first described by Kahlbaum, is characterised by profound mental withdrawal, accompanied by abnormal posturing, muscular rigidity and catalepsy (waxy rigidity), culminating in stupor, or conversely a state of excitement. Why catatonia is now so uncommon in the West is not adequately explained. It is still seen in developing communities.

What do these schizophrenic movement disorders mean? One hypothesis is that they are indeed the result of a functional disturbance of motor control, paralleling that of mental activity. Originally, many classical writers drew analogies between them and the dyskinesias known to occur in visible basal ganglia disease. Indeed, they employed terms such as athetosis and chorea in their descriptions. Few would now be so bold! The problems are a) early descriptions of untreated schizophrenic populations probably were contaminated by individuals with recognised diseases, such as Huntington's chorea and encephalitis lethargica; b) later reports were confounded by the extrapyramidal side effects of antipsychotic drugs; c) there are no objective methods of defining athetosis, dystonia, chorea etc., which are 'all in the eye of the beholder'. A rigorous critic would have to conclude that the notion that schizophrenics exhibit movement disorders of the sort seen in basal ganglia disease is unproven at the present time. The concept may be valid, but there are neither the pure patient populations nor the diagnostic techniques to establish the point. However, the problem can be approached from the opposite direction — namely, do known brain diseases produce the movement disorders of schizophrenia? — and the answer is a qualified yes (see below).

An alternative serial, rather than parallel, hypothesis is that the motor disorders of schizophrenia are the consequence of the mental disturbance. This notion receives some support from the similarity of the motor and mental abnormalities. For example, motor blocking can be regarded as the equivalent of thought blocking, while stereotypies and mannerisms might be construed as motor responses to psychotic delusions. Indeed, some schizophrenic patients may explain their motor actions as driven by external agencies. Thus, these 'made' actions, along with 'made' thoughts and feelings, are considered to be passivity experiences, due to outside influences playing on the body. In this model, the abnormal thought processes are conceived as generating movement through normal motor mechanisms, without having to involve any parallel dysfunction of the motor regions of the brain. The movement disorders of schizophrenia then would become relegated to epiphenomena which give little insight into the abnormalities of the brain underlying schizophrenia.

How much effort should be devoted to understanding the movements of schizophrenia depends upon resolving which hypothesis is most likely to be valid. If such motor disorders are a parallel expression of a basic cerebral dysfunction, they may prove at least as amenable to investigate as the disorder of thought. If they are no more than a serial epiphenomenon, they are not of great interest.

At present it is not possible to decide between the two hypotheses, but there are possible ways of investigating the problem. One approach might be to employ positron emission tomography (PET) to assess whether the metabolic motor activity in the brain is normal or abnormal in schizophrenia. Another is to use the advanced techniques of event-related neurophysiology to analyse cerebral motor activity in the schizophrenic.

On balance, I would vote for the more exciting parallel hypothesis, on the grounds that patients with known brain disease may manifest movement disorders similar to those seen in schizophrenia.

PATIENTS WITH BRAIN DISEASES EXHIBIT MOVEMENT DISORDERS SIMILAR TO THOSE OF SCHIZOPHRENIA

Nowadays the syndrome of catatonia is as likely to be due to identifiable brain disease as to schizophrenia. The range of illness reported to cause catatonia is huge, but of particular interest is the observation that, occasionally, frontal lobe damage (resulting from tumour, infection or inflammation) may present with such a clinical picture. The neuroleptic malignant syndrome, a rare complication of medication with antipsychotic drugs that block cerebral dopamine receptors, also has similarities with catatonia. Indeed, a similar syndrome with intense rigidity, fever and metabolic disturbance was occasionally encountered in schizophrenics before the advent of neuroleptic drugs.

The inherited syndrome of George Gilles de la Tourette (chronic multiple tics with vocalisations) is now firmly believed to be due to some unidentified (possibly metabolic) abnormality of the brain. The motor features of Gilles de la Tourette's syndrome bear strong resemblance to those of schizophrenia. Indeed, there is a confusing overlap in terminology for the movement disorders of the two conditions. Simple tics in Gilles de la Tourette's syndrome are physically identical to simple stereotypies in schizophrenia. Complex tics in the former illness are sometimes called stereotypies. Voluntary movements in tiquers often are manneristic. Motor blocking, either of vocal or body action, are seen in both conditions. Why should apparently identical movements in Gilles de la Tourette's syndrome be called tics, while in schizophrenics they are termed stereotypies and mannerisms?

Drug-induced movement disorders may also resemble stereotypies and mannerisms. The movements seen in those with neuroleptic-induced akathisia often have the characteristics of stereotypies, as may some of the repetitive diphasic dyskinesias produced by levodopa therapy in Parkinson's disease.

It must be concluded that visible brain disease, inherited metabolic conditions such as Gilles de la Tourette's syndrome, and bombardment of the brain by drugs, may all produce the abnormal movements that characterise the schizophrenic. Accordingly, such schizophrenic movement disorders may well be due to disorganised cerebral motor function and therefore worthy of close attention.

To prove the point, it is necessary to establish beyond doubt that schizophrenic movement disorders and similar motor phenomena caused by cerebral damage or drugs are identical. Again, the powerful technique of PET and clinical neurophysiology may help. In addition, a purely phenomenological analysis utilising digitised videotape recordings might prove valuable.

MOVEMENT DISORDERS IN DEPRESSION

The severely retarded depressive appears uncannily like the patient with Parkinson's disease. The face is expressionless, the posture is bowed, spontaneous motor action is reduced and voluntary movement is slow. The possibility of confusion is even greater, for about a third of those with Parkinson's disease are depressed. Furthermore, a sizeable proportion of those Parkinsonians who are not depressed exhibit a slowness of thought (bradyphrenia) superficially indistinguishable from that of depressives.

The inescapable conclusion is that motor changes in the severely retarded depressive may be due to some abnormality of cerebral metabolic activity in common with Parkinson's disease, such as reduced dopamine action in some critical brain area. PET utilising ^{18}F-dopa to measure cerebral dopamine synthesis, turnover and storage, ^{11}C-nomifensine to identify dopaminergic terminals, and ^{11}C-raclopride to identify postsynaptic dopamine receptors may unearth some defect of dopaminergic mechanisms in the brain of those with retarded depression.

What then distinguishes Parkinson's disease from severe retarded depression? Patients with the former illness, additionally, exhibit muscular rigidity and diagnostic rest tremor, and respond to treatment with levodopa or other dopamine agonists.

Depression, generally, is not responsive to levodopa treatment. However, it is not yet clear whether the motor sequences of retarded depression can be reversed by dopamine agonist therapy.

Rest tremor in Parkinson's disease may be due to more than just striatal dopamine depletion. At least in experimental studies in primates, it requires lesions of both nigrostriatal dopamine pathways and ascending cerebello-thalamic and cerebello-rubral pathways to produce rest tremor. If the same is true in Parkinson's disease, then the absence of rest tremor in depressives can be accounted for by the absence of the additional cerebellar pathway dysfunction.

Rigidity in Parkinson's disease, which is not characteristic of depression, may also be due to additional pathology in the former illness. Rigidity appears to be the consequence of both exaggerated long-latency (perhaps transcortical) stretch reflexes and enhanced tonic stretch reflexes (perhaps reflecting dysfunction of the spinal cord motor machinery). Both may be the result of defective striopallidal control of motor systems, other than those involved in the control of initiation and speed of movement. These other motor systems may not be compromised in depression.

Much effort has been expended in trying to analyse the pathophysiology of akinesia in Parkinson's disease. Methods have been devised to study simple and complex movements in the Parkinsonian. The application of similar clinical neurophysiological techniques to analyse movement in depression might reveal abnormalities similar to those in Parkinson's disease. If so, this would reinforce the notion that there exists some defect of motor control in the depressive. Experiments that might be rewarding include the study of simultaneous and sequential two-joint movements, which break down in Parkinson's disease, and long-latency stretch reflexes might be exaggerated in the depressive, even if clinical rigidity is not evident.

The link between depression itself and Parkinson's disease is also worthy of further exploration. While striatal dopamine depletion is the central and necessary biochemical pathology of the Parkinsonian, there are additional neurotransmitter defects in that condition. In particular, there are deficiencies of noradrenaline and serotonin, both of which are implicated in depression itself. Understanding of how these biochemical defects contribute to depression in Parkinson's disease may provide closer links to primary depressive illness.

Finally, slowness of thought (as well as movement) is characteristic of both Parkinson's disease and depression. The analysis of the pathophysiology and biochemical substitute of such bradyphrenia again may reveal shared abnormalities in the two conditions.

In conclusion, depressive mood, bradyphrenia and akinesia are common to both Parkinson's disease and depression. All may reflect similar dysfunction of specific cerebral mechanisms in the two illnesses. Understanding of these features in Parkinson's disease may give insight into depressive conditions, et vice versa — a fruitful field for further exploration.

MOVEMENT DISORDERS IN OBSESSIVE-COMPULSIVE NEUROSIS

While many have considered the significance of movement disorders in schizophrenia and depression, less attention has been given to the motor behaviour of the obsessional. Yet mere observation suggests that these individuals have a disorder of movement. The compulsions so characteristic of the obsessional are, superficially, normal motor acts driven to repetition by the abnormal thought. However, some affected individuals deny (or are unaware of) any mental drive to their motor rituals, which could be just as well described as stereotypies or tics. Indeed, recent evidence strongly links obsessional neurosis to Gilles de la Tourette's disease. About a third of patients with the latter illness exhibit an obsessional neurosis. Close analysis of large families with Gilles de la Tourette's disease, in which dominant inheritance is evident, has revealed that obligate carriers of the gene may exhibit an obsessional neurosis in the absence of the typical tics and vocalisations. Furthermore, the mental component of a tic, namely the urge to carry out the motor action which, if suppressed voluntarily, leads to mounting inner tension, is typical of the compulsion. Thus, the obsessional struggles against his motor rituals, and if the latter are constrained, mounting anxiety results.

The suspicion is that the motor rituals of the obsessional may share some pathophysiology with the complex tics of Gilles de la Tourette's syndrome. Neurophysiological analysis of at least the simple tics of the latter illness has revealed that they are not generated through the brain mechanisms responsible for normal voluntary movement. The Bereitschaftspotential, a negative brain wave in the electroencephalogram best recorded over the vertex region corresponding to the supplementary motor area, normally precedes the initiation of a normal voluntary movement. There is no Bereitschaftspotential prior to simple tics. Whether there is a Bereitschafts-potential prior to complex tics, or prior to the compulsive rituals of the obsessional, remains to be established.

There also is a subset of those with the obsessional neurosis who exhibit marked motor inhibition. Such obsessional slowness of movement is reminiscent of akinesia in Parkinson's disease, even to the extent of inability to initiate movement, and slowness in its execution. Some such individuals, like the Parkinsonian, resort to tricks to start a movement, such as walking on the spot or tapping with the hand.

As an hypothesis, it may be that obsessional rituals and obsessional slow-ness in those with obsessive compulsive neurosis have a pathophysiology similar to that responsible for analogous movement disorders in Gilles de la Tourette's syndrome and Parkinson's disease.

MOVEMENT DISORDERS IN HYSTERIA

Finally, we come to the most difficult but, perhaps, the most fascinating challenge of all. At least a third of those with conversion symptoms exhibit disorders of movement. It is easy to dismiss hysterical paralysis or weak-ness, or hysterical involuntary movements or muscle spasms, as involuntary (assumed) symptoms of secondary (interpreted) gain. Indeed, frequently it is impossible to be sure that there is not conscious motivation behind motor hysteria (malingering), particularly when compensation is involved. Yet, amidst the morass of those with motor hysteria are some whose motor disabilities appear unconstructive, and lead to disabling physical incapaci-ties. Such individuals appear unable, despite their wishes, to engage normal motor activities. Their inability to move is analogous to hysterical sensory deficit, where demonstrable sensory input to the brain (as evidenced by normal initial components of somatosensory evoked potentials) produces no conscious experience. In the motor sphere, a conscious attempt to move evokes no motor activity. It is as though consciousness of the motor attempt or sensory reception, is divorced from the next stage of cerebral function, be it generation of movement or interpretation of sensory signals.

Clinical neurophysiology is gradually disentangling consciousness from the final motor output, or the initial sensory input into the brain. For example, the initiation of the Bereitschaftspotential may precede conscious appreciation of the desire to move; likewise, motor response to external stimuli may occur in advance of perception of the sensory event, either in consciousness or as evidenced by late cognitive evoked potentials such as the P300. Such evidence, gradually being accumulated in contemporary experiments, increasingly divorces consciousness from action or unconscious perception. Such data is not the proof of a dualistic philosophy, but the beginnings of an experimental analysis of the classical components of 'mind' and 'brain'. The hysteric may have a dissociation between the cerebral mechanisms of the will (the 'mind') and those responsible for action and perception (the 'brain'). In the motor sphere, this represents the paralysis of the idea expressed by Russell Reynolds.

Freud was an inspired neurologist, whose forays into the mind may have been misinterpreted by subsequent generations. It is worth recalling that he established the origin of mammalian posterior root ganglia from their homologous components in the spinal cord of fish; that he unravelled the fibrillary structure of nerve fibres from studies of the crayfish; that he disintangled the inter-relations of the posterior columns of the spinal cord with the accoustic and vestibular inputs to the brainstem, and its cerebellar connections, using a technically sophisticated method of gold staining of nerve tissue; and that he predicted the use of cocaine as a local anaesthetic. His monograph on aphasia in 1891 was, and is, a landmark in that subject. Less well-known is his treatise on infantile cerebral paralysis of 1897; this stands as an unrivalled and monumental description of the morass of motor syndromes originating in infancy and childhood, which Strumpell had attributed to encephalitis. It was from this base that Freud attacked hysteria, and some would say became diverted from his solid scientific grounding. Yet Freud was intrigued by the manifestations of hysteria as an expression of the separation of the brain mechanisms responsible for consciousness from those responsible for subconscious mental activity. Movement spans both Russell Reynolds' conscious 'idea' and subconscious execution. Freud explored, in his own way, the pathophysiology of the subconscious, and the reasons why ideas can be divorced from the performance. Janet, too, was grappling with the same problem; how can those with hysterical anaesthesia (or amnesia) have no consciousness of sensation, but yet all the elements of sensation are present, except the personal perception of it. Hysterical movement disorders present the same problem in reverse; how can those with hysterical paralysis have the personal perception of the desire to move, and normal executive motor output pathways from the brain, yet be unable to link the two into action.

Modern neurophysiology and imaging of brain function are developing the tools to attack these problems. Denis Hill would have approved — he knew that the EEG held the promise of understanding the mind.

Hysteria

INTRODUCTION

It is generally acknowledged that hysteria is one of the oldest conditions described in medicine (Veith 1965), and yet definitions are difficult to find. It is rather as if everyone knows what they mean by using the term and assume it has some conformity with the thoughts of others, yet are afraid to proffer a definition lest they find out the fragility of their own conceptions. Further, any definition bound on the printed page will be there for all time as a possible subject for criticism. While some authors confidently predict the value and survival of hysteria as a diagnosis (Lewis 1975), others refer to it as 'a label assigned to a particular relationship between the observer and the observed' (Slater 1961).

As a diagnosis, hysteria is generally considered a problem for psychiatry and yet the historical and contemporary associations are largely neurological. In this chapter, some of these issues are explored and an attempt to organise some thoughts about the current status of hysteria will be made.

HISTORICAL ASSOCIATIONS

The associations between the brain and hysteria probably began with Willis (1622–75), the first British neurologist. He declined to accept the view, popular from ancient times, that hysteria was a disease of the uterus, stating, 'this passion comes not from the vapours rising into the head from the uterus or spleen, nor from a rapid flow of blood into the pulmonary vessels, but has its origin in the brain itself' (Dewhurst 1980, p 87). Further, for Willis the condition was primarily a convulsive condition, emphasising another historical trend, namely the close association between epilepsy and hysteria (Trimble 1986). It should be recalled that at the time that Willis was writing, 'nervous diseases' represented a protean group of conditions that somehow were related to disturbed nerve function, a theme elaborated by Sydenham (1624–89) who described the morbid type 'hysteria', recognising it as one of the commonest chronic diseases encountered in practice. Whytt (1714–66) defined nervous as follows (Whytt 1765, p 93):

> . . . those disorders may, peculiarly, deserve the name of nervous, which, on account of an unusual delicacy, or unnatural states of the nerves, are produced by causes, which, in people of sound constitution, would either have no such effects, or at least in a much less degree.

The 19th century saw a rapid explosion of knowledge regarding the pathogeneses of many conditions that a century earlier were called 'nervous', rechristened 'neuroses' by Cullen. This reflected the success of anatomo-clinical medicine and the localisation of pathology in discrete organs of the body including the brain. However, such methods failed to clarify the origins of hysteria. It was mainly the French neurologists of the second half of the century who re-emphasised the nosological boundaries of hysteria and considered it a condition, as any other in medicine, in which observation should precede speculation.

Briquet (1796–1881) defined hysteria as a 'neurosis of the brain . .' (Briquet 1859, p 3) and made careful observations on 430 patients. He noted the premorbid characterological predispositions of patients and reflected that anything that may disturb the equilibrium of the nervous system may provoke the condition. In particular, marital and family afflictions were important, especially grief. Charcot (1825–93), following Briquet, felt that hysteria, like other medical conditions, was 'governed by rules and laws, which attentive and sufficiently numerous observations always permit us to establish' (Charcot 1889, p 13).

In England there appears to have been much less interest in hysteria (Wilson 1910), but Gowers (1845–1915), in his well known text book (1893), wrote of hysteria that 'the primary derangement is in the higher cerebral centres . . . the malady is a real one, and to a large extent beyond the direct influence of the patient's will' (vol 2, p 984).

The story of how another neurologist, Freud (1856–1939), after a brief spell under the tuteledge of Charcot, returned to Vienna and, initially with Breuer (1842–1925), developed the psychology of hysteria and ultimately the technique of psychoanalysis is well known. However, often less appreciated is the role given to psychologically stressful events by preceeding authors. Certainly Sydenham referred to 'violent perturbations of the mind from some sudden assult, either of anger or grief, or such like passions', and similar antecedents were discussed bv Baglivi (1668–1706) and Briquet, among others.

The advent of psychoanalysis, and the subsequent era in psychiatry, dominated as it was by psychological speculations of supposed aetiologies of mental illness, led to a diminution of interest among neurologists in hysteria, although there were exceptions such as Wilson, Head, Walshe and Symonds. For these authors, the presence of hysteria had been magnified by the large numbers of acute presentations seen in various war settings, and the suggestions of the Freudians that sexual repression and trauma lay

at the seat of hysterical phenomena were untenable. Head (1922) emphasised the importance clinically of establishing 'positive signs' of hysteria
and that it was not a diagnosis simply to be made by exclusion. Walshe
(1965) reaffirmed the unitary nature of the condition and Symonds (1970)
agreed that 'hysteria is not a myth but a reality'.

DEFINITIONS

The ICD 9 definition of hysteria refers to a mental disorder 'in which
motives, of which the patient seems unaware, produce either a restriction
of the field of consciousness or disturbances of motor and sensory function
which may seem to have psychological advantage or symbolic value' (WHO
1980). This immediately introduces the idea of a mechanism into the diagnostic criteria, an unusual step in medicine generally. Although similar
definitions were given in earlier editions of the American Psychiatric Association's DSM 1 and 11, the DSM 111 made a significant departure in
removing the term neurosis entirely. This was done on the assumption that
the term is associated with certain theories of pathogenesis. In DSM III,
hysteria is fragmented under somatisation disorder and conversion disorder.
Nonetheless, the criteria still insist on the disorder being 'medically unex-
plainable'. Further, 'a temporal relationship between symptom onset and
some external event or psychological conflict, or the symptom allows the
individual to avoid unpleasant activity or the symptom provides opportunity
for support which may not have been otherwise available' must be present
(APA 1980). The insistence on the condition being medically inexplicable
seems extraordinary, if psychiatry is a branch of medicine. The other
inclusions rely entirely on subjective opinions of the examining physician
— secondary gain, in other words, being usually in the eye of the beholder.
   More pragmatic definitions are those of Walshe (1965):

> Hysteria shows the presence of signs which cannot originate from nervous
> system dysfunction, an absence of signs of nervous system disease [and]
> . . . patterns of disorder that plainly arise from mental disposition . . .
> [reflecting] . . . the subject's notions about his bodily arrangements and his
> functioning.

This to some extent follows Head (1922) in emphasising the disparity
between neurological signs and symptoms in making the diagnosis, but falls
down on two counts. First, as noted below, hysteria is commonly seen
in the presence of neurological disease and, secondly, it again relies on a
subjective impression, this time relating to the patient's 'mental
disposition'.

DEVELOPMENTS SINCE THE 1950s

An important step forward was made by Chodoff & Lyons (1958). They
highlighted the problem that, historically, two potentially independent

aspects had been confused, namely the distinction between a personality style, referred to as hysterical, and certain symptoms, referred to as conversion or dissociative.

The hysterical personality

This personality style has certain features that are instantly recognisable in its fully fledged form. These include a dramatic and emotional style of presentation, with excessive gestures and exaggerated imprecise verbal responses. The affect is shallow and labile, but without the emptiness of that of a person with a pseudobulbar palsy. Patients are both seductive and demanding in their interpersonal relationships and there is a tendency to both drug abuse and suicidal behaviour. Jaspers (1963), who also suggested a division such as that advocated by Chodoff and Lyons, referred to those with the hysterical personality as craving 'to appear, both to themselves and others, as more than they are and to experience more than they are ever capable of' (p 443).

The hysterical personality is recognised by the ICD 9, while DSM 111 refers to it as the histrionic personality, the features of which are given in Table 12.1. In DSM 111 this is grouped in Axis 2, while somatisation disorder and conversion disorder are under Axis I. This distinction gives further credence to the separation of personality from illness, a principle first clearly elaborated by Jaspers.

The hysterical personality style has been shown, by factor analysis, to be reliably identified and separate from both obsessional and 'oral' personalities

Table 12.1 Features of the histrionic personality disorder (American Psychiatric Association 1980)

Diagnostic criteria
The following are characteristic of the individual's current and long-term functioning, are not limited to episodes of illness, and cause either significant impairment in social or occupational functioning or subjective distress.

A. Behaviour that is overly dramatic, reactive, and intensely expressed, as indicated by at least three of the following:
1. self-dramatization, e.g. exaggerated expression of emotions
2. incessant drawing of attention to oneself
3. craving for activity and excitement
4. over-reaction to minor events
5. irrational, angry outbursts or tantrums

B. Characteristic disturbances in interpersonal relationships as indicated by at least two of the following:
1. perceived by others as shallow and lacking genuineness, even if superficially warm and charming
2. egocentric, self-indulgent, and inconsiderate of others
3. vain and demanding
4. dependent, helpless, constantly seeking reassurance
5. prone to manipulative suicidal threats, gestures, or attempts

---

(Lazare et al 1970). Further, both males and females with hysterical personalities show greater variability of mood, even on a day-to-day basis, than controls (Slaveney & Rich 1980). Their cognition may be referred to as 'global, relatively diffuse, and lacking in sharpness . . . in a word, impressionistic' (Shapiro 1965). This has several consequences, leading to poor concentrating abilities, distractability and an impressionistic cognitive style lacking attention to detail, and susceptible to accidental influences (Shapiro 1965).

Conversion symptoms

The precise origin of the word conversion in relation to symptoms is unclear, although according to Hunter & MacAlpine (1963) credit is given to Ferrier (1761–1815), physician to the Manchester Infirmary. He actually referred to cases of 'hysterical conversions', the term being used to explain how symptoms of a disease could affect apparently unconnected regions of the body, based on earlier theories of 'sympathy' between organs.

Freud reintroduced the term conversion to refer to somatic changes of physical functions which occur 'unconsciously and in a disorted form [and which] give expression to instinctual impulses that previously had been repressed' (Fenichel 1946, p 216). However, this was not conceived of as a simple somatic representation of an affect, but as 'very specific representations of thoughts' which could be retranslated back to the original by the method of psychoanalysis. Engel (1970) gives a more contemporary psychoanalytic definition of conversion symptoms (p 650–651) which:

> . . . originate in the mind but are experienced as bodily (physical in origin). They derive from stored mental representations (memories) of bodily activities or functioning which are utilised to express symbolically unconscious wishes or impulses as a means of coping with psychological conflict. Hence the conversion symptom is completely intrapsychic in nature:

In contrast, Ziegler & Imboden (1962) noted (p 283)

> [we] know of no scientific evidence that would warrant further delay of the long overdue abandonment of the libidinal, energetic and 'instinctual' implications connoted by the term 'conversion'. We do, however, retain the term 'conversion', used in a metaphorical sense, because no better term immediately suggests itself to denote the observable alteration of function.

In their conceptual model, they use the term conversion reaction, as opposed to hysteria, and refer to the symptoms and signs as 'symbols of somatic symptoms' (p 286). One major difficulty of defining conversion symptoms in the ways already given is that their demonstration depends on eliciting the relevant symbolism and conflict from a patient prior to diagnosis and, in seeking this from patients, the latter reach the conclusion that their problem 'is all in the mind'.

The association between the hysterical personality and conversion symptoms

The ideas of Charcot, while acknowledging the influence of emotional factors in relation to hysteria, were essentially based on a disease model, influenced by Morel's theory of degeneration. The search was not for unconscious conflicts, but for stigmata of the condition, elicited by sound clinical examination and observation. Janet (1859–1947) conceived of the importance of subconscious fixed ideas caused by traumatic events, which were replaced by symptoms, but emphasised the dissociation to be spontaneous and to be linked fundamentally to the underlying constitution, ascribed to hereditary factors. The patient with the hysterical personality was unable to perceive all phenomena and demonstrated a narrowing of consciousness, the unwanted phenomena developing independently with the patient unaware of them. Here the psychical and neurological blend, as do the patient's personalities and their symptoms.

In contrast, the psychoanalysts, as noted, developed their theories emphasising the symptom, the patients' experiences, and such mental mechanisms as symbolism and repression. Others, such as Kretschmer (1926) gave greater emphasis to underlying constitutional factors, but emphasising the hysterical form of reaction as 'ontogenetically preformed . . . arising from the impulsive psychic subsoil' (p viii): a biological propensity available to all. In these latter views, the concept of an altered central nervous system as the fundamental problem underlying the symptoms of hysteria was lost, as was the nucleus of the hysterical personality.

Following the developments suggested by Chodoff & Lyons (1958), several groups have examined the relationship between conversion symptoms and underlying personality. Chodoff and Lyons themselves, in a small study of 17 patients with conversion phenomena without known neurological disease, noted only 3 (17.6%) to conform to the hysterical personality style. Ljungberg (1957), in a larger study of 381 patients, noted only 20.7 to have this style, while Merskey & Trimble (1979), using a control population of psychiatric patients without conversion symptoms, gave a figure of 19%, which was greater than the frequency in the control group.

These estimates were all based on clinical impressions, but do have some conformity. Wilson-Barnett and Trimble (1985) assessed 79 patients with conversion symptoms using the Hysteroid-Obsessoid Questionnaire of Foulds. No overall difference was found between the hysteria patients and a control group of psychiatric patients, and 19% of the hysteria sample was regarded as scoring in the range showing the most florid elements of the hysterical personality.

The conclusions from these studies is that the hysterical personality may be marginally over-represented in patients diagnosed as hysteria, but the association is by no means inevitable. Certainly the clinician should not be misled into assuming that a diagnosis of hysteria is appropriate based on personality features alone.

Association with organic disease

Several investigators have reported a high association between hysteria and organic neurological disease. Gowers (1893) noted, 'there is hardly a single disease of the nervous system by which such symptoms [hysteria] may not be evoked in predisposed subjects' (p 988). Tissenbaum et al (1951) reviewed 395 patients with neurological disease and found 13% who were diagnosed as 'functional' for up to 8 years before pathology was recognised. Whitlock (1967) reported that 62.5% of patients with hysterical symptoms had significant coexistant or preceding histories of organic disorder, compared with 5% of a control group. Merskey & Buhrich (1975) reported that organic disease was present in 68% of patients with conversion symptoms, athough this did not differ from a control group. Epilepsy and disorders of higher brain function were particularly involved.

Others have highlighted a relationship with multiple sclerosis. This was implied by Charcot and most clearly stated by Brain (1930) and Langworthy (1948). However, the link was investigated by Pratt (1951) who failed to note any differences between an index and a control group for either hysterical manifestations or premorbid personalities.

The high frequency of later development of organic disease found in a follow-up study by Slater (1965) was the reason for his suggestion that hysteria was 'a myth'. He obtained follow-up information on 85 of 89 patients seen at the National Hospitals and diagnosed as hysteria. Four had committed suicide and 8 had died of natural causes. Of the remaining 73 cases, nearly 60% had either an associated recognisible disease at the time of the diagnosis of hysteria, or developed one during the follow up interval. Of the remaining cases, 31% had developed a recognisable psychiatric disorder. In a further study, Slater (1961) failed to find a genetic or familial bias for the development of conversion phenomena, including data from a study comparing monozygous and dizygous twin pairs. This was evidence for him against the consideration of hysteria as an illness. Slater (1965) was led to the conclusion that 'all the signs of "hysteria" are the signs not of disease but of health . . . one cannot build up a picture of an illness out of elements which are severally the evidence of absence of illness' (p 1396). He went on to state, 'the diagnosis of "hysteria" is a disguise for ignorance and a fertile source of clinical error' (p 1399).

In order to explore the organic factors further and their relationship with personality variables, Merskey & Trimble (1979) clinically assessed the personality style of patients with conversion hysteria of which 40% had a known neurological condition. Obsessional personalities were more likely to have such an association, although the differences were not significant. Their conclusion was that personality variables and underlying neuropathology, in association with situational factors, all played a role in the manifestation of conversion phenomena.

One of the arguments for assuming an underlying neurophysiological abnormality in hysteria relates to the persistent reporting of an over-representation of symptoms on the left side of the body. Briquet (1859) reported that of 400 cases of hysteria, 93 had an anaesthetic area, which was left-sided in 70. In addition, this lateralisation was found for a variety of other symptoms. These observations have been consistently replicated, both with regards to anaesthetic areas (Gowers 1893, Purves Stewart 1920) and other symptoms such as pain (Merskey and Boyd 1978). Stern (1977) reported on the lateralisation of conversion symptoms in 191 patients, taking account of their handedness: 45 had sensory loss and in 37 this was unilateral. Of these, both right- and left-handed patients reported more anaesthesia on the left. Keshaven et al (1979) and Galin et al (1977) reported this association mainly in women, which may explain one of the few contradictory reports, that of Fallik and Sigal (1971), who reported an excess of dominant-sided symptoms, but their sample contained 90% males.

The anaesthesia may affect all modalities, is frequently on the left side, and may be associated with diminished taste, smell and hearing on that side. Further examination may reveal a restricted visual field and the motor reflexes may also be diminished on the side of the anaesthesia.

Several authors have speculated on the mechanism of the unilateral anaesthesias. Galin et al (1977) implicated the special properties of the non-dominant hemisphere in the processing of unconscious information. Flor-Henry (1983) emphasised the link to gender, noting that the pyramidal tracts are asymmetrically distributed, the left being larger than the right with more ipsilateral connections. Thus, a lesion of the left side is more likely to provoke bilateral symptoms, whereas a non-dominant hemisphere lesion will lead only to unilateral symptoms. It is certainly of interest that disorders of body image that occur after a lesion to the non-dominant parietal cortex, such as anosognosia, are unilateral, while those occurring after lesions of the dominant parietal cortex, such as autotopagnosia and finger agnosia, are bilateral in their representation. Further, anosognosia and its milder variant anosodiaphoria, denial of illness and hemiplegia, seen after a non-dominant lesion, have some resemblance to the intense denial so often reported in association with hysteria, referred to as 'la belle indifference'.

Association with psychopathology

In Slater's follow-up study there was a high incidence of suicide. In addition, he reported two cases that developed schizophrenia, and eight with an affective disorder. The association of conversion symptoms and affective illness has been reviewed by others (Klerman 1982) and been the subject of several investigations. Ziegler et al (1960) noted 'depressive features . . . although overshadowed by conversion symptoms, in 40 of 134 patients' (p 904). These were of a higher age and often presented with a pain syndrome. Roy (1980) examined a consecutive series of patients diagnosed as conversion hysteria, and compared them with a control psychiatric population diagnosed as depressive neurosis. They were given various standardised rating scales and their past history reviewed; 88% of the probands were clinically rated as having a depressive syndrome. The mean length of the history of the hysterical symptoms was significantly longer in the non-depressed subgroup, in which males were over-represented.

A more recent extensive investigation, using several standardised rating scales as well as clinical evaluation, has been carried out by Wilson-Barnett and Trimble (1985). Data from 79 patients with conversion symptoms were compared with both a psychiatric and a neurological control group. The former were free of somatic symptoms and the latter had no evidence of psychopathology. Depression, as rated on the Beck Depression Inventory (BDI), differed across the groups. Thus, the psychiatric controls scored highest, then came the conversion patients, followed by the neurological controls with the lowest score of all. In the hysteria patient group, 35% were rated as mildly or moderately depressed and 24% as extremely depressed. In this study, subjects were also given a rating scale which assessed the patients' denial of their life problems. Denial was significantly negatively associated with scores of anxiety and depression. These data imply the existence of a subpopulation in whom denial is high, but expression of affective symptoms is low, one superficial manifestation of what has been termed 'conversion'.

The relationship to psychosis has been less studied. Clinically, it is not uncommon for conversion phenomena to be the initial presenting symptoms in early schizophrenia, or in an evolving dementia, although the quality of the presentation is often different to that of the neurosis. In psychosis the underlying delusional system may be clear and, far from being associated with 'la belle indifference', the associated anxiety may be high. Ziegler et al (1960), in their series of 134 patients, noted an 'underlying or incipient schizophrenic process' in 19, the mean age of this group being significantly lower than for an affective disorder group.

The other main psychopathology noted is anxiety. This is particularly evident in settings of acute stress, notably seen at times of war or following military or civilian disaster. Such presentations have, however, been the subject of very few systematic studies. Wilson-Barnett and Trimble (1985) rated anxiety in their patients with a mood adjective check list and noted high scores in the conversion patients compared with neurological controls.

Briquet's syndrome:

The syndrome of stable hysteria has been defined by Guze and colleagues in the following way (Woodruff et al 1982, p 117):

> Hysteria is a polysymptomatic disorder that begins early in life (usually in the teens, rarely after the 20s), chiefly affects women, and is characterised by recurrent multiple somatic complaints, often described dramatically, characteristic features, all unexplained by other known clinical disorders, of varied pains, anxiety symptoms, gastrointestinal disturbances, urinary symptoms,

menstrual difficulties, sexual and marital maladjustment, nervousness, mood disturbances and conversion symptoms. Repeated visits to physicians and clinics, the use of a large number of medications . . . and frequent hospitalisations and operations result in a florid medical history.

In DSM 111 this is referred to as somatisation disorder, and the diagnostic features are shown in Table 12.2. While many question the validity or the merit of this diagnosis, and certainly using the strict criteria of DSM 111 renders this quite a rare diagnosis, in practice such patients are not hard to discern. It is reported in 1–2% of consecutive female patients attending hospital for investigation and in 10% of psychiatric inpatients. It is a rarity in males, and 1st degree female relatives have a 10-fold increase in the same syndrome. Male relatives show a proponderence of antisocial personalities and alcoholism. Monozygotic twins have a greater concordance rate (29%), compared with dizygous pairs (10%) (Torgersen 1986).

It assumes importance among patients presenting with neurological symptoms, as such problems as fits, faints, convulsions, loss of consciousness, visual symptoms, weakness, headaches, anaesthesias and paralyses are all commonly reported by patients with Briquet's syndrome (Woodruff et al 1982). However, the diagnosis has prognostic validity, and individual symptoms can only be assessed in the full knowledge of the

Table 12.2 Somatisation disorder (American Psychiatric Association 1980)

Diagnostic criteria
A. A history of physical symptoms of several years' duration, beginning before the age of 30

B. Complaints of at least 14 symptoms for women and 12 for men from the 37 symptoms listed below. To count a symptom as present the individual must report that the symptom caused him or her to take medicine (other than aspirin), alter his or her life pattern, or see a physician. The symptoms, in the judgement of the clinician, are not adequately explained by physical disorder or physical injury and are not side effects of medication, drugs or alcohol. The clinician need not be convinced that the symptom was actually present, e.g. that the individual actually vomited throughout her entire pregnancy; report of the symptom by the individual is sufficient
Sickly: believes that he or she has been sickly for a good part of his or her life
Conversion or pseudoneurological symptoms: difficulty swallowing, loss of voice, deafness, double vision, blurred vision, blindness, fainting or loss of consciousness, memory loss, seizures or convulsions, trouble walking, paralysis or muscle weakness, urinary retention or difficulty urinating
Gastrointestinal symptoms: abdominal pain, nausea, vomiting spells (other than during pregnancy), bloating (gassy), intolerance (e.g. gets sick) of a variety of foods, diarrhoea
Female reproductive symptoms: judged by the individual as occuring more frequently or severely than in most women: painful menstruation, menstrual irregularity, excessive bleeding, severe vomiting throughout pregnancy or causing hospitalisation during pregnancy
Psychosexual symptoms: for the major part of the individual's life after opportunity for sexual activity: sexual indifference, lack of pleasure during intercourse, pain during intercourse
Pain: pain in back, joints, extremities, genital area (other than during intercourse); pain on urination; other pain (other than headaches)
Cardiopulmonary symptoms: shortness of breath, palpitations, chest pain, dizziness

overall medical and psychiatric history of patients. In any one patient at a point in time, concentration only on presenting symptoms will lead to errors in diagnosis and a failure to recognise this syndrome.

Abnormal illness behaviour (AIB)

Pilowksy (1975) introduced the concept of AIB based on the ideas of Mechanic (1962). For the latter, illness behaviour refers to 'the ways in which given symptoms may be differentially perceived, evaluated and acted (or not acted) upon by various kinds of persons' (p 189). AIB is therefore defined (Pilowsky 1971, p 136) as:

> . . . the persistence of an inappropriate mode of perceiving, evaluating, acting in relation to one's state of health, despite the fact that a doctor has offered a reasonably lucid explanation of the nature of the illness, and the appropriate course of management to be followed, based on a thorough medical examination.

This broad definition covers a number of other states, such as hypochondriasis, hysteria, malingering and the Münchausen syndrome, in which a disturbance of illness behaviour is a common feature, and places the understanding of these phenomena at the interface of sociology and medicine. Pilowsky noted that these diagnoses are usually made by non-psychiatrists on the basis of a discrepency between detectable somatic pathology and the patient's reaction. In other words, 'the doctor does not believe that the sick role the patient assumes is appropriate to the objective pathology detected' (Pilowsky 1975, p 142). He recognised psychotic and non-psychotic forms, and those where motivation is predominantly either conscious or unconscious. Another dimension relates to illness affirming or illness denying characteristics of the AIB. Anosognosia is a neurological variant of the latter.

To explore further the nature of AIB, Pilowsky devised a questionnaire (the IBQ) which has been given to various populations of patients, but validated mainly on chronic pain patients. On this, seven factors were identified:
1. Generalised hypochondriasis
2. Disease conviction
3. Psychological vs somatic perception of illness
4. Affective inhibition
5. Affective disturbance
6. Denial of life problems
7. Irritability.

In general, AIB patients are more likely to be convinced that they have something seriously the matter with their bodies and would not believe a doctor if he told them that they had nothing wrong. They tend to deny problems in their lives and to express their feelings poorly, especially those of anger. In the only investigation to date of this inventory in a neurological

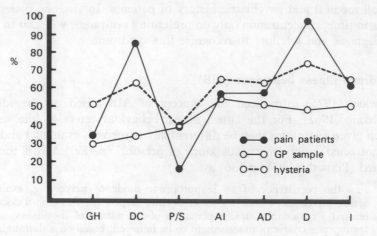

Fig. 12.1 Showing the IBQ profiles of three groups of patients. Pain patients and GP sample are from Pilowsky (IBQ manual, Adelaide) and the hysteria sample from Wilson-Barnett & Trimble (1985). The seven factors are given in text. The hysteria sample is less somatically orientated and shows less disease conviction than the pain sample.

setting, Wilson-Barnett and Trimble (1985) reported on the responses of 79 patients clinically diagnosed as hysteria or conversion, in whom underlying neurological illness had been rigorously excluded. The IBQ profiles of these patients was compared with a non-somatising psychiatric group and non-psychiatrically ill neurological controls. The profile of the index group on the seven factors was interestingly different from the controls and also differed from Pilowsky's pain patients (see Fig. 12.1). Thus, the hysteria group reported significantly more affective inhibition than neurological controls and greater denial than the psychiatric patients. Scores on depression rating scales correlated positively with all of the IBQ items, except denial, which, however, was correlated positively with the extraversion dimension of the Eysenck personality inventory and a somatic perception of disease on the IBQ. In other words, these patients tend to deny their life problems, poorly express affects and have a tendency to minimise the possibility of some psychological problems. In contrast to chronic pain patients, however, the hysteria group report less disease conviction and denial (see Fig. 12.1), suggesting that they may be more amenable to therapeutic intervention. The IBQ has been used in another setting of interest to neurologists and psychiatrists, namely with compensation cases. Clayer et al (1984) asked people to fill out the IBQ as if they were malingering and compared the responses to a chronic pain patient group. From the results they developed a new 21 item scale (The Conscious Symptom Exaggeration Scale) to detect malingering, although this has yet to be validated in alternative settings.

MECHANISMS

A number of authors in recent times have attempted to understand hysteria in a useful clinical and conceptual way. None has returned to the more exacting medical model of the late 19th century and few have supported Slater's contention that the condition does not exist. Straddling the interface between neurology and psychiatry were the ideas of Schilder (1939). His definition of hysteria was of 'psychological processes which lead to symptoms of physical suffering which are not accompanied by severe physiological and organic changes' (p 1391). He emphasized the motoric aspects of emotional life, preceding ideas currently in vogue today, notably those based on the known association between the neuroanatomical representations of both motor and emotional behaviour, the basal ganglia and the limbic system respectively (Nauta & Domesick 1982).

Schilder recognised that hysteria was facilitated by organic disease, although this was usually not severe, and developed the theme of 'organic repression', the idea that there are structural as well as psychological mechanisms of repression. Brain lesions thus do not create new material, but, 'from the moment a brain lesion occurs we live our life at a more primitive level' (Schilder 1951, p 33). One consequence, however, was that in cases of organic, as opposed to psychogenic, repression the motives for the repression remain obscure.

Barham Carter (1972) referred to hysteria as 'a condition in which patients respond to stress by converting their emotional problems into physical disabilities' (p 1241). He then discussed four main forms: simple hysteria, hysteria complicating organic illness (mainly related to over-reaction and worry about their lives or illness), self poisoning and chronic hysteria. In the latter were included writer's cramp and spasmodic torticollis. While seemingly simple, this outline leaves the mechanism of the conversion completely unexplained and fails to differentiate the personality aspects of the problem from hysteria per se.

Merskey (1979), in a series of publications, has given considerable thought to the problem largely based on his experience with neurological patients. He distinguishes seven different uses of the term:

1. Hysteria with one or two symptoms usually motor or dissociative (as in amnesia) and sometimes pain.

2. Polysymptomatic hysteria, especially hypochondriasis and Briquet's syndrome.

3. Hysterical elaboration of organic complaints.

4. Symptoms of self-induced illness or self-damage in abnormal personalities, ranging from anorexia nervosa to hospital addiction.

5. Psychotic or pseudopsychotic disorders (such as Ganser's syndrome and hysterical psychosis).

6. Hysterical personality.

7. Culturally sanctioned endemic or epidemic hysteria.

From the point of view of this review, it is the first three that are most relevant, although, like others, he also defines a separate heading for the hysterical personality. He distinguishes a monosymptomatic condition from the polysymptomatic Briquet's syndrome and includes a category of hysterical elaboration of organic complaints. Although this has a ring of clinical pragmatism, the evidence for such clustering from anything but clinical impression is meagre. With regard to mechanism, Merskey places much emphasis on the symptoms being dependent on an idea, a concept attributed originally to Russell Reynolds (1828–96). The writings of the latter heralded a tradition of looking at the symptoms of hysteria solely as the outcome of psychological processes, culminating with the psychoanalytical views of Freud some 70 years later. Essentially, the reason the symptoms did not correspond to expected patterns of neurological illness was that they represented, not a damaged set of nerves, but an idea. This could be supplied to a patient by suggestion and likewise removed through the influence of hypnotism. Some objections to this theory were well presented by Wilson (1910), noting cases where hysteria developed independently of suggestion, especially acutely after trauma. Further, defining what to be 'suggestible' means, both in neurological and neurophysiological terms, has not been attempted. If it is a general property of the human mind, then it is hardly specific to hysteria; if it is specific, then it must be so for certain individuals and be recognised by defining characteristics. This essential dilemma was well recognised by both Charcot and Janet and is easily obscured by glibly citing suggestion as the simple solution.

A related theme that evolves from this is that hysteria reflects on the relationship between the observer (usually the doctor) and the observed (the patient). Thus, suggestion emanates from the one to the other, especially in the therapeutic arena of hypnotism. The symptoms of hysteria become gestures of communication and for some, such as Szasz (1972), hysteria is the non-discursive language of illness.

An alternative but related way of looking at hysteria incorporated the views of social science and the concept of the sick role with the development of theories of illness behaviour, normal and abnormal. Disease which doctors identify and is grounded in somatic pathology, is contrasted with illness, the symptoms that patients bring to doctors. In medical school we are taught that disease and illness are synonymous, but a brief contact with clinical work reveals the obvious, yet poorly discussed, disparity between them. Abnormal illness behaviour defines one aspect of this difference, filled as it then becomes with medical terms such as hypochondriasis and hysteria. For symptoms to manifest, Taylor (1986) requires the presence of a predicament with blocked solutions, Freud's conflicts with repression. The choice of symptoms relates to symbolism or identification, or merely experience with illness from a personal encounter (Ziegler & Imboden 1962). Kendell (1982), adopting the ideas of Pilowsky and a behavioural model, relates illness behaviour to either fear of disease, or reinforcement provided by the advantages of the sick role. The former relates to hypo-chondriasis, the latter to hysteria. Yet, this is only one step away from acknowledging the potential financial advantages of the sick role for the development of symptoms, and the equating of hysteria with malingering. To rely on some subtle differentiation between conscious and unconscious motives to distinguish the two is a hazardous exercise, the answer to which will be in the eyes of the beholder.

CONCLUSIONS

Hysteria will not go away. In spite of the definitive pronouncements of Slater, the diagnosis is still made regularly, especially at certain specialist centres (Trimble 1981, Marsden 1986). Although it is often stated that hysteria is disappearing in the modern world with increasing sophistication of both patients and medicine, the rate of diagnosis remains fairly constant and the pattern of the symptoms hardly alters in neurological settings. It is diagnosed in some 1% of neurological admissions and must be a tempting diagnosis for a much higher proportion of those 25% of outpatients for whom no diagnosis is possible, excluding those receiving such epithets as tension headache (Perkin 1986). In the series reported by Trimble (1981), the only symptom category to diminish in frequency recently was that of movement disorders, notably in the late 1960s and 1970s, following the discovery of L-dopa and its influence on behaviour. Marsden (1986) forcibly makes the point that patients with now recognised neurological conditions, such as dystonia musculorum deformans, blepharospams and spasmodic torticollis, were at one time and often still are diagnosed as hysteria. Viewed historically, however, hysteria was firmly a neurological, if not gynaecol-ogical condition, with the exception of the last 70 years.

The speculated pathogeneses have varied and to supplant one based on complexes, conflict and repression with one that adopts learning theory, or neurotransmitters, reflects the passage of progress in medical thought. It is not clear, however, how supplanting the theoretical constructs of the id and ego with those of dopamine has influenced the prognosis or treatment of these conditions, or necessarily provided more direct as opposed to circumstantial evidence for their aetiology.

Any theory of hysteria has to embrace multiple potential pathogeneses for the final common outcome and recognise the different settings in which it occurs. Hysteria in the setting of the battle front may be different in many ways from that developing following trauma in a civilian compen-sation setting, which again differs from Briquet's hysteria. Learning theory is not enough, although symbolism, identification and past illness experi-ence may all account for the location and pattern of symptoms in selected patients. Abnormal illness behaviour, often representing a variant of personality disorder with a propensity to seek medical help, is another variant, but the cultural, genetic, familial and ontogenetic factors that feed into the final exotic clinical pattern have been poorly investigated.

Physiological factors cannot be discounted. The persistant observations of anaesthesias in patients are not to be dismissed as suggestion. Although attempts to use electrophysiological techniques, such as evoked potentials, have failed to reveal much about such clinical signs, their persistent recording over several hundred years, and documentation by naive physicians, such as the houseman in his first week of neurology, as well as by the great masters such as Briquet and Charcot, implies their significance. The over-representation of left-sided symptoms is also of significance, suggesting some functional disturbance of the non-dominant hemisphere in patients where this is found. It may be more than coincidence that damage to this hemisphere is linked with indifference, disturbances of arousal and attention, and contralateral syndromes of neglect. The non-dominant hemisphere relates to performance in the non-verbal sphere and is said to be synthetic, using holistic images as opposed to analysing details.

The relationship of hysteria to affective disorder seems well established and has both clinical and theoretical importance. Practically, identifying this leads to potential treatments; thus, careful clinical evaluation, including third-party accounts of any change of the patient's behaviour which may reflect a depressive illness, is mandatory. A low-dose dexamethasone suppression test may provide a useful clue if abnormal. From the theoretical point of view, there is some evidence linking the non-dominant hemisphere to affective syndromes, and the underlying neurotransmitter changes in depressive illness, especially serotonin deficits (Trimble 1987), may provide clues to some aspects of somatisation.*

Hysteria then has been viewed variously as an idea, as a relationship, as a non-entity and as a syndrome with appropriate qualities to rank as a medical diagnosis. For patients who suffer, and for those working in neurological settings, hysteria is a reality. It is for Briquet to have the last word:

> Placed by force of circumstances at the head of a clinical unit which had an established tradition for managing those with hysterical conditions, I felt that I should, to relieve my conscience, devote all my attention to this type of patient, for which I felt but little inclination. Treating these was for me a most unpleasant task, but I resigned myself and set to this work. Before long I had discovered that hysteria had never been studied like other diseases, by observing first and concluding thereafter. It was not theories which were lacking, but facts.

*Interestingly, Briquet made the following observation: 'Pleuralgia is found on the left side 19 times in 20: hyperaesthesias and anaesthesias are 5 times more frequent; convulsions are at least twice as frequent; and paralysis is 3 times more common on the left side. No other affection has this peculiarity . . . to what reason can we attribute this characteristic? It is probable that in the manifestation of the passions, the right side of the brain is more active than the left . . .' (Briquet 1859, p 557; quoted from the translation of Mai & Mersky 1980).

REFERENCES

American Psychiatric Association 1980 DSM 111. APA, Washington
Barham Carter A 1972 A physicians view of hysteria. Lancet ii: 1241–1243
Brain W R 1930 Critical review: disseminated sclerosis. Quarterly Journal of Medicine 23: 343–391
Briquet P 1859 Traite de l'hysterie. Balliere et fils, Paris
Charcot J M 1889 Clinical lectures on diseases of the nervous system, vol 3. New Sydenham Society, London
Chodoff P, Lyons H 1958 Hysteria, the hysterical personality and 'hysterical' conversion. American Journal of Psychiatry 114: 734–740
Clayer J R, Bookless C, Ross M W 1984 Neurosis and conscious symptom exaggeration: its differentiation by the IBQ. Journal of Psychosomatic Research 28: 237–241
Dewhurst K 1980 Willis's Oxford lectures. Sandford, Oxford
Engel G L 1970 Conversion symptoms. In: MacBryde and Blacklow Signs and symptoms, 5th edn. Pitman, London, p 650–668
Fallik A, Sigal M 1971 Hysteria — the choice of symptom site. Psychotherapy and Psychosomatics 19: 310–318
Fenichel O 1946 The psychoanalytic theory of neurosis. Kegan Paul, Trench and Trubner, London
Flor Henry P 1983 Cerebral basis of psychopathology. J Wright, Bristol
Galin D, Diamond R, Braff D 1977 Lateralisation of conversion symptoms: more frequent on the left. American Journal of Psychiatry 134: 578–580
Gowers W R 1893 A manual of diseases of the nervous system, 2nd edn. J & A Churchill, London
Head H 1922 The diagnosis of hysteria. British Medical Journal i: 827–829
Hunter R, Macalpine I 1963 Three hundred years of psychiatry. Oxford University Press, Oxford
Jaspers K 1963 General psychopathology. Trans Hoenig and Hamilton. Manchester University Press, Manchester
Kendell R E 1982 A new look at hysteria. In: Roy A (ed) Hysteria. J Wiley, Chichester, p 27–40
Keshavan M S, Asok D A, Channabasavanna S M 1979 Laterality and hysterical conversion symptoms. Indian Journal of Psychological Medicine 2: 29–33
Klerman G L 1982 Hysteria and depression. In: Roy A (ed) Hysteria. J Wiley, Chichester, p 211–228
Kretschmer E 1926 Hysteria. Trans Boltz O H. Nervous and Mental Disease Publishing Co, New York
Langworthy O R 1948 Relation of personality problems to onset and prognosis of multiple sclerosis. Archives of Neurology and Psychiatry 59: 13–28
Lazare A, Klerman G, Armor D J 1970 Oral, obsessive and hysterical personality patterns. Journal of Psychiatric Research 7: 275–284
Lewis A J 1975 The survival of hysteria. Psychological Medicine 5: 9–12
Ljungberg L 1957 Hysteria; a clinical, prognostic and genetic study. Act Psychiatrica Scandanavica 32: suppl 112
Mai F M, Merskey H 1980 Briquet's teratise on hysteria. Archives of General Psychiatry 37: 1401–1405
Marsden C D 1986 Hysteria: a neurologists view. Psychological Medicine 16: 277–288
Mechanic D 1962 The concept of illness behaviour. Journal of Chronic Disease 15: 189–194
Merskey H 1979 The analysis of hysteria. Balliere Tindall, London
Merskey H 1983 The history of an idea. Canadian Journal of Psychiatry 28: 428–433
Merskey H, Boyd D B 1978 Emotional adjustment of chronic pain. London Psychiatric Hospital Bulletin 1: 111–112
Merskey H, Buhrich N A 1975 Hysteria and organic brain disease. British Journal of Medical Psychology 48: 359–366
Merskey H, Trimble M R 1979 Personality, sexual adjustment and brain lesions in patients with conversion symptoms. American Journal of Psychiatry 136: 179–182
Nauta W J H, Domesick V B 1982 Neural associations of the limbic system. In: Beckman A (ed) Neural basis of behaviour. Spectrum, New York, p 175–206

Perkin G D 1986 Pattern of neurological outpatient practice: implications for undergraduate and postgraduate teaching. Journal of the Royal Society of Medicine 79: 655–657

Pilowsky I 1971 The diagnosis of abnormal illness behaviour. Australian and New Zealand Journal of Psychiatry 5: 136–138

Pilowsky I 1975 Dimensions of abnormal illness behaviour. Australian and New Zealand Journal of Psychiatry 9: 141–147

Pratt R T C 1951 An investigation of the psychiatric aspects of disseminated sclerosis. Journal of Neurology Neurosurgery and Psychiatry 14: 326–225

Purves-Stewart J 1920 The diagnosis of nervous diseases. Butler and Tanner, London

Roy A 1980 Hysteria. Journal of Psychosomatic Research 24: 53–56

Schilder P 1939 The concept of hysteria. American Journal of Psychiatry 98: 1389–1409

Schilder P 1951 Brain and personality. International University Press, New York

Shapiro D 1965 Neurotic Styles. Basic Books, New York

Slater E 1961 Hysteria 311. Journal of Mental Science 107: 359–381

Slater E 1965 The diagnosis of hysteria. British Medical Journal i: 1395–1399

Slaveney P R, Rich G 1980 Variability of mood and the diagnosis of hysterical personality disorder. British Journal of Psychiatry 136: 402–404

Stern D B 1977 Lateral distribution of conversion reactions. Journal of Nervous and Mental Disease 164: 122–128

Symonds C 1970 Address given at the National Hospital, Queen Square, 27th February

Szasz T S 1972 The myth of mental illness. Paladin, London

Taylor D C 1986 Hysteria, play acting and courage. British Journal of Psychiatry 146: 37–41

Tissenbaum M J, Harter H M, Friedman A P 1951 Organic neurological syndromes diagnosed as functional disorders. Journal of the American Medical Association 147: 1519–1521

Torgersen S 1986 Genetics of somatoform disorders. Archives of General Psychiatry 43: 502–505

Trimble M R 1981 Neuropsychiatry. J Wiley, Chichester

Trimble M R 1986 Hysteria, hystero-epilepsy and epilepsy. In: Trimble M R, Reynolds E H (eds) What is epilepsy? Churchill Livingstone, Edinburgh, p 192–205

Trimble M R 1987 Biological psychiatry. J Wiley, Chichester

Veith I 1965 Hysteria: the history of a disease. University of Chicago Press, Chicago

Walshe F M R 1965 Diagnosis of hysteria. British Medical Journal ii: 1451–1454

Whitlock F 1967 The aetiology of hysteria. Acta Psychiatrica Scandanavica 43: 144–162

Whytt R 1765 Observations on the nature, causes and cure of those disorders which are commonly called nervous, hypochondriacal or hysteria. Becket and Du Hondt, Edinburgh

Wilson S A K 1910 Some modern French conceptions of hysteria. Brain 33: 293–338

Wilson-Barnett J, Trimble M R 1985 An investigation of hysteria using the IBQ. British Journal of Psychiatry 146: 601–608

Woodruff R A, Goodwin D W, Guze S B 1982 Hysteria (Briquet's syndrome). In: Roy A (ed) Hysteria. J Wiley, Chichester, p 117–143

World Health Organisation 1980 Mental disorders: glossary and guide to their classification. 9th revision of the ICD. WHO, Geneva

Ziegler F J, Imboden J B 1962 Contemporary conversion reactions. Archives of General Psychiatry 6: 279–287

Ziegler F J, Imboden J, Meyer E 1960 Contemporary conversion reactions: a clinical study. American Journal of Psychiatry 116: 901–909

Anxiety and phobic states*

INTRODUCTION

The growth of scientific interest in the anxiety disorders in recent years has brought to light a large body of factual information about their neurobiological concomitants and generated fresh enquiries into the effects of pharmacological and behavioural treatments. Agoraphobic neurosis and the panic attacks which are often a prominent feature has been the subject of particular interest. Having regard to the clearly defined features and course of this syndrome, it may be regarded as something of a paradigm of neurotic disorders as a whole. The result of the extensive enquiries undertaken into it therefore have wide implications for understanding and further investigation of this whole group of conditions. This chapter will be devoted to a review of some of the new observations and to evaluate the theories of causation that have been derived from them.

RECENT DEVELOPMENTS IN THE NEUROBIOLOGICAL ASPECTS OF AGORAPHOBIC-PANIC DISORDER

As biological enquiries have yielded the most impressive new observations, they will be considered first together with the theories that have emanated from them.

The neurobiological theory of this group of disorders leans on the evidence that agoraphobia is a genetically determined metabolic disorder with a specific and consistent symptomatology and a number of psychological correlates that responds to treatment with biological therapies such as tricyclic antidepressants, monoamine oxidase inhibitors and the triazolobenzodiazepine Alprazolam.

As far as the clinical picture is concerned there is a striking consistency in terms of sex distribution, age of onset, the uniformity of the situations liable to generate avoidance behaviour (distance from home, shops, travel

*Some sections of this paper are revised and updated versions of 'Agoraphobia, panic disorder and generalized anxiety disorder: some implications of recent advances' from *Psychiatric Developments*, Vol 2, No. 1, Spring 1984, and appear with permission of Oxford University Press.

in public transport, attendance in church, theatre or at other public gatherings, waiting in queues or at traffic lights while driving in a car). The factors that serve to mitigate or completely control symptoms (presence of spouse, relative or friend) and the thought content, which is concerned with fears of losing control, making a scene, going berserk, fainting in public, and becoming insane, are also closely similar from case to case.

Many other clinical features are manifest in unvarying form across different social classes, personalities and cultures so as to suggest the presence of some unitary biological disturbance as the underlying explanation for the phenomenon.

This impression is heightened by the presence of a range of perceptual disturbances in the most severe forms of agoraphobic disorder. Examination will bring to light experiences such as depersonalisation, derealisation often heightened by light intensity, visual distortion, deja vu and jamais vu, panoramic memory and the experience of a division of the self into an observing self and an affectless passive observed component of it (Roth 1959, 1960, Uhde et al 1982).

These phenomena are reminiscent of the aura of temporal lobe epilepsy. The perceptual phenomena in this latter condition are more vivid and wide ranging, the march of symptoms is swift, consistent and orderly whereas in agoraphobic states they vary from one attack to the next, chaotic in sequence and sustained over much longer time periods than is the case in temporal lobe epilepsy. Yet the resemblance is close enough to suggest that a similar cerebral functional pathway, possibly in the limbic system, is being affected in different ways by the two phenomena. The studies of Jeffrey Gray (1982) have led him to conclude that underlying all anxiety states there is deranged activity within a specific subsystem in the cerebrum; the structures involved include the septohippocampal system, the entorhinal, cingulate and prefrontal cortex and the ascending noradrenergic and serotonergic pathways arising in the brain stem to project to these regions in the forebrain.

There is a large body of evidence that lesions in the temporal lobe or limbic system are particularly liable to be associated with symptoms of anxiety and attacks of panic. Williams (1956) has described ictal fear as being a more common affective experience and more brief in duration than ictal depression. Ictal fear can occur alone in temporal lobe epilepsy, or be accompanied by terrifying hallucinations, automatisms, or symptoms of autonomic disturbance, sensations such as tachycardia, palpitations, flushing, sweating, itching and vomiting.

Malamud (1967), reporting on 18 patients with temporal lobe tumours that had been surgically removed, found a case with 'disproportionately marked emotional reactions of anxiety with episodes of unmotivated fear'. The tumour occupied the entire hippocampal formation on the right side. In the other cases with a neoplasm in the mesiobasal part of the temporal lobe, anxiety and depression were prominent in the symptomatology.

Ictal anxiety is particularly liable to be misdiagnosed when it is of sudden onset and brief duration. In a proportion of cases of agoraphobia with panic disorder the EEG may be abnormal (Trimble 1981), although the changes are generally non-specific, exhibiting no indubitable epileptic features (Harper & Roth 1962). When a full history and psychiatric examination has been carried out, difficulties in diagnosis are uncommon.

In patients in whom panic attacks, or an agoraphobic syndrome with panic, arise without any antecedent neurotic symptoms or previous history of emotional disorder or situational factors which shed light on the sudden appearance of agoraphobia, full investigations for exclusion of an organic lesion should be undertaken. A problem of particular difficulty for diagnosis is presented by the rare cases with tumours at the tip of the temporal lobe which may develop slowly over a period of years. The main forms of growth are gliomas, meningiomas and oligodendrogliomas. Blustein and Seeman (1986) have drawn attention to the presentation of many of these patients with a long neurotic prodromal stage during which psychopathological symptoms may dominate the picture to the exclusion of physical signs.

Strian & Ploog (1988) have recently described success in detecting these elusive growths with the aid of nuclear magnetic resonance imaging. The syndromes discussed here exemplify a general phenomenon. In the borderlands of all forms of 'functional' psychiatric disorder there is a small marginal group of cases in which cerebral or other organic factors contribute in causation. The clinical features of one of the main 'functional' groups of mental disorders are simulated (Roth 1963). But it is rare for the mimicry to be so close that comprehensive clinical evaluation will fail to raise a suspicion that there may be a concomitant organic lesion. Redmond and his colleagues (Redmond & Huang 1979) have adduced evidence that the nucleus locus coeruleus, which contains the cells of origin of noradrenergic projections to cerebral cortex, limbic system and brain stem, may constitute a central part of the functional anatomical circuit that subserves the biological activities of anxiety, fear and arousal. Activation of this noradrenergic nucleus in monkeys generates fear behaviours that closely resemble those observed on exposure to threat in humans (Redmond, 1979). It is also associated with increased levels of NA and MHPG in the brain, CSF and plasma. Further, plasma MHPG and state anxiety are positively correlated during anxiety-provoking situations in both normal volunteers (Uhde et al 1982) and patients with panic disorder (Ko et al 1983).

Attempts to relate the symptoms of agoraphobic disorder to abnormal functioning of neurotransmitters, however, are approaching an unmanageable complexity. For, in addition to noradrenergic mechanisms, serotonin, benzodiazepine receptors and GABA are all being involved in theories of causation. Both the central and peripheral noradrenergic systems are considered in the light of the evidence to be linked to each other and to the hypothalamo-pituitary-adrenal axis in the genesis of the underlying physiological activities. It is difficult to submit hypotheses of this complexity to experimental investigation.

There is evidence to suggest that the unitary factor underlying the varying neurobiological disturbances may be an hereditary predisposition to panic-agoraphobic disorder. The morbid risk for anxiety neurosis among first relatives appears in a number of studies and has been found to be approximately 15/100 (Noyes et al 1978, Carey & Gottesman 1981). There is also confirmatory evidence for a hereditary contribution in panic disorder from twin concordance studies (Torgersen 1983). However, in the absence of results from adoption studies, there should be caution in drawing conclusions regarding the extent of the role played by heredity in causation.

Kandel's experimental model of anxiety

There is a great deal about agoraphobic disorder that biological theories, in their simplistic forms, cannot explain. But the experiments of Kandel and his colleagues (Kandel & Schwartz 1982) in the marine snail *Aplysia* have led him to formulate a comprehensive theory of anxiety, the implications of which are of considerable interest. He has succeeded in generating a response which he regards as having a kinship with human anxiety. A parallel phenomenon for anticipatory or 'signal' anxiety is to be found, he believes, in the increased aversive behaviour manifest in the form of defensive responses, such as head withdrawal escape locomotion in response to a conditioned stimulus. Chronic anxiety is paralleled by a lasting state of sensitisation to stimuli (Kandel 1983).

The form of anxiety which develops in *Aplysia* following long-term sensitisation and which Kandel regards as possibly homologous with chronic anxiety in man, is associated with amplification of the strength of the connections made by the sensory synapses onto the motor neurons and interneurons within the neural circuits that subserve defensive responses. The expression of such chronic anxiety, which is the most relevant in the present context, is associated with enhancement of transmitter release, promoted by cyclic AMP-dependent phosphorylation of a potassium channel protein. The effect of this is to close the potassium channel and reduce the potassium currents that normally produce repolarisation, thus permitting more calcium to flow into the terminals. In consequence, more vesicles bind to release sites, more transmitter is released and the responsiveness of the animal is enhanced in a manner that characterises sensitisation of chronic anxiety in *Aplysia*.

The acquisition of new learning, as in chronic anxiety, causes morphological as well as functional changes. In particular, the number and distribution of synaptic vesicles and the size and extent of the active zones on them has been found to be increased. Kandel & Schwartz (1982) suggest that underlying chronic anxiety there may be a specific mode of alteration in gene expression, namely, one that induces the gene to provide a new protein kinase which ensures lasting phosphorylation of the potassium channel.

Kandel's hypothesis is speculative and extrapolations from a model in a sea snail to man, though bold, have to be treated with reservation. Its interest resides in the farther experimental enquiries in higher animals, including man they suggest. Its synthesis of behavioural, neurochemical and molecular biological data provides a model which neurobiologists, armed with an adequate body of data, could attempt to replicate in human forms of chronic anxiety with avoidance behaviour.

Biological theories of causation of the agoraphobic-panic group of disorders have to be set in the context of the relevant phenomenological and developmental data to evaluate their validity and promise. These aspects are considered in the two sections that follow.

THE EPIDEMIOLOGY AND PHENOMENOLOGY OF AGORAPHOBIA

In an epidemiological enquiry in Greater Burlington, Vermont, Agras et al (1969) estimated the total prevalence of phobias at 76.9 per 1000 of the normal population, but only 2.2 per 1000 were severely disabled. Hare (1961–63) found that 2–3% of the patients treated by psychiatrists were diagnosed as phobic neuroses and others have arrived at similar figures (Errera & Coleman 1963). Having regard to the tendency of agoraphobic patients to be ashamed of their humiliating dependence and to conceal symptoms over long periods, these figures may underestimate the true prevalence. In more recent enquiries prevalence rates for panic disorders (1 month–1 year) have varied between 0.4 per 100 and 1.2 per 100 and for agoraphobia (6 months–1 year) between 2.5 per 1000 and 5.8 per 100 (Weissmann 1988).

In most cases, a long period of general anxiety over months or years precedes the emergence of specific agoraphobia or panic symptoms. The first experience of panic or situational anxiety may be followed rapidly, and often in stepwise fashion, by a complicated network of avoidance behaviours. There may have been a sudden surge of terror in a crowded store, or a near-syncopal attack in church, in a queue, in the WC of a friend's house. Within a few weeks the patient may have difficulty in leaving her home, being unable to walk further without experiencing imminent panic.

The mean age of onset has varied in different studies between 24 years (Marks & Gelder 1965) and 31–32 years (Shafar 1976 and Buglass et al 1977). There is some evidence that age of onset may be significantly earlier in men, 24–25 years as against 28.5 years (Burns & Thorpe 1977). In the National Survey of 1963 of agoraphobics, 88.16% of the sufferers were female and a similar degree of female preponderance has been reported in most groups of patients investigated in a clinical setting (Roth 1959, Marks & Gelder 1965 and Shafar 1976). In this and in certain other respects, the contemporary agoraphobic neurosis departs in its features from that for which Westphal (1871) coined the term 'agoraphobia'. His paper described three male subjects with fear of certain streets or squares; but it is not streets, squares or empty open spaces that the modern patient fears.

Anxiety and panic are aroused by crowded shops and streets, in queues, public transport and any setting in which large numbers of people gather. There is a special terror in situations that entail minimal physical activity under the scrutiny of strangers. Visits to the hairdresser, the dentist, a cinema, theatre or church, from which quick escape may prove difficult in the event of panic, arouse anticipatory anxiety so severe that they have to be avoided. The most intense anxiety is felt in anticipation of the ordeals to come.

The physical symptoms cover the entire repertoire of those found in ordinary anxiety; weakness of the legs, pounding of the heart, overbreathing, dizziness, perspiration, dry mouth, visual distortion and feelings of impending fainting are prominent. In walking there is a sense of imbalance and the ground feels like 'cottonwool'. Fears of fainting are far more common than frank syncopal attacks, though these occur in rare instances. Feelings of depersonalisation and the experience of a divided self, one part observing the other occur in 30–40% of cases. The fear of lying prostrate and helpless and being the object of curiosity and attention by strangers causes particular embarrassment and distress. Others live in terror of losing their reason or running beserk.

The main situations for which the patient is phobic may be elaborated into a complicated repertoire of avoidance behaviours with consequent limitations of activity that render many patients virtually housebound. The housebound housewife is completely unable to leave her home to go shopping, visit friends or relatives, get to work if she has a job, or to collect her children from school. Relatives, friends and neighbours are enlisted to run errands, shop and fetch children from school. Social engagements are avoided and the patient becomes isolated. A proportion of severely disabled subjects are unable, owing to anxiety and panic, to remain in their own homes alone. The presence of a familiar supportive figure, mother, husband, daughter, will usually alleviate and sometimes completely control anxiety in all situations. A number of devices may serve to keep anxiety in check; wheeling a child in a pram, taking a dog on a lead or wearing dark glasses, may make it possible to venture into the street or into shops. Some patients will have strained their powers of endurance to their limits and beyond in attempts to control irrational fears. Failure causes them remorse, diminished self-esteem, depression and a decline in motivation. The associated depressive syndrome may be much more specific than such depressive colouring and in some cases it is the primary disorder. There is considerable variation in the severity of symptoms in agoraphobia of long standing and, for a few days at a time, patients manage to function normally, though rarely with complete freedom from anxiety.

Continuity and discontinuity in the evolution of agoraphobic disorder

The first attack of severe phobic anxiety or panic often develops abruptly against a background of neurotic symptoms or personality difficulties. It may present as a disproportionately severe response to some adverse life event, or appear at first examination for no apparent cause. Within a few weeks, a woman who may have previously appeared confident, energetic, high spirited and successful may be reduced to a helplessly housebound state. The course of events in the early phase of illness often conveys a strong impression of some stepwise shift in mental life, followed by a qualitative change in patterns of behaviour and adaptation. Even when seen in the early stages of their illness, such patients may prove as resistant to treatment as chronic cases. However, more detailed investigation will usually reveal that the disorder has not emerged out of an entirely clear sky and that the complex repertoire of avoidance behaviours and helpless dependence on others were not entirely without premorbid antecedents. That there is continuity as well as discontinuity in respect of the disabilities presented by agoraphobic patients is illustrated by the following case.

Mrs M. C. was aged 32 when her symptoms began. She had previously been energetic, efficient, conscientious and highly successful as a buyer of women's clothes for a large local store. She had been a reticent woman, but considerate of others, reliable and well-liked by her colleagues and employers. She and her husband had, over a period of eight years, shared an apartment with the patient's mother, a masterful and overbearing woman towards whom the patient's feelings were ambiguously poised. Although her husband had often tried to prevail on the patient to find other accommodation in which they could live with their 8-year-old son, she had been very reluctant to move. Her symptoms began abruptly. Her mother dropped dead from myocardial infarction in the street and the news was first conveyed to the husband at his place of work. He returned home immediately and gently informed his wife that her mother had died an hour previously.

The patient responded with an immediate attack of severe panic, she rushed out of the flat and across the road into her mother-in-law's house suffering from severe anxiety symptoms interspersed with bouts of weeping. The task of removing their possessions from the flat had to be undertaken entirely by the husband. The patient never set foot in her mother's apartment again. She continued to suffer from anxiety and insomnia in the week that followed, but thereafter made an attempt to return to work. She suffered a severe attack of panic while walking to the bus stop and was compelled to return home. At first she would not leave the house even with her husband, but within a month she recovered enough confidence to walk a short distance from her home when accompanied by her husband or a friend.

In the acute stage, feelings of unreality comprising a sense of great distance from the outside world which appeared remote, alien and lifeless, were prominent. They occurred mainly in the form of short episodes but occasionally they would last for hours or an entire day. While walking in the street she experienced giddiness, lightness in the head, unsteadiness in the legs as people or vehicles moved past. There was severe tension and apprehension in shops, streets and vehicles, particularly when they were crowded. She frequently experienced a sense of imminent collapse, feelings of impending death, a dread of drawing attention to herself, losing control, making a scene, going mad or falling unconscious and being observed in a helpless state. Derealisation symptoms faded after a few months but short-lived feelings of moving like a puppet and finding her voice strange and distant returned before and during bouts of acute anxiety for a further period.

Depressive symptoms with loss of pleasure in all things and a decline of self esteem and energy occurred intermittently and were manifest at the time she presented for examination. This woman had been wholly housebound unless accompanied during the eight years before she sought medical advice. In this period she had displayed a wide range of symptoms, but the most constant feature of the illness was the agoraphobic syndrome which showed limited fluctuations in severity.

Comment

Although the symptoms had evolved in this case in an abrupt manner, they ushered in a period of qualitative change in the patient's mode of life. Further investigation showed that neither panics nor phobias had emerged out of an entirely clear sky. She had experienced brief periods of moderate to severe anxiety over four to five years before phobic symptoms began. She also reported mild surges of anxiety when standing in queues or when she was about to set out on shopping expeditions or journeys that took her some distance from home. These she had previously surmounted by an effort of will and they were well camouflaged from her employers to whom she had always seemed confident, masterful and in complete control. In some respects, the patterns of behaviour that entered with the onset of agoraphobia were therefore new. But in other respects they seemed no more than an exaggeration or parody of long-established personality traits accentuated during transient periods to cause more severe bouts of fear previously regarded by the patient as normal for her. That agoraphobic patients differ from patients with other forms of affective disorders and normal controls, in respect of a wide range of features that characterise their pre-morbid state, is suggested by many lines of evidence. The facts suggest that these antecedent characteristics contribute to the aetiological process that culminates in the housebound state. If this conclusion is valid, the agoraphobic stage of the process cannot be regarded as the whole illness. The evidence bearing on these points will be summarised in the following section.

DEVELOPMENT AND PERSONALITY IN AGORAPHOBIC AND PANIC DISORDERS

Developmental history

It is a part of psychoanalytic teaching that starting points of neurotic disorders in adult life should be sought in the emotions and conflicts engendered during the early formative years. Klein (1981) has interpreted his data as consistent with the view that adult agoraphobia represents a recrudescence and intensification of a separation anxiety first manifest in childhood in the form of school phobia and kindred phenomena. In more recent investigations (Gittleman & Klein 1984, 1985) no significant differences were found in respect of a history of childhood separation between 77 adult patients with agoraphobia and 81 simple phobic patients, although agoraphobics had been drawn from more close-knit protective families. Another study has reported a higher incidence of school phobia with the childhood histories of patients with agoraphobia than in those with panic disorders uncomplicated by phobic avoidance (Deltito et al 1986). Harper & Roth (1962) found 60% of their agoraphobic patients to have a history of phobias in childhood, a prevalence significantly in excess of that found in control subjects. However, as Snaith et al (1971) have pointed out, most of these symptoms are in the form of transient fears of specific objects or circumscribed situations, such as the dark, thunder, certain animals, heights, water, which differ from the fears of adult life. They are benign, short-lived and, once having subsided in childhood, do not recur among agoraphobics in adult life.

School phobia bears a little more resemblance to agoraphobia. There is evidence to suggest that this is a benign disorder confined to childhood when it commences below the age of 11. It is only cases which commence late, at the age of 12–13, that develop a chronic disorder which evolves into a severe form of agoraphobia in adult life (Warren 1965, Tyrer & Tyrer 1974). The severely disabling agoraphobias of early onset are relatively rare. They constituted less than 2% of the 135 agoraphobic patients described in an early comparative study (Roth 1959). The outcome of school phobias of the first decade, which constitute the majority of cases, is consistent with the transient nature of the majority of neurotic disturbances in childhood and their low predictive value as far as the development of neurosis in adult life is concerned.

Early family background and child/parent relationship

Having regard to the difficulty of obtaining reliable information in retrospect, it is not surprising that the available evidence on this subject should show some contradictions. A number of investigators have described family ties of agoraphobics as strong and stable (Roth 1959, Marks & Gelder 1965). The unstable family background described by Snaith et al (1971) emerged from a comparison with other phobics: the latter were found to have had the more favourable family environment. In early comparative studies with controls, the agoraphobics were judged to have had a more closely knit and coherent family background. But in a later comparative study (Buglass et al 1977) it was found that step-parents, step-siblings or adopted sibs and other anomalies were commoner in the families of agoraphobics than those of control subjects. Some of these inconsistencies stem from differences in the type of comparison made and in the methods of investigation used. Perhaps the conclusion most consistent with the available evidence is that some agoraphobics may be drawn from markedly well knit and inward looking families, others from divided unstable ones. It is not difficult to see how either type of setting might form the starting point for maladaptive behaviour.

The mothers of agoraphobic patients have been described as overprotective (Solyom et al 1976), but some of the available evidence is in conflict with this claim (Snaith et al 1971). In the national survey sample of agoraphobic subjects (Burns & Thorpe 1977) 36.7% described their mothers as having been overprotective; significantly more female subjects had described their mothers in these terms. Forty-three per cent of the mothers were seen as being overanxious and 11.2% to have been rejecting. About 40% described their fathers as strict and a third as unaffectionate.

Later developmental history

Patients with anxiety neuroses in adult life experience some accentuation of their tendency to respond with anxiety in the later part of the second decade. In a comparative investigation of anxious and depressed patients (Roth et al 1972) anticipatory anxiety prior to examinations, social gatherings and other ordeals were significantly more often reported by the anxious patients. Agoraphobic subjects were most markedly affected. Sixty per cent of these patients reported anxiety to the point of marked discomfort or minor disability at this time. Such symptoms are masked and concealed at this stage, although in retrospect they appear to have been the probable cause of unexpected examination failure in gifted and intelligent young people. In the middle or late 20s increased tension with anticipatory anxiety is common and manifest in overapprehensive preoccupation with everyday difficulties. In a study by Argyle & Roth (1989) of 90 patients with panic disorder, about half the patients with agoraphobic symptoms who comprised 85% of the cases, began in the second decade to suffer from a social phobic neurosis of a severely incapacitatory nature in most cases.

It is of interest that the mean age of onset of agoraphobia is in the late 20s and that the majority of patients who present clinically are married. In an early enquiry, a group of 135 (Roth 1959) agoraphobic patients were compared with a general population of comparable age and sex in respect of the proportion married. It was found that the proportion of female agoraphobic subjects married was significantly greater and the proportion of single patients lower than in the general population of Northumberland of comparable age, a difference that may reflect a more determined quest for security among the patients. The men did not differ significantly from the normal population in respect of frequency of marriage. Agoraphobic neurosis commences in most patients after they have established themselves in an independent home with a husband or consort and the term 'house-bound housewife' has been translated into many languages.

Anxiety, not so much about the bearing of children as the maternal role and the responsibility for rearing them, is common. In a recently studied group of anxious and depressed patients (Gurney et al 1972), 12% of the agoraphobics had developed their symptoms during the first year after childbirth. Agoraphobic patients would appear therefore to suffer from non-specific anxiety symptoms more often than control subjects over a period of years before the onset of their disabling agoraphobic symptoms usually in the mid- or late 20s. The data available about the premorbid personality of agoraphobic patients are consistent with this conclusion. Investigations into the premorbid emotional stability and adaptation of agoraphobic and related subjects with the aid of modern standardised and reliable methods are needed.

The premorbid personality

As school refusal, often regarded as a form of separation anxiety, nearly always subsides without a trace when it commences as it usually does under the age of 11 years, there is no sound evidence for regarding agoraphobic illness as a recrudescence of some similar disorder in childhood. But there are observations that suggest that agoraphobic patients are vulnerable to breakdown on account of specific personality traits before symptoms make their appearance.

'Dependence' is an important variable in that certain features of the agoraphobic syndrome can be regarded as an exaggerated or parodied form of dependence on others. In a comparative study of patients with anxiety neuroses and depressive states, the former proved more hypersensitive to criticism and socially anxious, the agoraphobic patients having been most severely affected in these respects (Roth et al 1972). In a study by Buglass et al (1977), no significant differences were found between agoraphobic and control subjects using an inclusive set of indices. However, 17% of the agoraphobic patients were described as having reported a combination of dependency on others and resentment about it. This describes rather well the ambiguously poised attitude towards parents and others on whom they are dependent to be found in agoraphobic subjects in the course of system-atic clinical evaluation. It is difficult to obtain reliable information since patients employ well developed strategies to conceal dependency on others and feelings of being beholden to them; revelation of these tendencies engenders shame and impairment of self-esteem.

In more recent enquiries Reich et al (1986) noted that the most frequently noted diagnosis among a group of 88 patients with panic disorder was an axis 2 diagnosis (in DSM-III) of dependant personality disorder. Those with phobic avoidance were significantly more often classed as 'dependant' personalities. A later study of 36 recovered patients reported them as showing less emotional stability and greater interpersonal dependence than others. Specially designed measures are required to circumvent the tendency of these patients to camouflage dependent and related personality traits.

Enquiries with the aid of the standardised clinical interview (Roth et al 1972, Gurney et al 1972) showed agoraphobic patients have higher scores on anxiety proneness and neuroticism than patients with non-phobic anxiety and depressive illness. Anxious patients have been found to register significantly higher scores than depressive patients on the Maudsley Personality Inventory both during the presenting illness ($p<0.02$) and at follow up ($p<0.01$). The agoraphobic patients had the highest neuroticism scores. At the follow-up examination, the neuroticism scores of male patients had declined markedly, but no comparable fall in the scores of female agoraphobics was found. The anxious group also had the lowest scores for extraversion and, among women who had recovered from agoraphobic general anxiety states, these scores remained significantly below the norms recorded in the general population. In contrast, the scores of endogenous depressive patients were found to be significantly above normal levels, even after recovery from illness. The higher neuroticism and introversion of patients with agoraphobic states is therefore exaggerated by illness. But the deviations from the norm in respect of scores on these measures are still present in those who have recovered and may reflect inherent personality traits.

THE IMPLICATIONS OF RECENT ADVANCES IN TREATMENT

The behavioural therapies

The behavioural treatments of agoraphobia developed during the past decade constitute a significant advance in the management of this group of conditions. Controlled investigations reported from different parts of the world (Marks 1981a, Matthews et al 1976, Emmelkamp 1982) have established exposure in vivo over an adequate period of time, that is until subjective fear begins to decline, to be the most effective form of behavioural treatment. Practice between treatment sessions and exposure in real life to the situations for which there is a phobic aversion has been shown to make a significant contribution to the success of treatment (McDonald et al 1979). There are a number of self-help manuals which provide detailed instructions regarding the steps to be adopted (Marks 1981b, Matthews et al 1976). A long period of exposure has proved to be superior to a number of separate sessions in which agoraphobics were exposed for the same total length of time (Stern & Marks 1973).

Among the few discrepant bodies of observation, that of Klein et al (1983) is noteworthy. In an enquiry into 218 patients no significant differences were observed between results of behaviour therapy and supportive, dynamically oriented psychotherapy. It was suggested that the increased motivation generated had perhaps led patients in both groups to practice real life exposure to feared situations. But most of the evidence appears to be consistent with the view that the effects of those behavioural therapies that utilise real life exposure are beneficial and specific. A number of follow-up studies have established that the improvements achieved in the course of behavioural treatment can endure over periods as long as 2–7 years (Marks 1971, Munby & Johnson 1980, McPherson et al 1980). Evidence has recently been adduced to suggest that the results of exposure may be enhanced by the addition of cognitive methods which aim to modify attitudes, understanding and beliefs in respect of illness (Cobb 1983).

However, certain gaps in knowledge remain to be filled and therefore certain reservations enter. Little information is provided about the method by which patients are selected for treatment in centres engaged in behavioural therapies. Nor is there information on record regarding the extent to which those submitted to trials for treatment represent the total population of agoraphobic subjects who seek help in psychiatric departments. The improvements registered on existing scales, which grade the severity of phobias fail to provide an adequate picture of the extent to which the lives of some patients remain limited and constrained. Many psychiatric clinics have a substantial burden of agoraphobic patients who remain disabled and require long-term support and supervision. Some have been judged unsuitable for behavioural treatment on account of too extensive a range of phobic symptoms, concomitant personality disorder, insufficient motivation and co-operation or other reasons. A proportion have relapsed after one or more courses of behavioural treatment. More observations are therefore needed to define more precisely the limitations and failures as well as the successes of behavioural treatments.

Pharmacological treatment

There is some evidence from double-blind and placebo-controlled investigations in favour of the efficacy of both tricyclic compounds and monoamine oxidase inhibitors in the treatment of panic disorders. The investigation by Zitrin and his colleagues (1981), comparing the results of imipramine with behaviour therapy, imipramine with supportive psychotherapy, and placebo with behaviour therapy over a 26-week period is well known. Each method that incorporated a tricyclic compound proved significantly superior to methods without an active pharmacological agent. The results were attributed to the beneficial effects of imipramine on spontaneous panic, causing anticipatory anxiety and avoidance behaviour to recede. However, as the effects of tricyclics are judged to be confined to panic anxiety and without direct effect on avoidance behaviour, the failure to demonstrate any advantage of behaviour therapy over supportive psychotherapy is surprising; that exposure is effective in some measure in the treatment of avoidance behaviour is well established.

In one enquiry, phenelzine has proved superior to imipramine (Sheehan et al 1980). But in another investigation imipramine was found ineffective in the treatment of agoraphobia when compared with placebo, where exposure in vivo produced significant improvement (Marks et al 1983). McNair & Kahn (1981) reported that imipramine had brought about a significant reduction in panic attacks. But it had also proved effective in the alleviation of depression and the greatest reductions in agoraphobic symptoms were observed in the most depressed, who were also the most phobic cases. The observations of Zitrin's group are clearly important and call for replication in other centres. Certain problems are in particular need of attention in future investigations. Drop-outs in the main enquiry (Zitrin et al 1981) ranged from 20–26% in the agoraphobic cases and 22% of the patients were in relapse at the end of the year. Follow-ups over longer periods have been few, and, on the whole, suggest that the effects of treatment with tricyclic compounds are not well sustained (Cloninger et al 1981). There is also a need for more information about the disabilities that continue after pharmacological treatment. At the end of the clinical trials, ratings in the published accounts tend to show agoraphobic patients to be substantially above the bottom of the ordinates that represent their scores on severity scales.

Having regard to the conflicting claims made by those who employ behavioural treatments on the one hand and pharmacological therapy on the other, as also the drop-out rate reported in both, and taking account also of the proportion of patients that relapse, the possibility arises that the successes reported by these rival groups of therapists may be related to different populations of agoraphobic patients. These issues can be settled only by a fresh generation of controlled trials in which patients are selected by strict criteria to take account of such controversial points as the degree of depressive colouring, the definition of panic and the severity of phobic disability, and are allocated at random to groups in which (1) behavioural therapy, (2) pharmacological treatment, (3) a combination of both forms of therapy would be administered. Moreover, although psychotherapy used as a sole form of treatment has for the present proved to be inferior to other methods of treatment, trials are also needed to ascertain whether employed as an adjunct to other therapies, it improves the results, or makes no significant addition to what is achieved.

CURRENT THEORIES REGARDING THE AETIOLOGICAL BASIS OF AGORAPHOBIC AND RELATED NEUROSES

Many of the controversial issues regarding the classification of treatment of agoraphobia stem from difference in theory regarding the nature and origin of this disorder.

Psychoanalytic and related theories

Psychoanalytic theories trace the symptoms to the conflicts engendered in early childhood which give rise to a defective character structure. As the conflicts remain unresolved they are repressed along with the anxiety they engender into the unconscious. The anxiety is displaced on to situations that symbolically represent the real sources of fear and avoidance. The patient deals with his unresolved problems vicariously by escaping from the symbols that represent them while the real origins of his difficulties, which are sexual and aggressive drives that cannot be given direct expression, remain unaffected. It is inherent in the psychoanalytic view that the repression, displacement and regression to an earlier stage of development should be manifest not only in neurotic symptoms and behaviour but in sexual, marital, interpersonal relationships and in social adaptation.

Klein (1981) and Gittleman & Klein (1985) have adduced evidence that separation anxiety in the form of school avoidance and phobia is a common childhood antecedent of the panic-agoraphobic group of disorders. Psychoanalysts construe this finding as evidence that the agoraphobic syndrome represents a recrudescence of anxieties experienced in early life in the context of a complex — laden parent/child relationship. The evidence about separation anxiety is inconsistent and uncertain. In some enquiries it has been found only in the agoraphobic group of patients and not in those with panic disorder (Deltito et al 1986). The specificity of the connection between childhood separation, anxiety and agoraphobia is difficult to reconcile with the recent finding of some association with simple phobia (Gittleman & Klein 1984, 1985). Behavioural and cognitive treatments do not promote cures for agoraphobic disorders, but their value in management is supported by strong evidence (Marks 1981, Cobb 1983). Comparable testimony in favour of psychoanalytic methods of treatment in this group is lacking. Moreover, psychoanalytic theories view agoraphobia as evolving in a continuous linear fashion from the early formative years into adulthood. But the development of agoraphobia is explosive rather than continuous. There are step-like shifts in psychic functioning before symptoms make their appearance, and some of the changes in mental life, behaviour and adaptation are qualitative in character. Psychodynamic theories rooted in infantile conflicts cannot explain such discontinuities and the chronic neurotic disorders that so often follow.

Learning theories

A second group of theories postulates Pavlovian conditioning, learning and cognitive distortion of perception or varying combinations of these psychological processes in the genesis of phobic avoidance. In theories that have their starting point in Pavalovian conditioning, the chance association of certain environmental situations with an attack of anxiety is held to create classically conditioned fear responses so that previously neutral environments are converted into conditional stimuli which generate escape behaviour. As successful escape reduces anxiety, avoidance behaviour is reinforced and becomes resistant to extinction. Another version views the panic attack as a powerful conditioning stimulus. Patients seek to escape, not from certain conditioned environmental stimuli, but from settings in which they have learned that they are at high risk of developing panic.

Conditioning and learning theories have difficulty in accounting for the absence in a high proportion of cases of any fearful event or circumstance that could have served as the conditioned stimulus. The setting in which the first panic or phobic experience occurs bears no resemblance to the situations that subsequently evoke avoidance. There is also a remarkable measure of consistency among agoraphobic patients in respect of the types of situation that generate phobic conduct; more individual variation would have been predicted from learning theories.

The persistence of anxiety and signs of autonomic arousal, including physiological concomitants of panic in patients who successfully overcome phobias by means of real life exposure, is also difficult to reconcile with conditioning and learning concepts alone.

In recent years cognitive therapies have been introduced which seek to modify the symptoms of agoraphobics by direct approach to their inner thoughts and attitudes and beliefs about the disorder. There is some evidence (Emmelkamp & Mersch 1982) that this helps to sustain the improvements achieved with the aid of behavioural techniques using in vivo exposure.

Theories of causation of a disorder such as agoraphobia (or indeed of any psychiatric or somatic illness) cannot be validly deduced from results of the effects of specific forms of treatment. And those who interpret the results of behavioural and cognitive theories as justifying the view that the symptoms are the disease overlook the constrained and disabled lives of many of the patients who have derived some measure of symptomatic relief from such treatment.

Neurobiological theories

A third type of theory regards panic disorder and its sequel in agoraphobia as a genetically determined medical condition expressed as an endogenous biochemical disorder of the central nervous system. The successes achieved with the aid of drugs in the treatment of panic disorder and subsequently of agoraphobia are cited as validating evidence for this hypothesis (Sheehan & Sheehan 1982, Sheehan et al 1980). And pure panic disorder which does not advance to agoraphobic or other neurotic illness is a well-established phenomenon.

The fact that tricyclic compounds were found by Klein to be specifically effective against panic attacks was judged by him to signify that these and the phobic disorder which followed were mediated by specific cerebral mechanisms, the clearer definition of which might promote major advances in the understanding of the origins of panic-agoraphobic disorders. However, the specificity of imipramine is called in question by the efficacy of some benzodiazepines such as alprazolam. And imipramine seems also to be an effective therapeutic agent in general anxiety disorder. Finally, phobic symptoms do not go into abeyance when panic attacks are brought under control.

Klein (1981) and Klein & Klein (1988) are leading exponents of the theory that it is the 'spontaneous' panic attack that emerged out of a clear sky in the absence of all stressful antecedents that is the specific aetiological starting point from which all features of the agoraphobic syndrome evolve as a secondary development. Moreover, when panic attacks are controlled by treatment with imipramine the agoraphobic symptoms recede.

The theory is attractive for a number of reasons. The attacks are similar to the apparently spontaneous episodes in the form of 'ictal anxiety', that arise in epileptic disorder due to a temporal lobe lesion. Klein advances a clear and testable hypothesis that can be investigated with the tools of modern neurobiology and has some heuristic value.

But the evidence held to favour this theory can be called into question at several points. Closer examination of ostensibly spontaneous panic attacks and the psychological and physiological settings in which they arise sheds light on the primary causes of the panic in a high proportion of cases (Barlow et al 1985). Panic attacks of all kinds also occur in association with social phobia, obsessive compulsive disorder and major depressive episodes, among other emotional disorders. It is implausible that panic can be the primary cause of all these conditions, or that it is the starting point for agoraphobia but without causal relationship to the other conditions mentioned.

CONCLUDING REMARKS

There is, for the present, no plausible synthesis that will accommodate all three of the aetiological theories for the agoraphobic and panic group of disorders which have been summarised here. Each accounts for a certain body of observations on theories, but fails to explain their findings. There is insufficient knowledge to enable us to detect connecting links between the three main types of causal explanation. The phenomenal and behavioural treatments are far from providing cures for these disorders, but their efficacy in alleviating distress has been established by systematic enquiries. Psychiatrists who are increasingly utilising such treatments must, however, bear in mind the contribution made by experience during development and by the personality profile of the individual. For these rarely fail to impart some understanding and insight into the reasons for the development of anxiety neurosis in individual patients. The neurobiological investigator is compelled to concentrate his efforts on some limited aspects of the problem if he is to make any progress. But he will be wise to avoid the simplistic reductionism which may cause him to ignore dimensions beyond the compass of his narrow interests. Tunnel vision will be liable to lead him into error in pursuit of his own enquiries.

Neurobiological research is the most active and promising growing point within the range of enquiries into agoraphobia and other anxiety disorders at the present time. Progress may enable this line of enquiry to provide a more precise and detailed account of the cerebral functional mechanisms underlying this group of disorders and to pave the way for methods of treatment of unprecedented effectiveness, even though such achievements may appear out of reach in the foreseeable future. Should they materialise, our concepts, not only about neurotic disorder but the intention and motivation in normal human beings, may require radical revision.

REFERENCES

Agras S, Sylvester D, Oliveau D 1969 The epidemiology of common fears and phobias. Comprehensive Psychiatry 10: 151–156

Argyle N, Roth M 1989 A phenomenological study of 90 patients with panic disorder and its relationship with other anxiety and affective disorders. In press

Barlow D H, Vermulyea J A, Blanchard E B, Vermulyea B R, De Nardo P A, Carney J A 1985 The phenomenon of panic. Journal of Abnormal Psychology 94: 320–328

Blustein J, Seeman M V 1986 Brain tumors presenting as functional psychiatric disturbances. Canadian Psychiatric Association Journal 17: 59–65

Buglass D, Clarke J, Henderson A S, Kreitman N, Presley A S 1977 A study of agoraphobic housewives. Psychological Medicine 7: 73–86

Burns L E, Thorpe G L 1977 The epidemiology of fears and phobias (with particular reference to the National Survey of Agoraphobics). Journal of International Medical Research 5: Suppl 5, 1–7

Carey G, Gottesman I I 1981 Twin and family studies of anxiety, phobic and obsessive disorders. In: Klein D K, Rabkin J (eds) Anxiety: new research and changing concepts. Raven Press, New York

Cloninger C R, Martin R L, Clayton P, Guze S B 1981 A blind follow-up and family study of anxiety neurosis: Preliminary analysis of the St Louis 500. In: Klein D F, Rabkin J G (eds). Anxiety, new research and changing concepts. Raven Press, New York, p 137–154

Cobb J 1983 Behaviour therapy in phobic and obsessional disorders. Psychiatric Developments 1: 351–365

Deltito J A, Perugi G, Maremmani I, Miagnani V, Cassano G B 1986 The importance of separation anxiety in the differentiation of panic disorder from agoraphobia. Psychiatric Developments 3: 227–236

Diagnostic and Statistical Manual of Mental Disorders (DSM-III-R). 1980. American Psychiatric Association, Washington DC

Emmelkamp P M G 1982 Phobic and obsessive compulsive disorders, theory, research and practice. Plenum Press, New York

Emmelkamp P M G, Mersch P 1982 Cognition and exposure in vivo in the treatment of agoraphobia. Short-term and delayed effects. Cognitive Therapy and Research 6: 77–88

Errera P, Coleman J V 1963 A long-term follow-up of neurotic phobic patients in psychiatric care. Journal of Nervous and Mental Disease 136: 267–271

Gittleman R, Klein D F 1984 Relationship between separation anxiety and panic and agoraphobia disorders. Psychopathology 17: (suppl 1) 56

Gittleman R, Klein D F 1985 Childhood separation anxiety and adult agoraphobia. In: Tuma A Y, Maser J D (eds) Anxiety and the anxiety disorder. Erlbaum, Hillsdale N J, p 389

Gray J A 1972 The neuropsychology of anxiety: an enquiry into the functions of the septo-hippocampal system. Oxford University Press, Oxford

Gurney C, Roth M, Garside R F, Kerr T A, Schapira K 1972 Studies in the classification of affective disorders. The relationship between anxiety states and depressive illness II. British Journal of Psychiatry 121: 162–166

Hare E G 1961–63 Triennial statistical report. Bethlem Royal and Maudsley Hospital, London

Harper M, Roth M 1962 Temporal lobe epilepsy and the phobic anxiety depersonalisation syndrome. Comprehensive Psychiatry 3: 129–151

Kandel E R 1983 From metapsychology to molecular biology: exploration into the nature of anxiety. American Journal of Psychiatry 140: 1277–1293

Kandel E R, Schwartz J H 1982 Molecular biology of an elementary form of learning: modulation of transmitter release by cyclic AMP. Science 218: 433–443

Klein D F 1981 Anxiety reconceptualised. In: Klein D F, Rabkin J G (eds) Anxiety, new research and changing concepts. Raven Press, New York, p 235–262

Klein D F, Klein H M 1988 The nosology of anxiety disorders: a critical review of hypothesis testing about spontaneous panic (in press)

Klein D R, Zitrin C M, Woerner M G, Ross D C 1983 Treatment of phobias II Behaviour therapy and supportive psychotherapy: are there any specific ingredients? Archives of General Psychiatry 40: 139–145

Ko G N, Elsworth J D, Roth R H et al 1983 Panic-induced elevation of plasma MHPG levels in phobic-anxious patients. Archives of General Psychiatry 40: 425–430

McDonald R, Sartory G, Grey S J, Cobb J, Stern R, Marks I 1979 The effects of self exposure instructions on agoraphobic out-patients. Behaviour Research and Therapy 17: 83–85

McNair D M, Kahn R J 1981 Imipramine compared with a benzodiazepine in agoraphobia. In: Klein D F, Rabkin J G (eds) Anxiety, new research and changing concepts. Academic Press, New York, p 69–80

McPherson F M, Brougham L, McLaren S 1980 Maintenance of improvement in agoraphobic patients treated by behavioural methods — a four-year follow-up. Behaviour research and Therapy 18: 50–152

Malamud N 1967 Psychiatric disorders with intracranial tumors of the limbic system. Archives of Neurology 17: 113–118

Marks I M 1971 Phobic disorders four years after treatment: a prospective follow-up British Journal of Psychiatry 118: 683–688

Marks I M 1981a Behavioural treatment plus drugs in anxiety syndromes. In: Klein D F, Rabkin J G (eds) Anxiety, new research and changing concepts. Raven Press, New York, p 265–289

Marks I M 1981b Care and cure of neurosis. New York, Wiley

Marks I M, Gelder M G 1965 A controlled retrospective study of behaviour in agoraphobic patients. British Journal of Psychiatry 111: 561–573

Marks I M, Gray S, Cohen D, Hill R, Mawson D, Ramm E, Stern R S 1983 Imipramine and brief therapist aided exposure in agoraphobic having self-exposure homework. Archives of General Psychiatry 40: 153–162

Matthews A M, Johnston D W, Lancashire M, Munby M, Shaw P M, Gelder M G 1976 Imaginal flooding and exposure to real phobic situations: treatment outcome with agoraphobic patients. British Journal of Psychiatry 129: 362–371

Munby M, Johnson D W 1980 Agoraphobia: the long-term follow-up of behavioural treatment. British Journal of Psychiatry 137: 418–427

Noyes R Jr, Clancy J, Crowe R R, Slymen D J, Ghoneim M M, Hinrichs J F 1978 The familial prevalence of anxiety neurosis. Archives of General Psychiatry 35: 1056–1059 35: 1056–1059

Redmond D E 1979 New and old evidence for the involvement of a brain norepinephrine system in anxiety. In: Fann W E, Karacan I (eds) Phenomenology and treatment of anxiety. Spectrum Publications, New York, p 153–203

Redmond D E Jr, Huang Y E 1979 New evidence for a locus coeruleus-norepinephrine connection with anxiety. Life Science 25: 2149–2162

Reich G, Noyes R G, Troughton E 1986 Dependent personality disorder associated with phobic avoidance in patients with anxiety disorder. American Journal of Psychiatry 144: 323–326

Roth M 1959 The phobic anxiety depersonalisation syndrome. Proceedings of the Royal Society of Medicine 52: 587–595

Roth M 1960 The phobic anxiety-depersonalization syndrome and some general aetiological problems in psychiatry. Journal of Neuropsychiatry 1: 293–306

Roth M 1963 Neurosis, psychosis and the concept of disease in psychiatry. (Celebration volume for Torsten Sjogren, C H Alstom & E Stromgren. Munksgaard), Copenhagen. Acta Psychiatria Scandinavica 39: 128–145

Roth M 1984 Agoraphobia, panic disorder and generalized anxiety disorder: Some implications of recent advances. Psychiatric Developments 2: 31–52

Roth M, Gurney C, Garside R F, Kerr T A 1972 Studies in the classification of affective disorders. The relationship between anxiety states and depressive illness I. British Journal of Psychiatry 121: 147–162

Shafar S 1976 Aspects of phobic illness — a study of 90 personal cases. British Journal of Medical Psychology 49: 211–236

Sheehan D V, Sheehan K H 1982 The classification of anxiety and hysterical states. Part I. A historical review and empirical delineation. Journal of Clinical Psychopharmacology 2: 235–243

Sheehan D V, Sheehan K H 1982 The classification of anxiety and hysterical states. Part II. Toward a more heuristic classification. Journal of Clinical Psychopharmacology 2: 386–393

Sheehan D V, Ballenger J, Jacobsen G 1980 Treatment of endogenous anxiety with phobic, hysterical and hypochondriacal symptoms. Archives of General Psychiatry 57: 51–69

Snaith R P, Ahmed S N, Mehta S, Hamilton M 1971 A clinical investigation of phobias. Psychological Medicine 1: 143–149

Solyom L, Silversfeld M, Solyom C 1976 Maternal overprotection in the aetiology of agoraphobia. Canadian Psychological Association Journal 21: 109–113

Stern R, Marks I M 1973 Brief and prolonged flooding: a comparison in agoraphobic patients. Archives of General Psychiatry 28: 170–176

Strian H, Ploog D 1988 Anxiety related to central nervous system dysfunction. In: Handbook of anxiety, vol II, ch. 19. Elsevier Science Publishers, Amsterdam, in press

Torgersen S 1983 Genetics of neuroses: The effects of sampling variation upon the twin concordance ratio. British Journal of Psychiatry 142: 126–132

Trimble M R 1981 Neuropsychiatry. John Wiley, Chichester

Tyrer P, Tyrer S 1974 School refusal, truancy and adult neurotic illness. Psychological Medicine 4: 416–421

Uhde T A, Siever L J, Post R M, Jimerson D C, Boulenger J P, Buchsbaum M S 1982 The relationship of plasma-free MHPG to anxiety and psychophysical pain in normal volunteers. Psychopharmacology Bulletin 18: 129–132

Warren W 1965 A study of adolescent psychiatric in-patients and the outcome six or more years later II: Follow-up study. Journal of Child Psychology and Psychiatry 6: 141–160

Weismann M M 1988 Anxiety disorders and epidemiologic perspective. In: Handbook of anxiety, vol 1. Elsevier Science Publishers, Amsterdam, in press

Westphal C 1871 Die agoraphobie; eine neuropathische erscheinung. Archiv für Psychiatrie u. Nervenkranheiten 3: 138–161

Williams D 1956 The structure of emotions reflected in epileptic experiences. Brain 79: 29–67

Zitrin C M, Klein D F, Woerner M G 1980 Treatment of agoraphobia with group exposure in vivo and imipramine. Archives of General Psychiatry 37: 63–72

Zitrin C M, Woerner M G, Klein D F 1981 Differentiation of panic anxiety from anticipatory anxiety and avoidance behaviour. In: Klein D F, Rabkin J G (eds) anxiety, new research and changing concepts. Raven Press, New York, p 27–42

A psychobiological view of depression

Based on the seventh Shorvon Memorial lecture delivered at The National
Hospital, Queen's Square, London WC1 on Thursday 24 January 1985 and
published in a slightly modified form in the *Postgraduate Medical Journal*
1986, 62: 179–185.

INTRODUCTION

The melancholy mind has been recognised throughout recorded history. It
was given a medical context by the ancient Greeks who claimed for it a
relationship with constitution in the form of physique, body chemistry and
temperament. It was subject to scholarly analysis by Burton (1927) over 300
years ago and within, and perhaps despite, the potentially smothering
context wherein the puritanical and dualistic thinking of the time perceived
the mind as corruptible by the evil body. The disorder has not always been
medicalised and some cultures have tended instead to recognise it as a
proper and sometimes creative state of mind. It was through the English
translation of Kraepelin's writings (1921) that the word 'depression' entered
the main present day medical arena. Subsequently Meyer (1934) emphasised the notion that depression was a psychobiological reaction to adverse
events. This view has found more recent expression in the writings of
Schmale and Engel (1975) in particular.

In this country the debate concerning the nature and subclassification of
depressive illnesses has become a major preoccupation of psychiatry. The
long-standing concept of 'endogenous depression' is handicapped by
implying aetiological understanding to what is essentially a phenomenological approach. Protagonists of the various views have sometimes seemingly
forgotten that in an analysis of such data you only get out what you have
put in in terms of patient subgroups and symptoms. For instance, the large
group of depressed people lurking in medical wards and outpatient clinics
has seldom been incorporated into studies of other patients attending
hospitals and labelled with the diagnosis (Crisp 1976, 1983). Nor has the
rich range of feeling states and their disturbances been incorporated into
the symptomatology. These have usually been excluded in favour of appar-

ently hard data such as the presence or otherwise of psychotic phenomena, appetite and weight and sleep changes, all of which can in fact be difficult and elusive features in terms of meaning and measurement. To tap this wide spectrum of potentially relevant feeling states and moods one only has to read Burton or *Roget's Thesaurus* (1953). Roget would surely be of great help to us today in our attempts to understand the disorder. He was a physician and an engineer. He was fascinated, in his search for meaning, by the crevices of language and, at the same time, capable of inventing a system of sand filtration for London's water supply which is still operative. Recently, Paykel (1983) has expressed a measured view about our present state of knowledge in respect of phenomenology and classification. Not much more can be said than that a previous history of a manic episode is probably important prognostically; the presence of anxiety is more common in moderate depressive illness, whilst agitation is more common in severe depression. Furthermore, these categorisations may have therapeutic relevance. Meanwhile, there is now a new, elaborate classification DSM III (APA 1980), based strictly on observation and description.

Why has the word 'depression' prevailed for so long? As a word borrowed from physics it seems liable to obscure rather than clarify the nature of the states of mind in question, perhaps bringing to them a spurious sense of understanding in physical terms. In medicine in connection with brain function, we already talk about 'depression of consciousness' and 'CNS depressant drugs' and so it could be muddling also to apply the word to disordered mood. If, however, one turns to the Concise Oxford Dictionary then the definitions there seem possibly to be of some relevance. Depression is a *lowering* or a *sinking*, a *reduction in vigour, especially of trade*, the *centre of minimum atmospheric pressure* and so on, whilst to depress means *to lower*, *to reduce the activity of* or *to push down* or *to pull down*. These last two alternative ways of looking at the concept are perhaps amongst the most arresting, although some of the other definitions invite psychological parallels. Could the word, for instance, all these years have embodied this compelling and pervasive idea that, in a mentally depressing process, both *push* and *pull* can be involved? Could the push derive from *avoidance* of painful experience and the pull from the potential *rewards of helplessness* and fulfilled dependency needs? Could the depressed state, or for that matter the long ignored concept of *inertia* described by Freud and amplified by Schur (1970), comprise either one such process or both processes facilitating each other?

Furthermore, if the variety of distorted moods such as anger, envy, discontent, hatred, sadness, despair, hopelessness, anxiety, that Burton describes and which Engel (1962) attempted to identify as discrete psychobiological entities, are considered as part of and operating within depressed states, then one has a recipe for great complexity and variation within these syndromes. This would be so without taking into account their further distortion when displayed, described or expressed within the doctor/patient relationship and the context of individual personality. Some of these psychobiologically rooted mood states will contain important elements that are incompatible with each other, for instance when anxiety and anger coexist. Some will contribute predominantly to vectors which are part of the depressing mechanism whether of the push or pull kind. Others will reinforce vectors generating engagement with the outside world and associated affective reactivity.

SLEEP PATTERNS AND DEPRESSION

The model which I wish to endorse posits man as a prospecting, problem-solving organism with long-established biological goals and more recently acquired complex social needs and goals, some of an existential kind. First, let us look at early morning wakening which has for long been regarded as an important marker for severe depressive illness. Early morning wakening within severe depression is a salient complaint, often a bitter one. Many authorities regard it as a biological marker for depression, along with diurnal variation of mood, retardation and/or agitation; these latter disturbances being greatest in the morning. In this sense the phenomenon has often been contrasted with sleeping difficulties in the first half of the night, which tend to be more common in anxious subjects and which are often regarded as more likely to characterise mild depression and neurotic disorder. Certainly, it is easier for most of us readily to identify with initial insomnia and to consider it plausibly related to such feeling states as I have mentioned. But can waking early also be related to either normal mental states or else mental states not qualitatively different from the normal? As we get older, we waken earlier (Tune, 1968). Energetic, able and well organised people sleep less and waken earlier than their counterparts (Hartmann et al 1972) and perhaps we are all capable of this when at our most effective. Some people claim to be able to waken early if needs be, as if some internal alarm clock has been set the evening before. If our mind is active when we go to bed we may not only find it remaining so for the first hour or two thereafter, but we may waken with the same thoughts during the night and perhaps also awaken earlier the next day with the same association. Business has never really ceased. Perhaps such mechanisms also operate within psychiatric illness including severe depression.

Sleep studies

My own line of enquiry into early morning wakening initially appeared remote from depressive illness since it was concerned with anorexia nervosa. Such people, who are usually young and hence come from a population which sleeps well on the whole, often waken early in the morning but deny it (Crisp 1967).

The patient in Figure 14.1 with severe anorexia nervosa has much reduced 'polygraphic' sleep. She wakens finally just before 5 a.m. after

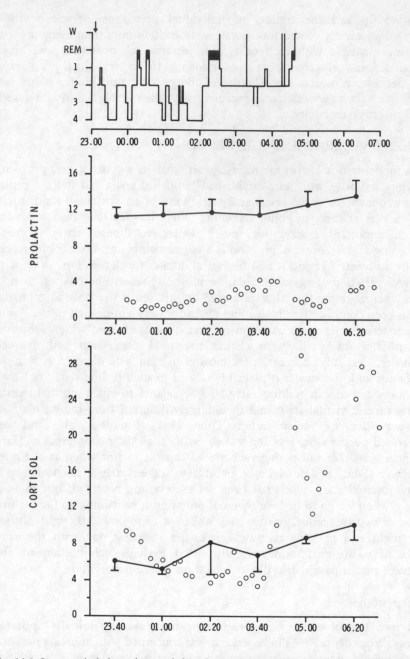

Fig. 14.1 Some typical sleep characteristics of anorexia nervosa in an 18-year-old female weighing 32.8 kg, height 1.58 metres. Light restless sleep with early final waking is evident in the EEG. This feature coincides with, and to some extent is even just preceded by, the beginnings of a massive increase of plasma cortisol levels (°), way above peak normal levels (●———● mean and standard deviation of plasma cortisol levels in 10 normal young adult females).

under six hours of total sleep, much of it light. Prior to wakening a major surge in her plasma cortisol level begins as part of the intense arousal about to overtake her. It was evident that the clinical features associated with such sleep patterns were nutritional rather than affective in kind. The more underweight and starved the individual the greater the sleep disturbance irrespective of mood. Perhaps we were witnessing the break up of the contrived eight hour or so long package of sleep induced in us in early life in temperate climates by our parents, themselves seeking uninterrupted sleep, and despite our own relatively unrequited hunger at the time. Most of us learn to do without this meal during the night even though, presumably, this step may distort our feeding patterns during the rest of the day. However, without nourishment to the extent found in anorexia nervosa there is little point in lengthy sleep. Some initial corrective to falling body temperature, such as bed warmth and perhaps also sleep itself under these circumstances, may be necessary; but thereafter it is more important, biologically, to waken, rise and forage. This erosion of sleep is only one aspect of the arousal experienced by the anorectic, the other being the high level of activity characteristically sustained during the day. Such intense arousal, eroding sleep and heightening restlessness during wakefulness, together with the associated plasma cortisol changes (presumably escaping dexamethasone suppression because of their high surge) it was thought might have implications for other conditions (vide infra).

Our next series of experiments also involved studies of sleep and mood in anorectics as they gained weight to normal levels and obese subjects as they lost substantial amounts of weight. In the former group normal sleep was reconstituted, whilst in the latter group it became eroded. These changes arose unrelated to changes in mood and appeared to be dependent upon weight change. It seemed possibly also to be a matter of available calories. Concurrently we (Crisp & Stonehill, 1973, 1976) tested the hypothesis that sleep disturbances in a variety of psychiatric disorders would be found to be related to weight changes, irrespective of diagnosis. Thus weight loss would be associated with reduced total sleep time, increased interruption of sleep and earlier wakening, whilst weight gain would be associated with the converse. We were aware, of course that such weight changes not infrequently occur in psychiatric illness, especially, it is said, depressive illness. Under these circumstances doctors duly note the weight change, perhaps most often weight loss, as indicative of the severity of the depressive disorder confronting them, but we do not often seem to stop and think of its biological consequences.

Most of us have great difficulty in losing weight. For the most part we maintain a steady state and this self regulation of shape and weight seems to be governed by both biological and social factors. Social and psychological factors include the reactions of those around us, our appearance in the mirror, the tightness of our clothes and how we feel about our bodies and about being in them. Biological factors are ill understood. They may include a central mechanism governing calorie intake. For instance, our own group (Phillips et al 1975) has shown that high carbohydrate intake one day is associated with increased REM sleep during the subsequent night whilst Siegel (1975) has shown that amount of REM sleep in small mammals is inversely related to the next day's carbohydrate intake. Any such regulatory mechanism, discernible within the architecture of sleep, could supposedly operate either directly through, say, blood glucose levels or perhaps indirectly through plasma free and bound tryptophan levels or tryptophan/tyrosine ratios, according to the Wurtmann and Fernstrom (1975) hypothesis. Tryptophan is a precursor of 5HT, which itself is thought possibly to mediate REM sleep (see Crisp 1980). We should remember that the brain probably processes all kinds of information and perhaps can get overloaded with nutritional information just as much as with 'social' information and perhaps can even get 'depressed' (the inertia of satiation) as one stance open to it in relation to its regulation of food intake. It seems likely then that the architecture of sleep, and perhaps also its experience, is sensitive to aspects of daily diet as well as to the impact of sustained starvation and weight loss. It would certainly seem that any such biological regulatory mechanisms may be over-ridden, and even severely distorted at times, by the kind of 'depression' under consideration here together with its contributory and corporate affects, the disturbances of which may have social origins. The major impact which consequent weight loss might then have in biological terms — its impact on the body's chemistry and its behaviour — has been largely ignored within psychiatric syndromes.

In our study of psychiatrically ill patients, therefore, we developed standardised questionnaires and assessed aspects of sleep, weight and mood and changes in them in a series of 375 new psychiatric outpatient referrals, examining these phenomena in relation to the various psychiatric diagnoses. Some of our principal findings relevant to the present matter were as follows:

A history of obesity confers a propensity for major weight change (increase or decrease) during the illness, whatever its nature, and has no specific association with a current diagnosis of endogenous depression or manic depressive psychosis. A history of having once been thin is associated with a current diagnosis of neurotic depression and/or very disturbed mood, especially tension. A history of weight loss during present illness is more likely to have arisen in neurotic depression and anxiety state than in endogenous depression.

A present state of thinness is more likely amongst those with the diagnosis of personality disorder and who are tense/angry rather than those who are anxious/sad. Most broken sleep and least total sleep characterises those who are angry. A population of psychiatrically ill people overall display a tendency to report having not changed their time of going to bed or time of waking, but to take longer to go to sleep, have more broken sleep and less total sleep than before the illness. Moreover, time of going to bed and falling asleep is earlier in endogenous depression than in other diagnoses. Time of waking is early in endogenous depression and late in anxiety state compared with the total population. Total sleep is less amongst patients with neurotic depression than the other diagnoses, and greatest in those having endogenous depression. The sleep period in endogenous depression occurs earlier within the 24-hour cycle than is the case with the overall population and this contrasts with the later sleep periods of subjects with neurotic depression and anxiety state.

Finally, within the total population and irrespective of diagnosis, there is an important association, especially in relation to the previous few weeks, between changes in weight and changes in sleep. Weight loss is associated with a reduction of total sleep, compounded of more broken sleep and earlier waking. Weight gain is associated with an increase in total sleep compounded of less broken sleep and later waking (see Table 7.1, p. 78 and 79).

The conclusion from our study in respect of so-called 'endogenous' depression was that people with such severe depression do not necessarily waken all that much earlier than before their illness. Moreover, they sleep for quite a long while. Firstly, they go to bed earlier and go to sleep earlier than others, so it would not be surprising if they wakened earlier. Thus it would seem that the hallmark of severe depression is, in fact, often not so much reduced sleep in the second half of the night but complaint about waking too early.

Discussion and hypothesis

Why do severely depressed people complain about waking early when patients with anorexia nervosa minimise it? Many normal people waken quite early and are delighted so to do. People with severe depression waken to find they are overwhelmed by gloom and despair. They have no solutions to the problems surrounding them and from which they may believe themselves to have been protected during sleep. Therefore, they complain of wakening early and often seek further oblivion in the form of CNS depressant drugs. It is this diurnal variation of mood in which despair and other features of the depressive syndrome are worse in the early part of the waking day which seems to me to be one of the real puzzles.

What do we wake from and wake to? Let us revert to the concept of ourselves as problem-confronting, solution-seeking creatures needing to prospect through the day in our search for food and security and its trappings. Oswald (1970) proposed that REM sleep, in particular, might reflect CNS restorative processes, perhaps also including updating and reprogramming of the CNS data bank and related to such sociobiological purposes, preparing us thereby for this task each day: 1. The individual can then take the best possible action, given his/her basic coping capacities, and the external and internal (personal) contexts of the problem. I emphasise the word *action* at this point so that I can later set it conceptually against the *inaction* that characterises us in severe depression. 2. Depression, in evolutionary terms, may be nature's way of discarding those who, in later life, are unable to continue to adapt. Equally, such a challenge in terms of survival may provide the pivot for real change so long as there is inner potential and complementary assistance from without. Meanwhile, the REM process is not conceived of as simply one of message processing. It is perhaps also one of problem-solving at these times when the system is especially capable of modification through learning.

REM sleep is a cerebrally active state. Cerebral blood flow is relatively high at this time. There is special activity in the autonomic nervous system, including for instance such 'instinctual' activity as penile erection, perhaps as part of the reprogramming exercise. Meanwhile, the musculoskeletal system, the rest of the body, is disengaged, the muscles are flaccid. During REM sleep especially it seems that we dream. Dreaming may reflect this process within which the memory stores are mobilised in their coded form thus enabling them to be more receptive to the latest information input both in terms of processing it and being modified by it. Freud, with his conviction of the basic relevance for human experience of the clash between biological and social needs, claimed that dreaming was a prime arena for this encounter. Furthermore, he claimed that memories, not usually accessible to awareness during the day, seemed to arise during the night and could then be accessed with certain techniques. It was Jung who considered that these memories were not only those of the individual himself or herself, but were also the genetically transmitted memories of evolutionary time. Presumably the latest information is necessary for the organism to cope best with the next day's task. However, it must be set against the enormous background of previous experience. Thus dreams, as many have claimed, may be as close as we come to prophesy — on waking the future, good or bad, is perceived most starkly.

Supposing the information coming into the system is presenting insoluble problems to the individual, yet the information is important. Such problems might reflect inability to fulfill one's potential, achieve one's goals or measure up to someone else's expectations of one, providing an overwhelming challenge to personal integrity or competence, or the enforced adoption of an unacceptable role. Such experiences will usually only be understandable, in terms of their personal meaning for the individual, through a deep knowledge of that person and might take many forms such as failure in academic performance, birth of a baby, retirement, rupture of a major bond within family or other relationships. Initial responses may have included the experience of such feelings as anxiety or anger. Grappling with this task of assimilating such information with a view to effective action and fulfilment is ultimately beyond the system and the outcome is defeat. The individual wakens in the morning with no problems solved and with no new resources to tackle the tasks which were overwhelming the previous day. Lewin (1950) described the 'blank dreams' which, as a psychoanalyst, he recognised as the harbingers of depression in his patients with cyclical affective illness. Inaction prevails. The reduced REM latency claimed by some as a feature of people with depression could, if it exists, perhaps reflect an attempt by the organism to embark afresh each night on the necessary tasks that I have just described, given the previous failure. The possible relationship of this to the phenomenon described earlier of the severely depressed person retiring to bed and going off to sleep earlier than before remains unclear. Retirement to bed may simply be another facet of the need to avoid the pain of wakefulness.

If, within sleep, no solution can be found to a problem, whether related to realistic or unrealistic goals, then it might seem natural for inertia, retardation, loss of drive, loss of libido, to result. The problem-solving system has ground to a halt and with it the drive which is normally reprogrammed regularly within REM sleep. This would not perhaps be all that different from the protective conservation-withdrawal stance. Alternatively, or in association, there might also be agitation or agitated stupor if anxiety and arousal is still being generated within the system. Gloomy, non-productive thoughts then become the substance of the next night's task and the state of mind is perpetuated. During the day there is some stimulation which tends to distract the individual but this may be insufficient to break the cycle. Then, during sleep, orientation to the outside world is reduced to memory once more. Orientation is now instead exclusively towards the self and preparation for the morrow. Irrelevant input from the previous day is discarded and the problem that won't go away and cannot be solved again prevails. Once again it proves overwhelming and on waking the individual is again inert — there is no direction in which he can go. Neither flight nor fight, manipulation nor negotiation is possible. Such inertia as a major feature each morning will attract our label of severe 'depression' and indeed may then be cardinal evidence of a need for re-evaluation, for instance of relationships, and a redirection of purpose for the individual. Inability to achieve this may prove a fatal flaw.

This model could plausibly accommodate hypomania as the expression of the organism's reaction to the threat of mounting inertia. Under such circumstances overdrive comes into operation in some individuals! Such a mechanism would have survival value if not excessive. The depressed person welcomes and endorses it — harnessing it as the last defence against depressive inertia and hopelessness. Such experientially driven endorsement might then contribute to florid hypomanic states. The basic mechanism, however, would reflect the biological potential and constitution of some individuals under such circumstances, perpetuated because of its advantage, at least when muted, beyond early and reproductive life. The cyclical nature of some patterns of manic depression might be accounted for by the cumulative effects of the cyclical problem-solving endeavours, which repetitively and successively lead to a point of release of the alternating mechanisms of inertia and exhausting overdrive, neither of which is capable of generating a solution to problems which, in humans, will often be existential in kind.

Other 'defences' against depression would include: mobilisation of any built-in propensities for somatisation — reflecting the strain but associated with denial of the problem, excessive commitment to 'neurotically' driven but goal-fulfilling activities such as work and achievement of high status, the mobilisation of relieving paranoid mechanisms, acting out behaviour often of an aggressive or other antisocial kind and drug dependence or one or other of the eating disorders, all depending on constitutional predispositions.

The relationship between this model of depression and the known effects of certain treatments invites consideration. For instance, if the individual is treated by sleep deprivation, either selectively or totally, and in order to achieve this there is a background of social stimulation throughout the night (e.g. 'occupational' therapy, playing games), then one would expect some remission of symptoms throughout the next day as found by Elsenga & Van den Hoofdakker (1982/83) but the effect would not extend beyond that. Treatments that did not allow, or even blocked the need, for problem-solving would sooner or later be counterproductive. However, there could be advantages for appropriate combinations of treatments capable of re-engaging or enhancing problem-solving resources. It has been argued (Crisp 1980) that some tricyclic 'antidepressant' drugs work by rekindling drive behaviour, perhaps at least in part through their impact on REM sleep which is not so much reduced as modified. Thus their effect would be to re-engage the person with the outside world and hence increase the opportunities of new and potentially therapeutic stimulation. Meanwhile, the basic problem-solving task in which the individual has failed can be taken up again within psychotherapy. Such psychotherapy could be both cognitive/behavioural as advocated by Beck (1976) and relationship oriented as advocated by Jacobson (1975), these processes facilitating each other.

The model also invites speculation as to how ECT works. Perhaps we should ask the question, 'Is there some biological purpose of epilepsy, which is inherent in us all?' Perhaps naturally and subliminally it reintegrates central nervous system functions when disorganisation has arisen or is threatening in response to intolerable arousal. Some epilepsy is perhaps restorative! If induced epilepsy was to operate similarly then it might best do so in those depressed subjects whose mental paralysis was the end product of overwhelming stimulation. High arousal is not always evident in depressive disorder itself but may potentially be there, and in my clinical experience this is often so if, for instance, the depressed individual is confronted with his psychological task. Hill (1954), whilst reviewing theories of mode of action of ECT suggested that it might work by reinforcing denial. In naturally occurring epilepsy there is memory loss, as with ECT. It seems to have been shown that memory loss as such is not the mechanism whereby ECT works. Nevertheless, I would think that disruption of recent memory processes, in the sense that I have been talking about, may be an important aspect of the therapeutic effect of ECT. Perhaps the abolition of recent memory is a minor aspect of the mechanism called into play and more relevant is the epileptic fit on the links between affect (in this case painful) and memory. Perhaps, as Hill proposed, we are physically mobilising the defensive effect of denial and dissociation. Any concurrent psychotherapy will then need to be sensitive to this renewed protective posture.

It has been argued here that some depressive states can provide the seedbed for personal growth. Some clinicians emphasise the therapeutic importance for patients who have become accustomed to complaining in physical terms, or who have developed even more global defences against the experience of 'depression', of being able instead to tolerate and express their underlying affective distress. This step is seen as a necessary enabling one if the individual is to regain awareness of the associated existential problem with the consequent potential to communicate that. The capacity to achieve these steps and then to solve the problem with psychological help will depend on such variables as age, personality resource and the nature of help available. People who can benefit from such an experience may ultimately emerge 'sadder but wiser' and freer from morbid depression. Others may remain condemned to some degree of chronic or recurrent disability.

In conclusion, so-called 'depression' is one of the most common syndromes of our time, but its full or direct expression may be heavily defended against. It is an unsatisfactory word. I, like others, prefer such words as dysphoria, dysphoric inertia, dysphoric agitation. Such dysphoric states can be related to real problems, real either in terms of their personal meaning or their more universal relevance, and demanding solutions. If tolerated and confronted, then with help they can sometimes teach us, both individually and as social groups, more about ourselves, thereby enhancing our capacity to survive both individually and collectively. Thus, 'depression', under these circumstances, may be the most mature of possible stances, particularly so when it arises in adolescence and when, with proper working through, alternative more viable solutions can be achieved which will enable the individual to survive or adopt a more robust adjustment than would otherwise be the case in later life. It is a good thing to have one's depression when young! The extent to which certain vegetative phenomena, such as appetite for food, bowel function, weight changes and physiological sleep changes arise, will depend upon the presence or otherwise of a relatively independent diathesis of appetitive sensitivity to emotional strain. However, early morning inertia is a more basic biological aspect of the syndrome in its severe form and is a particular indication of the need for outside help.

REFERENCES

American Psychiatric Association 1980 Diagnostic and statistical manual volume 3 (DSM III). American Psychiatric Press, Washington DC

Beck A T 1976 Cognitive theory and the emotional disorders. International University Press, New York

Burton R 1927 In: Dell F, Jordan-Smith P (eds) The anatomy of melancholy. Tudor Publishing Co, New York

Crisp A H 1967 The possible significance of some behavioural correlates of weight and carbohydrate intake. Journal of Psychosomatic Research 11: 117–131

Crisp A H 1976 Depression. In: Krauss S et al (eds) Encyclopaedic handbook of medical psychology. Butterworth, London, p 140–142

Crisp A H 1983 Symposium on the teaching of psychiatry to undergraduates: England: St George's Hospital Medical School, London. British Journal of Psychiatry 142: 345–349

Crisp A H 1980 Anorexia nervosa: let me be. Academic Press, London

Crisp A H, Stonehill E 1973 Aspects of the relationship between sleep and nurtrition: A study of 375 psychiatric outpatients. British Journal of Psychiatry 122: 379–394

Crisp A H, Stonehill E 1976 Sleep, nutrition and mood. Wiley, London

Elsenga S, van den Hoofdakker R H 1982/83 Clinical effects of sleep deprivation and clomipramine in endogenous depression. Journal of Psychiatric Research 17: 361–374

Engel G L 1962 Psychological development in health and disease. Saunders, Philadelphia

Hartmann E, Zwilling G R, Baekeland F 1972 Personality traits and life style data for long and short sleepers. Archives of General Psychiatry 26: 463–468

Hill J N D 1954 Psychotherapy and the physical methods of treatment in psychiatry. Journal of Mental Science 100: 360–374

Kraepelin E 1921 Manic depressive insanity and paranoia. E and S Livingstone, Edinburgh

Jacobson E 1975 The psychoanalytic treatment of depressed patients. In: Anthony E J, Benedek T (eds) Depression and human existence. Little, Brown, Boston

Lewin B D 1950 The psychoanalysis of elation. Norton, New York

Meyer A 1934 The psychobiological point of view. In: Bentley M, Cowdry E V (eds) The problem of mental health. McGraw-Hill, New York

Oswald I 1970 Sleep the great restorer. New Scientist 46: 170–172

Paykel E S 1983 The classification of depression. British Journal of Clinical Pharmacology 15: 155–159

Phillips F, Chen C N, Crisp A H et al 1975 Isocaloric diet changes and EEG sleep. Lancet ii: 723–725

Roget's Thesaurus of English Words and Phrases 1953 Revised by Dutch R A. Penguin Books, Harmondsworth, Middx, UK

Schur M 1970 A principle of evolutionary biology for psychoanalysis. Journal of the American Psychoanalytic Association 18: 442

Schmale A H, Engel G L 1975 The role of conservation-withdrawal in depressive reactions. In: Bentley E J, Benedek T (eds) Depression and human existence. Little, Brown, Boston

Siegel J M 1975 REM sleep predicts subsequent food intake. Physiology and Behaviour 15: 399–403

Tune G S 1968 Sleep and wakefulness in normal human adults. British Medical Journal ii: 269–271

Wurtmann R J, Fernstrom J D 1975 Control of brain monoamine synthesis by diet and plasma amino acids. Americal Journal of Clinical Nutrition 28: 638–647

M. A. Reveley

The brain in schizophrenia

INTRODUCTION

From the outset schizophrenia was conceived as a neurological disorder. Kraepelin (1896) brought together the illnesses catatonia, hebephrenia and paranoides into a unified disorder which he called dementia praecox. It was distinguished from manic depressive psychosis because of its tendency to chronicity and progression into a dementia like state. While Bleuler (1911) renamed the disorder the 'schizophrenias', because he believed it was several heterogenous conditions, he was even more pessimistic than Kraepelin about its inevitable deterioration. Kraepelin began the search for an organic cause; he established a department of psychiatry in which neuropathologists such as Alzheimer, Nissl and Brodman worked in search of lesions to explain dementia praecox and senile dementia. There was notably more success with senile dementia. The lesion or lesions of schizophrenia remain elusive to the present day.

Early researchers were limited to studies of neuropathology. As schizophrenia involved subtle disorders of thinking, feeling, volition and personality, early research focussed on the cerebral cortex. There were few studies of subcortical structures or the limbic system. While there were many positive findings, these were inconsistent, non-specific and often not replicated. These early studies had many methodological problems, such as inconsistencies in the selection of patients and controls, variation in the brain areas studied, type of preparation and stains used. Investigators further looked for a pathognomonic lesion and rejected variable findings without due regard for the clinical heterogeneity of the illness (Corsellis 1976).

At about this same time early neuroimaging studies were underway. The first pneumoencephalography study by Jacobi & Winkler (1927) found hydrocephalus in 18 of 19 chronic schizophrenic patients. While many of the subsequent studies were flawed by lack of controls, inadequate or incomplete diagnostic criteria and methodological problems in measurement, there were some relatively well designed studies. Lempke (1935) found ventricular enlargement in 50% of 100 chronic schizophrenics compared to 42 medical controls. Huber (1957) found enlargement of the third and/or lateral ventricles in 67% of schizophrenic patients diagnosed by the criteria of Schneider. Ventricular enlargement was associated with chronic illness and poor outcome. Storey (1966) compared 18 schizophrenics and 18 age-matched controls under age 40. Seven of the schizophrenics and 4 of the controls were abnormal by blind neuroradiologists' readings. This was not statistically significant.

Over the last decade, with the development of new neuroimaging techniques, there has been a resurgence of interest in the brain lesions which might be involved in schizophrenia. Studies using computerised tomography (CT) have demonstrated atrophy manifested by ventricular enlargement and sulcal dilatation. Studies using magnetic resonance imaging (MRI) have just begun to explore structural abnormalities. Positron emission tomography (PET) and single photon emission tomography (SPECT), including regional cerebral blood (rCBF) flow studies using xenon-133, have provided new information about the functional state of the brain in schizophrenia. Neuropathology studies using refined methodology have begun to explore subcortical and limbic regions following leads from the hypotheses generated from neuroimaging and neuropharmacology studies. The results of all these studies have implicated several different brain regions in schizophrenia, in particular the frontal lobes, left hemisphere, temporal lobes and limbic system, basal ganglia and corpus callosum.

FRONTAL LOBES

Clinical observations

One of the first observations to suggest that the frontal lobes might be involved in behaviour was that of Harlow in 1868. He described the case of Phineas Gage who suffered an accidental injury to the frontal lobe after an explosion drove an iron bar into his brain. Following the injury he had a personality change and began to behave in an inappropriate and impulsive manner. In the 1930s research showed that lesions to the frontal lobes could produce placid and carefree animals. This led to the introduction of frontal lobectomy by Egas Moniz in 1936 as a treatment for mental illness.

The frontal lobe syndrome consists of failure to plan ahead, stereotyped thinking, limitation of ability to think abstractly, lack of iniative, poor insight, social withdrawal and emotional changes such as flat affect, disinhibition, apathy, self-neglect, depression, euphoria and hostility. These symptoms are more characteristic of the schizophrenic defect state rather than acute psychosis. There are few case reports of frontal lobe injury leading to schizophrenic-like illness. However, Cox & Ludwig (1979) found more soft frontal lobe signs in schizophrenics than patient controls, but not more parietal, temporal or occipital signs. On psychological testing, patients with frontal lobe damage have difficulty with problem-solving tests, such as the Wisconsin Card Sort (Stuss & Benson 1984). This test involves the ability to anticipate and change cognitive set, and a deficit in this test would be reminiscent of the concreteness of schizophrenic thought disorder and the limitation in abstract thinking of the frontal lobe syndrome. Several studies have found schizophrenics to do poorly on the Wisconsin Card Sort (Kolb & Whisman 1983).

Neuroimaging studies

CT and MRI

Relatively few CT studies have examined the frontal lobes for atrophy. The width of the interhemispheric fissure (IHF) has been found to be widened in some studies (Weinberger et al 1979), but this is by no means a universal finding. CT is limited by the bone artefact in detecting small CSF spaces so close to bone, and this may account for the paucity of studies. MRI is not affected by bone artefact and any atrophy of the frontal lobes can be more accurately determined. Andreasen et al (1986) examined 38 schizophrenics and 49 normal controls with MRI using midsaggital cuts. They found that schizophrenics had smaller frontal lobes, as well as smaller cerebrums and craniums. However, while decreased cerebral and cranial size were associated with prominent negative symptoms, decreased frontal size was not, as might have been predicted by the clinical observations above. Still the results provided some anatomical evidence for the hypofrontality hypothesis.

rCBF

Ingvar & Franzen (1974) found that at rest several chronic schizophrenic patients showed a hypofrontal regional cerebral blood flow (rCBF) measured with xenon-133 which differed from the normal hyperfrontal distribution. This was interpreted to mean that there was a reduction of the frontal activity in the frontal cortex in schizophrenia, since cerebral blood flow is ultimately determined by the functional activity of neurons. Mathew et al (1982) found low flows in schizophrenia, but no regional reduction. However, both Ariel et al (1983) and Kurachi et al (1985) found a general reduction in rCBF in schizophrenia, which was most pronounced in the frontal regions. Weinberger et al (1986) found that with xenon-133 inhalation the rCBF of 20 unmedicated schizophrenics in comparison with 25 normal controls had a resting hypofrontal pattern with reduced relative, but not absolute flow, in the dorsolateral prefrontal cortex. Further, there was not a normal increase in flow during a test of frontal function, the Wisconsin Card Sort, so that both relative and absolute rCBF were reduced in schizophrenics compared with controls.

PET

Three PET studies using oxygen-15 were unable to demonstrate hypofrontality (Sheppard et al 1983, Gallhofer et al 1985, Early et al 1987), while the results from PET with 18-F-flurodeoxyglucose (18FDG) have been variable. Farkas et al (1984), Buchsbaum et al (1982), DeLisi et al (1985) and Wolkin et al (1985) did find reduced cerebral glucose uptake in schizophrenia, while Widen et al (1983), Kling et al (1986), Wiesel et al (1985) and Gur et al (1987) did not find definite evidence for hypofrontality in schizophrenia. The two studies of young, never-medicated schizophrenics (Sheppard et al 1983, Early et al 1987) found no evidence for hypofrontality, which suggests it may be a medication effect. Wolkin et al (1985) and Widen et al (1983) found that antipsychotic medication reduced the ratio of frontal/non-frontal blood flow and metabolism. Alternatively, chronicity of illness or negative symptoms may be additional factors contributing to hypofrontality, but these variables have not been fully explored in the small samples of patients used in PET studies.

Neuropathology studies

Many of the early studies of neuropathology of schizophrenia examined the cortex; however, because of the methodological problems the studies are inconclusive. There have been relatively fewer recent well-controlled studies. One of these is that of Benes et al (1986) who made quantitative morphometric determinations of neuronal and glial density, neuron-glia ratios and neuronal size in the prefrontal, anterior cingulate, and primary motor cortex of 10 controls and 10 schizophrenics diagnosed by the criteria of Feighner et al (1972) and examined under blind conditions. The study was particularly well carried out and statistical analysis used to control for the effects of age, postmortem interval, fixation effects, hypoxia, and neuroleptic exposure. Neuronal density was lower in layer VI of the prefrontal and layer III of the motor cortex. There was also a trend to fewer neurons in most layers, but this was significant only for the prefrontal area. The study did not support the hypothesis of neuronal degeneration, but did find variations in cytoarchitecture in schizophrenics compared with controls.

TEMPORAL LOBE AND LIMBIC STRUCTURES

Clinical observations

Some of the most characteristic symptoms of schizophrenia include abnormalities of language and perception. Formal thought disorder including loosening of associations with tangential or even incoherant speech are considered by some to be fundamental symptoms of schizophrenia. Damage to some areas of the temporal lobe produces language abnormalities, long recognized as the aphasias. Damage to Broca's area produces an ungrammatical speech, referred to as expressive aphasia, while damage to Wernicke's area produces an inability to comprehend, called receptive aphasia. While these classical neurological disorders are distinct from formal thought disorder, their similarities have provided a tantalising clue to the origin of some of the most characteristic schizophrenic symptoms.

Hallucinations, particularly auditory, are extremely common in schizophrenia, although they may occur in other mental illnesses. An association between temporal lobe epilepsy and schizophrenia has been found by several studies. Flor-Henry (1969) found that patients with a left temporal focus more often had a schizophrenia-like clinical picture. Trimble (1984) and Parnas et al (1982) also found an association of temporal lobe epilepsy with schizophrenia. The early literature has been reviewed by Stevens (1966). Davison and Bagley (1969) found, in their review of the literature, that when organic disorder was associated with schizophrenia-like psychoses, it most often involved the temporal lobes, particularly the left, or the diencephalon, particularly the hypothalamus.

Neuroimaging

CT and MRI

Because of bone artefact the temporal horns are difficult to visualise and brain density measures are subject to artefact. There have as yet been no MRI studies examining this area.

PET

Wolkin et al (1985) found lower absolute metabolic rates bilaterally in the temporal regions of 10 DSM-III schizophrenic patients before treatment versus 8 normal controls using 18FDG with a PET VI instrument. This result was not replicated by Early et al (1987), using oxygen-15 and even more precise measurement techniques.

Neuropathology

Stevens (1982) examined histological sections from 25 schizophrenics and 28 non-schizophrenic patients who died at St Elizabeth's hospital and 20 non-psychiatric patients from a general hospital. Using Holzer's stain for glial fibrils, Stevens found increased fibrillary gliosis affecting principally the periventricular structures of the diencephalon, the periaqueductal region of the mesencephalon, or the basal forebrain in three-quarters of the schizophrenics. The hypothalamus, midbrain tegmentum and substantia inominata were the most often affected. Gliosis was also found in the amygdala and hippocampus in 9 of 28 cases. The distribution and types of abnormalities found suggested an inflammatory process. However, Roberts et al (1987) could not confirm gliosis quantified using immunocytochemical techniques and densitometry in 20 areas of the temporal lobe from schizophrenics with demonstrated atrophy, in comparison with controls.

Kovelman and Scheibel (1984) found an apparently consistent alteration of pyramidal cell orientation in 10 chronic schizophrenics compared with 8 non-schizophrenic controls, particularly in the anterior and middle hippocampal regions. Only the left hippocampus was examined. The structural changes were postulated to occur during an early stage of nervous system development.

Bogerts et al (1985) examined the brains of 13 schizophrenic patients and 9 control cases and measured the volume of parts of the basal ganglia and the limbic system by planimetry of myelin-stained sections. The medial limbic structures of the temporal lobe (hippocampal formation, amygdala and parahippocampal gyrus) were significantly smaller in the schizophrenic group.

Jakob & Beckmann (1986) studied the brains of 64 chronic schizophrenic and 10 non-schizophrenic controls. Twenty cases had histologically defined cytoarchitectonic disturbances in the rostral entorhinal region and ventral insular cortex, which lie at the base of the hemisphere in the gyrus parahippocampalis. The changes were found mostly in hebephrenic or residual schizophrenics. These are two limbic regions in the temporal lobe. Histologically, there was poor development of the four upper layers in the entorhinal region. In layer II pre-alpha nerve cells were arranged irregularly in two rows, side by side and not in nodules, and were reduced in number. Also the number of neurons in layer III pre-beta and IV pre-alpha were reduced. In the ventral insular, the number of neurons in layers II and III were reduced in comparison with controls. The authors postulate a developmental abnormality, either genetic or environmentally induced, in the rostral entorhinal and ventral insular regions, occurring in the fourth to fifth fetal month when nerve cells migrate to form the cerebral cortex. If nerve cells are prevented in their migration, then heterotopic islands of cells and disorganised architecture in the cortex ensue.

Brown et al (1986) examined the brains of 41 schizophrenic and 29 patients with affective disorder matched for age, sex, and year of birth and carefully diagnosed by the criteria of Feighner et al (1972). Brains were assessed through the coronal section at the level of the interventricular foramina. Brains were photographed and measurements taken by planimetry of limbic and subcortical structures. The brains of schizophrenics were 6% lighter, had lateral ventricles that were larger in the anterior and temporal horns, and had significantly thinner (by 11%) parahippocampal cortices. These results suggest that the tissue loss is more prominent in the temporal lobes in schizophrenia.

BASAL GANGLIA

Clinical

The basal ganglia are primarily involved with motor control, but have been associated with catatonic symptoms.

Neuroimaging

PET studies

Early et al (1987) examined 10 never-treated schizophrenic patients diagnosed by DSM III and 20 healthy normal controls. A PETT VI system was used with $H_2^{15}O$ to measure regional cerebral blood flow. There was an abnormally ($p = .0012$) high ratio of left globus pallidus/whole brain blood flow in the schizophrenics (1.19) compared to controls (1.08). There were no other abnormalities in the other basal ganglia, the caudate or putamen, or in frontal or limbic structures. As there is close coupling of regional blood flow and neuronal activity, the globus pallidus abnormality is postulated to reflect increased activity in neurons with terminal fields in the globus pallidus. These projections originate from other limbic and subcortical regions, including the nucleus accumbens, which has been postulated to have a role in the pathophysiology of schizophrenia and the therapeutic action of neuroleptics (Crow et al 1977). Gur et al (1987) examined 12 schizophrenics and 12 controls with a PET-V scanner using 18FDG. Among the comparisons was a cortical/subcortical ratio, with subcortical being defined as caudate, lenticular nucleus, and thalamus. There was a relatively higher left hemisphere metabolism for subcortical than cortical regions. There was a diagnosis × region interaction, so that schizophrenics had a higher subcortical/cortical ratio than controls. Overall, schizophrenics had lower metabolism, both cortically and subcortically, analysis of region/whole brain ratios showed a relative hypercortical and hyposubcortical pattern. In contrast, Wolkin et al (1985) found greater relative right basal ganglia local cerebral metabolic rate of glucose metabolism in schizophrenics before treatment.

Neuropathology

Dom (1976) examined the brains from five catatonic schizophrenic cases selected from the C. and O. Vogt Institut für Hirnforschung. All cases had a positive family history for schizophrenia and a history of no somatic treatment. There was no loss of neurons, but he found significantly smaller microneurons (Golgi type II) in the caudate and putamen. The distribution suggested more hypotrophy rather than atrophy. In the posterior thalamus (pulvinar) Golgi type II neurons were 50% less numerous than in normal brain. As he did not find a reactive gliosis, Dom suggested that this represented a defect rather than atrophy.

While Stevens (1982) found widespread gliosis in periventricular structures of the diencephalon and mesencephalon, suggesting previous low grade inflammation, there were fewer findings in the basal ganglia. Of 25 schizophrenic brains from patients who died at St Elizabeth's Hospital, Washington DC, findings in the globus pallidus included 6 with gliosis, 4 with neuron loss, 9 with mineralisation and 3 with infarcts. The striatum had mineralisation in 4 cases and infarcts in 4 cases.

Bogerts et al (1985) found a moderate shrinkage of the inner pallidal segment (20% reduction) in schizophrenics compared with controls, while there were no significant volume differences in the outer pallidal segment, caudate, putamen or nucleus accumbens. However, Brown et al (1986) found no significant differences in basal ganglia structures between schizophrenics and controls with affective disorder.

CORPUS CALLOSUM

Clinical

Psychological and neurophysiological studies have suggested abnormalities in interhemispheric transfer in schizophrenia. Beaumont & Dimond (1973) suggested there was a functional abnormality in schizophrenia which led to a reduction in the passage of information between the two hemispheres when they found that comparisons across visual fields was poor in schizophrenics who were shown letters, digits or abstract shapes to one or both visual fields. Tress et al (1979) and Jones & Miller (1981) found synchronous somatosensory evoked potentials in both hemispheres after unilateral stimulation of the median nerve in the hand. The normal two millisecond delay was lost. The most plausible explanation for this, as Jones & Miller point out, is that the normal callosal conduction between the two cortices has been replaced by a direct pathway from brainstem to ipsilateral cortex.

Neuroimaging

Nasrallah et al (1986) used MRI to examine 38 schizophrenics and 41 healthy controls. There was a significant increase in mean callosal thickness in the middle and anterior, but not the posterior, parts of the callosal body in schizophrenic women, but not men, compared to controls. The authors suggest that this may reflect a lesser degree of cerebral asymmetry in schizophrenic, compared to control, women. Lewis et al (submitted) have reported a case of schizophrenia with an absence of the corpus callosum (but with anterior commisure present), as demonstrated with MRI.

Neuropathology

Rosenthal & Bigelow (1972) were the first to report increased thickening of the corpus callosum in schizophrenic postmortem brain. Bigelow et al

(1983) found increased thickness of the middle ($p = .004$) and anterior ($p = .042$) corpus callosum in 21 early-onset schizophrenics compared to late-onset schizophrenics and psychiatric and neurological controls. Nasrallah et al (1983b) examined histological sections of the corpus callosum, but found more severe gliosis in the callosi of the late onset schizophrenics, in comparison with the early onset schizophrenics and a control group. There were no significant differences in glial or myelinated callosal cell concentrations among groups.

LEFT HEMISPHERE

Clinical studies

Studies from several disciplines have implicated the left hemisphere in schizophrenia. There is extensive evidence from studies of normal brain of hemispheric specialisation of function. Many studies have shown that the left hemisphere is concerned with language, and the right, with non-verbal functions, such as spatial perception and musical ability (Geshwind & Galaburda 1985). Removal of the left temporal lobe results in impairment of verbal memory, and of right, non-verbal memory (Milner 1958).

Flor-Henry (1969) found a preponderance of left temporal foci (38% left, 18% right) in patients with temporal lobe epilepsy and schizophrenia-like psychoses. Davison & Bagley's (1969) review of the literature implicated organic damage to the left hemisphere, in particular, as associated with schizophrenia-like illnesses. These studies began an extensive literature examining the left hemisphere in schizophrenia. Gur (1977) reported an excess of sinistrality among 200 schizophrenics compared to 200 non-psychiatric patients and hospital workers on handedness, eyedness and footedness measures. Lishman & McMeekan (1976) found excess left handedness among young, male psychotics. Nasrallah et al (1982) found an excess of sinistrality in paranoid, but not non-paranoid, schizophrenics and and Taylor et al (1980) found that excess sinistrality was confined to an 'organic' subgroup of schizophrenics. However, excess sinistrality was not always demonstrated. Fleminger et al (1977) found more right handed female schizophrenics than expected.

An extensive literature on functional asymmetries has also developed, often implicating the left hemisphere in schizophrenia. Dichotic listening tasks depend on the simultaneous presentation of verbal and non-verbal stimuli to each ear. Normal subjects usually show an advantage for the ear contralateral to the hemisphere dominant for the task. Colbourn & Lishman (1979) found that schizophrenic patients in comparison with controls did not show the usual right ear advantage. On tachistostopic studies presenting information simultaneously to each half of the visual field, studies (Beaumont & Dimond, 1973, Gur 1978, Colbourn & Lishman 1979) have found defects in left hemisphere processing, although this was not always replicated.

Neuroimaging studies

CT studies

Computed tomography (CT) has been used to look for asymmetries in the brain by measuring the width of the frontal and occipital lobes and by examining the skull for petalia (indentations in the inner table of the skull). The normal pattern of asymmetry is that the right frontal and left occipital lobes are wider than those of the respective contralateral hemisphere. Further, there are petalia to coincide with the width asymmetry. Luchins et al (1979) found a significant reversal of the normal pattern of asymmetry in schizophrenics for both frontal and occipital lobes. However, this study was in general not replicated by subsequent researchers, and considerable methodological difficulties, particularly in establishing the mid-line, confounded these studies (Tsai et al 1983).

Studies using brain density measurements have implicated the left hemisphere as a site of abnormality in schizophrenia. Brain density, the degree to which brain tissue attenuates the X-ray beam in its path, is measured in Hounsfield Units (HU), on a scale from -1000 to $+1000$, with zero being the density of water.

The first study to examine brain density in schizophrenia was by Golden et al (1981), who examined 23 schizophrenic patients diagnosed by DSM-III (APA 1980) and 24 aged-matched medical control subjects. Density measurements were taken in the left, right, anterior and posterior regions on three separate scan levels. Of 6 measurements of anterior left hemisphere density, 5 showed lower density in schizophrenic brains as compared with normal brains. There was also a significant difference between the left and right hemisphere measurements for control subjects at all levels of brain. However, the schizophrenic patients showed significant differences for only 4 of 12 comparisons, suggesting the difference between the hemispheres was less pronounced in the schizophrenics than normals, especially in the anterior half of the brain. There was no age or medication effect. The study examined slice levels for the ventricles at their largest and at the next higher two slices. Whole-brain density was determined without correcting for ventricular or skull size. Portions of the brain which were known to contain ventricle or cisterns were included in the density measurements, on the assumption that partial volume artefact due to lower values of ventricular density would be negligible. However, it is not clear that such an assumption can be made in view of prior studies finding ventricular enlargement in schizophrenia.

Largen et al (1983) examined 16 schizophrenics and 6 schizoaffectives diagnosed by RDC criteria and compared them with 19 controls who had scans taken for headache. They found that the schizophrenics had significantly lower density in the left than right hemisphere in the posterior grey and anterior white matter on the single slice examined, which was 1.5 cm above the top of the lateral ventricle. There was no asymmetry of left versus right hemisphere density in controls, nor were the controls significantly different from schizophrenics in density in any area. Thus, unlike Golden et al, Largen et al found no absolute difference in density between schizophrenics and controls, but did find an asymmetry in schizophrenics and not in controls. These results are the opposite of those of Golden et al, who found less asymmetry across hemisphere in schizophrenics and more asymmetry in controls. Largen et al used a different technique in that a smaller region of interest marker was used, while Golden et al had examined the entire brain. Neither study took into account time of scan or apical bone artefact.

Coffman et al (1984) used a technique similar to that of Golden et al and examined 50 chronic schizophrenics and 24 normal controls. When density values for corresponding left and right hemisphere regions were compared, 11 of 12 comparisons showed the left hemisphere to be significantly more dense than the right for controls, while only 6 of 12 comparisons among schizophrenics showed left values significantly greater than right, suggesting an overall decreased relative density of the left cerebral hemisphere in schizophrenia. As the schizophrenics and control patients had been scanned on different machines, direct comparison between groups could not be made.

Coffman & Nasrallah (1984) compared brain density in 18 chronic schizophrenics and 11 manic males. The density measurements were similar to those of Golden et al. On level C (second slice above the slice showing the bodies of the lateral ventricles at their largest), the manics had significantly higher brain density than the schizophrenics in all four regions of both hemispheres. There was only one difference in the right hemisphere on level A and in the left hemisphere on level B, between schizophrenic and control; these were probably random findings. There were few significant left-right differences in either group. The schizophrenics had greater left than right hemisphere density on two of four comparisons each on the two highest slices. However, these were at low significance levels and would not have been significant if corrections for multiple comparisons had been made.

DeMeyer et al (1984) examined 8 schizophrenics, 7 mixed psychotics and 15 medically ill controls. The authors measured density using a series of circular regions of interest for four areas in the right and left hemisphere on three slices (the bodies at their largest and the next two above). When the psychiatric diagnostic groups were compared, on the basis of the numbers of left hemisphere density readings larger than, equal to, or less than right hemisphere density readings, the schizophrenic and mixed psychotic patients had significantly (Chi square) more right = left hemisphere densities and fewer left greater than right hemisphere densities than medical patients. There was no significant differences between the schizophrenics and the other psychotics.

Dewan et al (1983) found that in 23 chronic schizophrenics and 23 head-ache controls, the schizophrenics had significantly greater density than controls in both caudate and thalamus on both right and left sides. Lyon et al (1981) found that density values of the brain in posterior quadrants of both hemispheres on a single centrum semiovale slice were correlated with lifetime medication dosage, so that those with more medication had lower brain density.

Overall, the findings of studies of singletons support the hypothesis of relative left hemisphere hypodensity in schizophrenics. However, several of the studies failed to correct for partial volume artefact with ventricles and included areas containing ventricle or cistern in the analysis. Further, none of the studies corrected for beam hardening effects (Di Chiro et al 1978), which can influence density even in central brain regions (Coffman & Bloch 1984). Some studies used different scanners for different control and patient groups; most used medical controls; and none took into account the day of scan.

Reveley et al (1987) have examined brain density in pairs of identical (MZ) twins, discordant for schizophrenia selected from the Maudsley hospital twin register, and in pairs of age-matched normal volunteer MZ twins selected from the Institute of Psychiatry normal twin register. The brain density was measured on five CT scan slices, using a fully automated computer programme (Baldy et al 1986), which divided each slice into quadrants and removed CSF spaces, including ventricle, cistern, interhemispheric fissure and Sylvian fissures from the analysis. The outer five pixels around the cortex were removed from the analysis. Data were analysed by multivariate analysis of variance and covariance, using between-subjects factors of diagnosis (schizophrenic twin, well co-twin, or control twin), and within subjects factors of slice level (five slices from third ventricle towards the vertex), hemisphere (left-right) and region (anterior-posterior) with cranial and ventricular size as covariates.

The schizophrenic twins had significantly lower left relative to right hemisphere density than both their well co-twins and normal control twins (Reveley et al 1987). This was demonstrated by the presence of a hemisphere by diagnosis interaction. There was no region by diagnosis interaction and thus, no anterior-posterior difference in density across the diagnostic groups. The presence of left hemisphere hypodensity in the schizophrenic twin, but not in the identical cotwin, suggests that the effect is specifically related to the schizophrenic illness in these twins. This might have developed secondary to the illness, or more likely, predisposed to it. There was no overall diagnosis effect, demonstrating that there was no absolute difference in brain density between schizophrenics and controls or co-twins. These results therefore support those of Largen et al (1983), and Coffman et al (1984), but do not support those of other studies.

PET and rCBF

Recent work with positron emission tomography (PET) and Xe-133 regional cerebral blood flow (rCBF) also support a left hemisphere dysfunction. Gur et al (1983) found no difference in resting flows between schizophrenics and controls. They showed that in medicated schizophrenics, rCBF increased in the left hemisphere for spatial, but not verbal tasks, whereas in controls rCBF increased in the left hemisphere for verbal, and right hemisphere, for spacial tasks. Gur et al (1985) further found that resting rCBF was higher in the left hemisphere for unmedicated schizophrenics in comparison with controls, supporting the hypothesis of left hemisphere overactivation. Treatment with medication restored symmetric flows.

Sheppard et al (1983), using PET with oxygen-15, found that unmedicated schizophrenics differed from controls in laterality of flow in the direction of lower right relative to left hemisphere flows. Buchsbaum et al (1982) found diminished uptake in the left cortex and Gur et al (1987) found that, whilst unmedicated schizophrenics did not have significant asymmetry differences in comparison with controls, those schizophrenics with greater severity on the Brief Psychiatric Rating Scale had higher absolute metabolism and higher left relative to right hemisphere metabolism than patients with lesser severity. Wiesel et al (1985) found no hemisphere asymmetry. The conflicting results with laterality reflect differences in patient samples and PET technique.

Neuropathology

Brown et al (1986) found that schizophrenic brains were significantly lighter (by 6%) than brains from patients with affective disorder. The average parahippocampal cortical thickness was significantly reduced in the schizophrenic group. There was a significant diagnosis by hemisphere interaction, so that there was a greater difference between schizophrenia and affective disorder in parahippocampal cortex thickness in the left hemisphere. However, Jakob & Beckman (1986) found cellular abnormalities in both hemispheres in schizophrenics. Reynolds (1983) found that there was a specific increase of dopamine in the amygdalae in the left cerebral hemisphere in schizophrenic brains, in comparison with both the right hemisphere and controls, suggesting a neurochemical basis for left temporal lobe dysfunction in schizophrenia.

GENETIC VS ENVIRONMENTAL AETIOLOGY OF BRAIN ABNORMALITIES

Implications of CT scan studies

A large number of scan studies have examined the size of the lateral ventricles in schizophrenia. Most of the studies have found ventricular enlargement in varying degrees. Reveley et al (1982) have examined a group of (MZ) identical twins, discordant for schizophrenia, and normal MZ twin controls. The schizophrenic twins had significantly larger ventricular size than control twins, while their well co-twins were intermediate between the two, but not significantly different from either one. This suggested that ventricular enlargement in schizophrenia is an environmental rather than a genetic effect, as it was the schizophrenic twin, rather than both schizophrenic and co-twins, who were larger than controls. The intraclass correlation for ventricular size was high in normal control twins, but within the twins discordant for schizophrenia the intraclass correlation was significantly less, again demonstrating that environmental factors were operant in producing ventricular enlargement in the schizophrenic twins. In a subsequent study, Reveley et al (1984) compared a group of 21 schizophrenic twins to 18 normal control twins. Within the normal control twins, ventricular size was predicted by history of birth complications, while within the schizophrenics, ventricular size was predicted by having a negative family history for major psychiatric disorder. This led us to the hypothesis that various non-specific environmental events early in life, possible antenatally or perinatally, may contribute to the development of ventricular enlargement as an adult and may predispose towards schizophrenia in those with a lower genetic load for a psychiatric disorder. Thus there would be a continuum of liability to schizophrenia from the most environmental to the most genetic.

Weinberger et al (1981) examined Ventriculo-Brain Ratio (VBR) and cortical measures in patients with schizophrenia, their non-schizophrenic siblings and healthy siblings from normal sibships. Within the schizophrenic sibships the patients had significantly larger ventricles than siblings and in every sibship the schizophrenic had the larger ventricles even if his were in the normal range. Ventricular size in the schizophrenics and their siblings was much more variable than in the control sibships, as Reveley et al had found in twins. These results suggest that Ventricular Enlargement (VE) is a marker of the clinical illness and not a trait or genetic marker of vulnerability. Patients with atrophy had the same prevalence of schizophrenia in their families as patients with normal CT scans, weighing against a link between CT abnormalities and familial or genetic schizophrenia. Thus, VE is the result of environmental, not genetic, factors in schizophrenia.

In a larger family study, DeLisi et al (1986) examined brain lateral ventricular size in 26 schizophrenic subjects from 12 unrelated families, their available well siblings ($n = 10$) and 20 non-psychotic controls. The mean frontal horn VBR of the schizophrenic subjects was significantly greater than that of both controls, (2.82 vs 2.09, $p = .05$ by 1 tailed t-test), and their non-psychotic siblings (2.82 vs 1.83, $t = 2.2$, $p = .03$). The VBR, as measured through the bodies of the lateral ventricles, was also significantly greater in schizophrenics compared to controls (8.25 vs 6.39, $p = .05$), but not compared to their non-psychotic siblings.

Of particular interest is the high prevalence of adverse environmental events in this group selected for presumed 'genetic' schizophrenia. Four schizophrenic siblings had a history of obstetric complications and two of these had the largest frontal horn VBRs. Five schizophrenics and no controls had a history of significant head injury. One had a history of viral meningitis at age 5 years. Analysis of variance showed that for frontal horn VBR, age ($p = .004$), birth complication ($p = .0001$), and head injury ($p = .0009$) were significant sources of variance within the sample. After their variance was accounted for, family ($p = .031$) and diagnosis ($p = .052$) were still significant factors. For VBR through the lateral ventricles, age ($p = .05$), and head injuries ($p = .003$), were significant factors, while family ($p = .019$) remained significant after the effects of age, birth complications and head injuries were controlled. However, diagnosis, ($p = .87$), and birth complications ($p = .19$) were not significant predictors of VBR through the bodies.

The authors suggest that, as the increment in ventricular size is observed in families with multiple schizophrenic members, the data suggest that increased ventricular size could represent an inherited vulnerability towards schizophrenia. However, several considerations argue against these conclusions. (1) The most statistically significant effects were environmental. Taken together, history of birth complications or head injuries were present in all but one of the 8 schizophrenics with a frontal horn VBR greater than 1 standard deviation beyond the control mean. (2) There was no comparison of familial versus non-familial schizophrenics in this study. (3) If VE represented a genetic diathesis, one would have expected the non-psychotic siblings to have larger VBR than control, which was not the case at either level. The results could equally be interpreted that increased VBR is an illness, rather than a genetic, marker.

No significant diagnosis effect was found at the bodies of the lateral ventricles, and the authors suggest that technical difficulties with the scanning procedure may have accounted for this. However, Reveley (1985) demonstrated that computerised methods, mechanical planimetry and even Evan's ratio could distinguish schizophrenics from controls, regardless of slice, as long as comparable slices were used and controls and schizophrenics were randomly and blindly measured. Thus, measurement artefact is not likely to account for the findings, as the authors used similar settings and conditions for both patients and controls. Head injury appears to be more associated with VE than does schizophrenia in this sample.

While our findings on family history in schizophrenic twins were clear-cut, showing a clear distinction between familial and non-familial schizophrenia so that all the twins with a family history of major psychiatric disorder have ventricular size below the control mean, these results were not consistently replicated in singletons. This suggested that twins might not be a good model for singletons. Inspection of the data also appeared to show that singletons, obtained on the same scanner and measured in the same way, tended to have lower VBR and ventricular volume than twins. These results could not be explained on any methodological grounds and therefore we developed the hypothesis that twins, as a group, had a larger ventricular size than singletons. Reasons for this might be that low birthweight and complicated delivery are amongst the most important determinants of cerebral anoxia and haemorrhage in the newborn. As cerebral insults frequently give rise to ventriculomegaly, which may not be accompanied by neurological deficit, it suggested that twins who are particularly prone to such injury might therefore have mildly enlarged ventricles, even without neurological or behavioural deficit, as a result of adverse perinatal events or the complications of low birth weight. In that case, schizophrenic twins may have an even greater enviromental component and therefore the familial-sporadic distinction would be easier to demonstrate in twins than singletons.

Accordingly, Reveley & Reveley (1987) examined 25 schizophrenics of MZ twin birth, who were matched for age and severity of illness to 25 non-twin schizophrenics who were current patients at the Maudsley Hospital. All were interviewed using SADS L and were diagnosed as having schizophrenia by both RDC and DSM III. When a first- or second-degree relative had had a psychiatric hospitalisation for major psychiatric disorder, excluding alcohol or drug abuse, or had committed suicide, the family history was regarded as positive.

The VBR for the 25 schizophrenic twins was 7.2 ± 4.7, while that for the comparison group of schizophrenic singletons was 5.0 ± 2.8 ($t = 2.01$, $p < 0.05$, 2-tailed). Analysis of variance of VBR by twin birth and family history controlling for age showed that age ($p = .004$), twin birth ($p = .038$) and family history ($p = .035$) were significant main effects predicting VBR. In addition, there was a significant ($p = .028$) twin $\times$ family history interaction. This was because, when breaking the subjects down by family history, there was a much more striking difference in mean VBR between twins with a positive (4.15) vs negative (9.39) family history than between singletons with a positive (4.28) vs negative (5.77) family history.

Thus, a familial non-familial distinction resulted in a much clearer difference in VBR among the twin than among the singleton schizophrenics. However, there is a similar trend among the singleton schizophrenics. If these adverse environmental events were contributing to the development of schizophrenia in twins, one might expect a higher prevalence of schizophrenia among twins overall. However, prior studies have not found a higher prevalence of schizophrenia among twins than the general population rate. These studies can be criticised on the basis of having an artificially healthy sample, inadequate diagnostic criteria, heterogeneity and failure to achieve complete ascertainment. Further, there is an increased probability that the co-twin of twins who later developed schizophrenia will die at birth, further artefactually reducing the prevalence of schizophrenia in twins. Thus, more careful studies might be able to demonstrate an excess of schizophrenia in twins, which would be environmentally mediated, making the familial sporadic distinction easier to detect.

Three studies (Campbell et al 1979, Pearlson et al 1985, Farmer et al 1985) with small sample sizes found no relationship between ventricular size and family history of schizophrenia, while Nasrallah et al (1983a) are alone in reporting a higher rate of schizophrenia in the relatives of patients with large compared to those with normal ventricles. Four studies (Oxiensterna et al 1984, Reveley & Chitkara 1985, Cazzullo et al 1985, Turner et al 1986), in addition to the twin studies, have found an association of ventricular enlargement with negative family history. Owens et al (1985) found a curvilinear relationship between a definite family history of schizophrenia and VBR in 112 patients. They found that a positive family history of schizophrenia was associated with normal ventricular size and that extremes of large and small ventricles were less likely to have a positive family history. This introduces the interesting possibility that extremely small ventricles should be regarded as pathological, as well as extremely large ones.

A particularly unique study by Schulsinger et al (1984) examined ventricular size in a prospective longitudinal study of offspring of schizophrenic mothers. Schizophrenics exhibited larger ventricular size, and borderline schizophrenics (DSM III schizotypal), smaller ventricular size than mentally healthy controls. Ventricular size correlated with premorbidly attained obstetric data. There was no relationship between ventricular size and age, length of psychiatric hospitalisation, drug treatment or ECT. The results suggested support for the diathesis stress model, which considers schizophrenia as a result of deleterious environmental influences acting on a genetic predisposition. Thus, both the schizophrenics and borderline schizophrenics inherited a comparable genetic loading that was more severe than that of the no mental illness group. Those who remained at the borderline level appeared to have been exceptionally free from potentially detrimental stressors, e.g. perinatal complications, to which the schizophrenics had been exposed. In the absence of a schizophrenic genotype, such detrimental stressors will not produce schizophrenia, but given the necessary genetic predisposition, additional CNS insults increase the likelihood of psychosis, whether schizophrenia or affective disorders, developing.

Neuropathology

The presence of gliosis marks the site of the pathological process. Following brain injury of whatever cause (infections, toxins, trauma) astrocytes proliferate (seen as gliosis) forming scars. There have been several postmortem studies using stains for gliosis. Nieto & Escobar (1972) found gliosis in the diencephalon, reticular formation, septum, hypothalamus, and periaqueductal gray of schizophrenics. Stevens (1982) found widespread gliosis in schizophrenic brain using the Holzer stain for glial fibrils, particularly in the diencephalon and mesencephalon. These and other studies finding gliosis suggest that inflammation or other causes of neuronal damage may be causing cell loss and subsequent atrophy, reminiscent of the CT scan findings of atrophy.

In an attempt to find evidence for gliosis, Roberts et al (1986, 1987) examined the same brains in which atrophy had previously been demonstrated (Bogerts et al 1985, Brown et al 1986). Using the immunoreactivity to glial fibrillary acidic protein (GFAP) as a marker, they found no significant difference in gliosis between schizophrenics and controls, arguing against a process of continuing neuronal degeneration as an adult. However, brain damage to embryonic, newborn or immature animals results in cell loss, but not gliosis. These results support the hypothesis of Kovelman & Scheibel (1984) that brain injury in schizophrenia takes place at the embryonic stage (probably when the limbic system is developing during the second or third trimester) leading to atrophy or hypoplasia, but not reactive gliosis. Any of a number of aetiological agents, discussed above in this and in previous chapters, could be involved, including birth complications, infections, metabolic abnormalities, or immunological disorders.

CONCLUSIONS

Over the last decade a number of studies using a variety of techniques from the neurosciences have provided evidence for biological abnormalities in the brains of schizophrenics. It is clear that no one particular lesion is responsible for schizophrenia, and the answer probably lies in the complex interrelationships among the brain areas discussed above. These advances would not have occurred had not the bridge between psychiatry and the neurosciences been crossed. Further advances in the field will depend on the willingness of both researchers and clinicians to continue to cross that bridge, or perhaps even to realize that the gulf is not as wide as they had imagined.

REFERENCES

American Psychiatric Association 1980 Diagnostic and statistical manual volume 3 (DSM III). American Psychiatric Press, Washington DC
Andreasen N C, Nasrallah H A, Dunn V et al 1986 Structural abnormalities in the frontal system in schizophrenia: A magnetic resonance imaging study. Archives of General Psychiatry 43: 136–144
Ariel R N, Golden C J, Berg R A et al 1983 Regional cerebral blood flow in schizophrenics: Tests using Xenon Xe-133 inhalation method. Archives of General Psychiatry 40: 258–263
Baldy R E, Brindley G S, Ewusi-Mensah et al 1986 A fully-automated computer-assisted method of CT brain scan analysis for the measurement of crebrospinal fluid spaces and brain absorption density. Neuroradiology 28: 109–117
Beaumont J G, Dimond S J 1973 Brain disconnection and schizophrenia. British Journal of Psychiatry 123: 661–662
Benes F M, Davidson J, Bird E D 1986 Quantitative cytoarcitectural studies if the cerebral cortex of schizophrenics. Archives of General Psychistry 43: 31–35

Bigelow L B, Nasrallah H A, Rauscher F P 1983 Corpus callosum thickness in chronic
    schizophrenia. British Journal of Psychiatry 142: 284–287
Bleuler E 1911 Dementia praecox or the group of schizophrenias. Translated by J Zinkin.
    International Universities Press, New York, 1950
Bogerts B, Meertz E, Schonfeldt-Bausch R 1985 Basal ganglia and limbic system pathology
    in schizophrenia. Archives of General Psychiatry 42: 784–791
Brown R, Colter N, Corsellis J A N et al 1986 Postmortem evidence of structural brain
    changes in schizophrenia. Archives of General Psychiatry 43: 36–42
Buchsbaum M S, Ingvar D H, Kessler R et al 1982 Cerebral glucography with position
    tomography. Archives of General Psychiatry 39: 251–259
Campbell R, Hays P, Russell D B, Zacks D J 1979 CT scan variants and genetic
    heterogeniety in schizophrenia. American Journal of Psychiatry 136: 722–723
Cazzullo C L, Sacchetti E, Vita A et al 1985 Cerebral ventricular size in schizophrenia
    spectrum disorders: relationship to clinical, neuropsychological, and immunogenetic
    variables. Abstracts 4th World Congress of Biological Psychiatry, Philadelphia, 7–11 Sept
Coffman J A, Bloch S 1984 Interhemispheric differences in regional density of the normal
    brain. Journal of Psychiatric Research 18: 269–275
Coffman J A, Nasrallah H A 1984 Brain density patterns in schizophrenia and mania.
    Journal of Affective Disorder 6: 307–315
Coffman J A, Andreasen N C, Nasrallah H A 1984 Left hemispheric density deficits in
    chronic schizophrenia. Biological Psychiatry 19: 1237–1247
Colbourn C J, Lishman W A 1979 Lateralisation of function and psychotic illness: a left
    hemisphere deficit? In: Gruzelier J, Flor-Henry P (eds) Hemisphere asymmetrics of
    function in psychopathology. Elsevier, Amsterdam, p 539–560
Corsellis J A N 1976 Psychoses of obscure pathology. In: Blackwood H, Corsellis J A N
    (eds) Greenfield's neuropathology. Year Book Medical Publishers, Chicago, p 903–915
Cox S M, Ludwig A M 1979 Neurological soft signs and psychopathology. Journal of
    Nervous and Mental Disease 167: 161–165
Crow T J, Deakin J F W, Longdon A 1977 The nucleus accumbens — possible site of
    antipsychotic action of neuroleptic drugs? Psychological Medicine 7: 213–221
Davison K, Bagley C R 1969 Schizophrenia-like psychoses associated with organic disorders
    of the central nervous system: A review of the literature. In: Harrington R N (ed)
    Current problems in neuropsychiatry. British Journal of Psychiatry Special Publication
    no 4. Headley Brothers, Ashford, Kent, p 113–184
DeLisi L E, Buchsbaum M S, Holcomb H H et al 1985 Clinical correlates of decreased
    anteroposterior metabolic gradients in positron emission tomography (PET) of
    schizophrenic patients. American Journal of Psychiatry 142: 78–81
DeLisi L E, Goldin L R, Hamovit J R, Maxwell E, Kurtz D, Gershon E S 1986 A family
    study of the association of increased ventricular size with schizophrenia. Archives of
    General Psychiatry 43: 148–153
DeMeyer M K, Gilmor R, Hendrie H, DeMeyer W E, Franco J N 1984 Brain densities in
    treatment-resistent schizophrenic and other psychiatric patients. Journal of Operational
    Psychiatry 15: 9–16
Dewan M J, Pandurangi A K, Lee S H et al 1983 Cerebral brain morphology in chronic
    schizophrenic patients. Biological Psychiatry 18: 1133–1140
Di Chiro G, Brooks R A, Dubal L, Chew E 1978 The apical artefact: elevated attenuation
    values toward the apex of the skull. Journal of Computed Assisted Tomography 2: 65–70
Dom R 1976 Neostriatal and thalamic interneurons: their role in the pathophysiology of
    Huntington's chorea, Parkinson's disease and catatonic schizophrenia. Acco, Leuven
Early T S, Reiman E M, Raichle M E, Spitznagel E L 1987 Left globus pallidus
    abnormality in never-medicated patients with schizophrenia. Proceedings of the National
    Academy of Sciences of the USA 84: 561–563
Farmer A, McGuffin P, Jackson R, Storey P 1985 Classifying schizophrenia. Lancet i: 1333
Farkas T, Wolf A P, Jaeger J, Brodie J D, Christman D R, Fowler J S 1984 Regional
    brain glucose metabolism in chronic schizophrenia. A positron emission transaxial study.
    Archives of General Psychiatry 41: 293–300
Feighner J P, Robins G, Guze S, Woodruff R A, Winokur G, Munoz R 1972 Diagnostic
    criteria for use in psychiatric research. Archives of General Psychiatry 26: 57–63
Fleminger J J, Dalton R, Standage K F 1977 Handedness in psychiatric patients. British
    Journal of Psychiatry 131: 448–452

Flor-Henry P 1969 Psychosis in temporal lobe epilepsy: a controlled investigation. Epilepsia 10: 363–395

Gallhofer B, Trimble M R, Frackowiak R, Gibbs J, Jones T 1985 A study of cerebral blood flow and metabolism in epileptic psychosis using positron emission tomography and oxygen. Journal of Neurology, Neurosurgery and Psychiatry 48: 201–206

Geshwind N, Galaburda A M 1985 Cerebral lateralization — biological mechanisms, associations, and pathology: I. A hypothesis and a program for research. Archives of Neurology 42: 428–459

Golden C J, Graber B, Coffman J, Berg R A, Newlin D B, Bloch S 1981 Structural brain deficits in schizophrenia: Identification by computed tomographic scan density measurements. Archives of General Psychiatry 38: 1014–1017

Gur R E 1977 Motor laterality imbalance in schizophrenia. Archives of General Psychiatry 34: 33–37

Gur R E 1978 Left hemisphere dysfunction and left hemisphere overactivation in schizophrenia. Journal of Abnormal Psychology 87: 226–238

Gur R E, Skolnick B E, Gur R C et al 1983 Brain function in psychiatric disorders. I. Regional cerebral blood flow in medicated schizophrenics. Archives of General Psychiatry 40: 1250–1254

Gur R E, Gur R C, Skolnick B E et al 1985 Brain function in psychiatric disorders. III. Regional cerebral blood flow in unmedicated schizophrenics. Archives of General Psychiatry 42: 329–334

Gur R E, Resnick S M, Alavi A et al 1987 Regional brain function in schizophrenia I. A positron emission tomography study. Archives of General Psychiatry 44: 119–125

Huber G 1957 Pneumoencephalographische und Psychopathologische Bilder Bei Endogen Psychosen. Springer-Verlag, Berlin

Ingvar, D H, Franzen, G 1974 Abnormalities in cerebral flood flow distribution in patients with chronic schizophrenia. Acta Psychiatrica Scandinavia 50: 425–436

Jakob H, Beckman H 1986 Prenatal developmental disturbances in the limbic allocortex in schizophrenics. Journal of Neural Transmission 65: 303–326

Jacobi W, Winkler H 1927 Encephalographische studien au chronisch schizophrenen. Archiv für Psychiatrie und Nervenkrankheiten 81: 299–332

Jones G H, Miller J J 1981 Functional states of the corpus callosum in schizophrenia. British Journal of Psychiatry 139: 553–557

Kling A S, Metter E J, Riege W H, Kuhl D E 1986 Comparison of PET measurement of local brain glucose metabolism and CAT measurement of brain atrophy in chronic schizophrenia and depression. American Journal of Psychiatry 143: 175–180

Kolb B, Whisman I Q 1983 Performance of schizophrenic patients on tests sensitive to left or right frontal temporal parietal function in neurological patients. Journal of Nervous and Mental Disease 171: 435–443

Kovelman J A, Scheibel A B 1984 A neurohistological correlate of schizophrenia. Biological Psychiatry 19: 1601–1621

Kraepelin E 1896 Psychiatrie, 5th edn. Barth, Leipzig. Translated by R M Barclay. E & S Livingstone, Edinburgh, 1919

Kurachi M, Kobayashi K, Matsubara R et al 1985 Regional cerebral blood flow in schizophrenic disorder. European Neurology 24: 176–181

Largen J W Jr, Calderon M, Smith R C 1983 Asymmetries in the densities of white and gray matter in the brains of schizophrenic patients. American Journal of Psychiatry 140: 1060–1062

Lempke R 1935 Utersuchungen über die soziale prognose der schizophrenic unter besonderer Berücksichtigung des encephalographischen Befundes. Archiv für Psychiatrie und Nervenkrankheiten 104: 89–136

Lewis S W, Reveley M A, David T, Ron M A 1988 Agenesis of the corpus callosum and schizophrenia. Psychological medicine 18: 341–347

Lishman W A, McMeekan E R L 1976 Hand preference patterns in psychiatric patients. British Journal of Psychiatry 129: 158–166

Luchins D J, Weinberger D R, Wyatt R J 1979 Schizophenia: evidence for a subgroup with reversed cerebral asymmetry. Archives of General Psychiatry 36: 1309–1311

Lyon K, Wilson J, Golden C J, Graber B, Coffman J A, Bloch S 1981 Effects of long-term neuroleptic use on brain density. Psychiatry Research 5: 33–37

Mathew R J, Duncan G C, Weinman M L, Barr D L 1982 A study of regional cerebral blood flow in schizophrenia. Archives of General Psychiatry 39: 1121–1124

Milner B 1958 Psychological defects produced by temporal lobe excision. Research Publication of the Association for Research into Nervous and Mental Disease 36: 244–257

Nasrallah H A, McCalley-Whitters M, Kuperman S 1982 Neurological differences between paranoid and nonparanoid schizophrenia: I sensory-motor lateralization. Journal of Clinical Psychiatry 43: 305–306

Nasrallah H A, Kuperman S, Hamra B J, McCalley-Whitters M 1983a Clinical differences between schizophrenic patients with and without large cerebral ventricles. Journal of Clincal Psychiatry 44: 407–409

Nasrallah H A, McCalley-Whitters M, Bigelow L B, Rauscher F P 1983b A histological study of the corpus callosum in chronic schizophrenia. Psychiatry Research 8: 251–260

Nasrallah H A, Andreason N C, Coffman J A et al 1986 A controlled magnetic resonance imaging study of corpus callosum thickness in schizophrenia. Biological Psychiatry 21: 274–282

Nieto D, Escobar A 1972 Major psychoses. In: Minckler J(ed) Pathology of the nervous system, vol 3. McGraw-Hill, New York, p 2654–2665

Owens DGC, Johnstone E, Crow T J et al 1985 Lateral ventricular size in schizophrenia: Relationship to the disease process and its clinical manifestations. Psychological Medicine 15: 27–41

Oxiensterna G, Bergstrand G, Bjerkenstedt L, Sedvall G, Wik G 1984 Evidence of disturbed CSF circulation and brain atrophy in cases of schizophrenic psychoses. British Journal of Psychiatry 144: 654–661

Parnas J, Korsgaard S, Krantwald O, Jensen PS 1982 Chronic psychosis in epilepsy. Acta Psychiatrica Scandinavica 66: 282–293

Pearlson G D, Garbacz D J, Moberg P J, Ahn HS and De Paulo J R 1985 Symptomatic, familial, perinatal and social correlates of computerised axial tomography (CAT) changes in schizophrenics and bipolars. Journal of Nervous and Mental Disease 173: 42 50

Reveley A M, Reveley M A 1987 The relationship of twinning to the familial-sporadic distinction in schizophrenia. Journal of Psychiatric Research 21: 515–520

Reveley A M, Reveley M A, Clifford C A, Murray R M 1982 Cerebral ventricular size in twins discordant for schizophrenia. Lancet i: 540–541

Reveley A M, Reveley M A, Murray R M 1984 Cerebral ventricular enlargement in nongenetic schizophrenia: A controlled twin study. British Journal of Psychiatry 144: 89–93

Reveley M A 1985 Ventricular enlargement in schizophrenia: validity of computerised tomogaphic findings. British Journal of Psychiatry 147: 233–240

Reveley M A, Chitkara B 1985 Subgroups in schizophrenia. Lancet i: 1503

Reveley M A, Reveley A M, Baldy R 1987 Left cerebral hemisphere hypodensity in discordant schizophrenic twins: A controlled study. Archives of General Psychiatry 44: 625–632

Reynolds G P 1983 Increased concentrations and lateral asymmetry of amygdala dopamine in schizophrenia. Nature 305: 527–529

Roberts G W, Colter N, Lofthouse R, Bogerts B, Zech M, Crow T J 1986 Gliosis in schizophrenia. Biological Psychiatry 21: 1043–1050

Roberts G W, Colter N, Lofthouse R, Johnstone E C, Crow T J 1987 Is there gliosis in schizophrenia? Investigation of the temporal lobe. Biological Psychiatry 22: 1459–1468

Rosenthal R, Bigelow L 1972 Quantitative brain measurements in chronic schizophrenia. British Journal of Psychiatry 121: 259–264

Schulsinger F, Parnas J, Petersen E T et al 1984 Cerebral ventricular size in the offspring of schizophrenic mothers: A preliminary study. Archives of General Psychiatry 41: 602–606

Sheppard G, Gruzelier J, Manchanda R et al 1983 O^{15} positron emission tomographic scanning in predominantly never-treated acute schizophrenic patients. Lancet ii: 1448–1452

Stevens J R 1966 Psychiatric implications of psychomotor epilepsy. Archives of General Psychiatry 14: 461–471

Stevens J R 1982 Neuropathology of schizophrenia. Archives of General Psychiatry 39: 1131–1139

Storey, P B 1966 Lumbar air encephalography in chronic schizophrenia: A controlled experiment. British Journal of Psychiatry 112: 135–144

Stuss D T, Benson D F 1984 Neuropsychological studies of the frontal lobes. Psychological Bulletin 95: 3–28

Taylor P J, Dalton R, Fleminger J J 1980 Handedness in schizophrenia. British Journal of Psychiatry 136: 375–383

Tress K H, Kugler B T, Coudrey D J 1979 Interhemispheric integration in shcizophrenia. In: Gruzelier J, Flor-Henry P (eds) Hemisphere asymmetries of function in psychopathology. Elsevier/North Holland Biomedical Press, Amsterdam, p 449–462

Trimble M R 1984 Interictal psychoses of epilepsy. Acta Psychiatrica Scandinavica 69: (suppl) 9–20

Tsai L Y, Nasrallah H A, Jacoby C G 1983 Hemispheric asymmetries on computed tomographic scans in schizophrenia and maina. Archives of General Psychiatry 40: 1286–1289

Turner S W, Toone B K, Brett-Jones J R 1986 Computerised tomographic scan changes in early schizophrenia: preliminary findings. Psychological Medicine 16: 219–225

Weinberger D R, Torrey E P, Neophytides A N, Wyatt R J 1979 Structural abnormalities in the cerebral cortex of chronic schizophrenic patients. Archives of General Psychiatry 36: 935–939

Weinberger D R, DeLisi L E, Neophytides A N, Wyatt R J 1981 Familial aspects of CT scan abnormalities in chronic schizophrenic patients. Psychiatry Research 4: 65–71

Weinberger D R, Berman K F, Zec R F 1986 Physiologic dysfunction of dorsolateral prefrontal cortex in schizophrenia I. Regional cerebral bloodflow evidence. Archives of General Psychiatry 43: 114–124

Wiesel F A, Blomqvist G, Ehrin E et al 1985 Brain energy metabolism in schizophrenia studies with 11 C-glucose. In: Greitz T et al (eds) The metabolism of the human brain studied with positron emission tomography. Raven Press, New York, p 485–493

Widen L, Blomquist G, Greitz T et al 1983 PET studies of glucose metabolism in patients with schizophrenia. American Journal of Neuroradiology 4: 550–552

Wolkin A, Jaeger J, Brodie J et al 1985 Persistence of cerebral metabolic abnormalities in chronic schizophrenia as determined by positron emission tomography. American Journal of Psychiatry 142: 564–571

Epilepsy and mental illness

Although the association of epilepsy and mental illness is not as common as was believed by the ancients, modern epidemiological studies have revealed a high incidence of psychological disorder in patients with active epilepsy (Pond 1981, Edeh & Toone 1987). The study of epileptic patients continues to illuminate many aspects of neurology and psychiatry, and there is no subject that is more centrally placed on the bridge between the two disciplines (Hill 1964, Reynolds & Trimble 1981).

HISTORICAL BACKGROUND

There is an enormous historical legacy, stretching back to the earliest literature on the 'sacred disease', which has shaped public attitudes to epilepsy. This has been reviewed in the classic work of Temkin (1945) which covers the period until the end of the 19th century. Other more recent contributions have been those of Lennox & Lennox (1960). Guerrant et al (1962), Hill (1981) and Berrios (1984).

To the Greeks epilepsy appeared a sacred disease, i.e. due to the invasion of the body by a god. Only a god could deprive a healthy man of his senses, throw him to the ground, convulse him and then rapidly restore him to his former self again. The remarkable thing about Hippocrates' famous treatise on the 'sacred disease' was that it was his opinion that epilepsy was *not* sacred, that the human body could not be polluted by a god, and that the brain was the seat of this disease. He had to wait nearly 25 centuries for this latter hypothesis to be generally accepted!

The gods occupied heavenly spheres, one of which was the moon. Hence the word *lunatic* was first applied to sufferers of epilepsy. In contrast mad people were *maniacs* as a result of invasion of the body by devils or evil spirits. However, the distinction soon became blurred and epileptic patients were regarded as both lunatic and maniac. In the gospel account of St Mark (Ch.9, v. 17–27) it was a 'foul spirit' that was cast out of the young man with fits. The association of epilepsy and mental disturbance continued in the public mind right up to the 19th century.

The 19th Century

The process of separating epilepsy from madness began in the 19th century and was linked with the development of neurology as a new and independent discipline. At the beginning and throughout most of the century epilepsy was still primarily the concern of alienists, the forerunners of modern psychiatrists, in charge of institutions such as the Salpêtrière. French alienists, such as Morel and Esquirol, were influential in perpetuating the view that most epileptic patients were mentally disturbed, and indeed Morel's famous 'degeneracy' theory was applied to the mentally ill with and without epilepsy. According to Morel (1857) much mental illness, including epilepsy, was the result of a progressive hereditary degenerative strain in which the ultimate prognosis for the individual was dementia and for the family extinction through idiocy. Such views were apparently accepted by influential figures such as Kraepelin and Maudsley. Epilepsy remained an integral part of psychiatric nosology.

It was the new neurologists who began to challenge these deeply entrenched concepts as they saw much epilepsy without mental illness in their private practice. Table 16.1 contrasts the perspectives of Herpin (1852), Reynolds (1861) and Gowers (1881) with those of Esquirol (1838) and Morel (1857) on the association of epilepsy and mental change. Even though Gowers is often quoted as stating that the mental state of the epileptic is frequently impaired, in fact he found that this was conspicuous in only 7% of his large series, slight degrees of memory impairment being discounted.

Table 16.1 19th century views of mental disorders associated with epilepsy

Psychiatrists	N	% with mental disorder	Neurologists	N	% with mental disorder
Esquirol 1838	385	80	Herpin 1852	38	2.5
Morel 1857	?	100	Reynolds 1861	62	18
			Gowers 1881	1085	7

According to Berrios (1984), as the neurological perspective of epilepsy began to develop the 'psychiatrists' invented a new strategy for keeping epilepsy in the psychiatric camp. New and obscure forms of epilepsy, such as 'larval' or 'masked' epilepsy or 'epileptic equivalent' were hypothesised to embrace vaguely paroxysmal forms of psychological disorder in the absence of any overt seizures. The French 'psychiatrists' Morel (1860) and Falret (1860) were again in the vanguard of this movement. Amongst the 'insanities' which could be 'masked epilepsy' were attacks of mania, moral perversion and criminal behaviour. Morel (1860) defined larval epilepsy as:

> a variety of epilepsy not manifested in seizures but in accessory symptoms such as periods of excitation and depression, motiveless and explosive anger, irritability, amnesia for the aggressive episodes, gradual weakening of mental

faculties, principally memory. Patients may also experience sensory symptoms .... such as auditory hallucinations.

The tendency to see epilepsy underlying paroxysmal psychological symptoms in the absence of clinical seizures is still with us to-day, but following the discovery of the EEG by Berger, newer words such as 'subclinical' and 'subictal' have replaced the earlier inventions. Furthermore these concepts are advanced now not only by psychiatrists, but to some extent by neurologists, clinical neurophysiologists and paediatricians.

In the latter half of the 19th century views about epilepsy were radically changed by Jackson (1873) who suggested that the word should be redefined in *neurophysiological* instead of clinical terms — 'Epilepsy is the name for occasional, sudden, excessive, rapid and local discharges of grey matter'.

This was the first neuronal theory of epilepsy, the foundation stone of our modern understanding of epilepsy. However, it brought with it certain complications. Like the psychiatrists with their 'masked' or 'larval' epilepsy, Jackson began to see epilepsy everywhere. This is illustrated, for example, in his statement that 'a sneeze is a sort of healthy epilepsy'. To his credit, he recognised this problem and in his Lumleian lectures Jackson (1890) reverted to an earlier *clinical* definition of epilepsy: 'I formerly used the term epilepsy generically for all excessive discharges of the cortex and their consequences . . . . I now use the term epilepsy for that neurosis which is often called genuine or ordinary epilepsy, and for that only'.

This semantic retreat by Jackson is apparently not well known and it was later overtaken by the discovery of the EEG. Although Berger himself did not understand English and possibly had never heard of Jackson, much less read his papers, a later generation of clinical neurophysiologists were convinced that the 'spikes' and other 'epileptiform' tracings that Berger and his successors had discovered corresponded with Jackson's intuitive neurophysiological definition of epilepsy (Reynolds 1986).

One spin-off from Jackson's neurophysiological definition of epilepsy was that it was now possible to classify the mental accompaniments of epilepsy into ictal and interictal, and later peri- or postictal. Jackson's own descriptions of 'dreamy states' represented an early attempt at defining ictal mental states.

The 20th century

At the beginning of this century the psychiatrists views about epilepsy still dominated the literature. Guerrant et al (1962) describe three new phases of evolution of thinking since then. In the early part of this century the concept of the epileptic character held sway. According to this view the epileptic patient could be identified by certain personality traits, mostly of an unfavourable or antisocial nature. Later, with the studies of Lennox in the 1930s and 1940s (see Lennox & Lennox 1960), it became more widely accepted that most epileptic patients had normal mental states. This was really an extension of the observations first hinted at by the 19th century neurologists (Table16.1). The culmination of this process is that only in the last 30 years has the diagnosis 'epilepsy per se', finally been removed from national and international classifications of psychiatric illness (Hill 1981).

Then in 1948 the publication of a paper by Gibbs et al ushered in what Guerrant et al (1962) have called the era of 'psychomotor peculiarity'. In their electrophysiological study of patients with psychomotor seizures Gibbs et al were impressed with the association of EEG abnormalities in the anterior temporal area and disturbances in personality. Since then the concept has expanded and an enormous and controversial literature has evolved relating temporal lobe epilepsy not only to personality, but to aggression, schizophrenia-like psychoses and much else. In many ways the personality debate is a rerun of the early 20th century controversy about epileptic character, but this time applied only to patients with a specific type of epilepsy.

The latter period of this century has been characterised by steadily increasing scientific study of the relationship between epilepsy and mental disturbance of all kinds. Instead of all embracing 'degeneracy', 'personality' and 'temporal lobe' theories, recent research has begun to concentrate on the wide range of complex biological and psychosocial factors which exert their influence to varying degrees in children, adolescents or adults with epilepsy.

EPIDEMIOLOGY

Most of the extensive literature on psychiatric aspects of epilepsy has been built on the study of hospital- or institution-based populations, which are inevitably biased by the accumulation of more severe or chronic epileptic patients. Even the few epidemiological studies of the subject that have been undertaken have a number of methodological weaknesses, especially with regard to the careful characterisation and quantification of both the epilepsy and the psychiatric disorder (Pond 1981; Edeh and Toone 1987), All agree, however, that there is a high incidence of psychological disorder in patients with 'active' epilepsy in the community. In a survey of 14 general practices in the south-east of England, Pond and Bidwell (1960) found that 29% of 245 epileptic patients had psychological disorders of sufficient severity to seek psychiatric treatment, i.e. 'conspicuous morbidity'. Amongst 987 patients with epilepsy in Iceland, Gudmundsson (1966) reported that 52% had personality changes of various kinds. Graham and Rutter (1968) studied schoolchildren between the ages of 5 and 15 on the Isle of Wight. The prevalence of psychiatric disorder in children with uncomplicated epilepsy was 28.6% compared with only 6.6% in the general population. In the children with epilepsy together with other brain disorders, e.g. cerebral palsy, the prevalence rose to 58.3%.

The most recent general practice study has been that of Edeh & Toone (1987) who identified 103 epileptic patients aged 16 or greater, in 5 group practices in South London with a registered adult population of 29 822, giving a prevalence rate of 3.45/1000. Of the 103 patients, 88 agreed to psychiatric interview with the Clinical Interview Schedule (CIS) and to neuropsychiatric investigation. 31% had a history of previous psychiatric referral, i.e. conspicuous morbidity, remarkably similar to the observations of Pond & Bidwell (1960). However, according to CIS criteria 48% were classified as psychiatric 'cases', indicating a significant hidden morbidity.

It should be stressed that all the above studies have employed varying criteria of active or continuing epilepsy and thus by definition will have excluded large numbers of patients whose epilepsy is in remission. For example, Edeh & Toone (1987) defined epilepsy as 'a history of at least three epileptic attacks in any 2-year period and the continuation of anti-convulsant therapy, if the period did not immediately precede the time of examination'. As Goodridge & Shorvon (1983) have reported from a general practice in Kent, UK that at least half of the epileptic patients in remission had stopped their medication, the operational definition of Edeh & Toone will have excluded many such patients. This fact, together with the exclusion of children, accounts for the relatively low prevalence of epilepsy in Edeh & Toone's study. The *lifetime* prevalence of epilepsy (including single seizures) in the practice of Goodridge and Shorvon was as high as 2%. This is in keeping with other recent community and hospital-based studies of epilepsy *from its onset* which suggests that some three-quarters of all epileptic patients can expect to go into prolonged remission with current anticonvulsant therapy (Reynolds et al 1983, Reynolds 1987). It is thus apparent that even general practice or other community-based studies that only include patients with continuing epilepsy and treatment will be unrepresentative of all epileptic patients and will thus probably overestimate psychiatric morbidity.

PHENOMENOLOGY

It is customary to classify the psychiatric associations of epilepsy into ictal and interictal. The former can be defined as 'the complex behavioural and experiential manifestations of on-going epileptic discharge' (Lishman 1978). The fact that in clinical practice this theoretically useful distinction is often unclear is emphasised by the existence of other catagories, i.e. pre- and postictal psychiatric disorder, the pathophysiology of which is also far from clear. Fenton (1981) prefers a classification into 'disorders related in time to seizure occurrence', which includes pre and postictal phenomena, and 'interictal disorders unrelated in time to the seizures'. This is a convenient classification provided that the word 'seizure' is defined clinically (Reynolds 1986). It is unfortunately the case that following Jackson's neurophysiological definition of epilepsy and the later discovery of the EEG there is no general agreement as to whether the word 'epilepsy', much less 'seizure' should be regarded as a purely clinical, electro-physiological or clinico-electrophysiological entity (Trimble & Reynolds 1986). In the so-called interictal psychiatric disorders EEG abnormalities of various kinds are not uncommon and so there is no shortage of 'subclinical', 'subictal' and other vaguely epileptic theories (vide supra) to account for them.

The psychological manifestations of some overt clinical seizures, epecially those complex partial seizures presumed to arise in the temporal lobes, have been an understandable source of speculation in relation not only to the interictal psychiatric disorders, but also non-epileptic psychiatric disorders. The fact that complex psychosensory symptoms (hallucinations, illusions and perceptual disturbances), psychomotor symptoms (automatisms), as well as cognitive and affective symptomatology can occur briefly in the context of a seizure has naturally provoked questions, so far unanswered, about the possible role of such 'discharges' and of the limbic system, in the more prolonged psychiatric disorders, especially psychotic illness, in which such symptoms are also prominent in the absence of obvious clouding of consciousness.

The psychological presentations of prolonged ictal discharge detectable on surface EEG recordings, as in petit mal or temporal lobe status, have been well described by Fenton (1978) and Toone (1981). The difficulties of distinguishing such states from epileptic fugues, twilight states and postictal disorders has been discussed by Lishman (1978), who emphasises the wide variety of clinical phenomena, which are hard to classify, and their uncertain relationships to disturbances of the electrical rhythms of the brain. Little has been added to the review by Dongier in 1959, who summarised the combined experience of several authors who between them studied 536 'acute psychotic episodes' in 516 epileptic patients. Twenty-five per cent of the episodes were preceded by seizures and 10% ended in seizures. In the remaining 65% the relationship to seizures was questionable or lacking. This emphasises that at least with respect to acute psychotic episodes the distinction between ictal, periictal and interictal remains clinically as well as theoretically blurred.

The interictal psychiatric disorders of epilepsy include all those phenomena encountered in general psychiatric practice and in patients with other forms of brain disorder. Despite the attention given in the literature to schizophrenia or schizophrenia-like psychoses, these disorders are rare compared to depression of neurotic or endogenous types, anxiety, personality and behaviour disorders, hysterical phenomena and mild degrees of cognitive impairment.

Most of the literature on psychiatric disorder in epileptic subjects is based on selected populations studied by psychiatrists or neurologists working in hospitals or institutions, and there is surprisingly little information about the frequency of psychiatric disability in epileptic patients in the community. In Pond & Bidwell's (1960) general practice study in which

Table 16.2 Type of epilepsy and psychiatric diagnosis (from Edeh & Toone 1987)

Diagnostic category	PGE		Focal non-TLE		TLE		Total
	n	%	n	%	n	%	
Normal	26	63	10	46	10	40	46
Anxiety neurosis	6	15	3	14	4	16	13
Depressive neurosis	6	15	4	18	9	36	19
Other neurosis	1	2	0	0	0	0	1
Schizophrenia	0	0	1	5	0	0	1
Affective psychosis	0	0	0	0	1	4	1
Organic psychosis	0	0	1	5	1	4	2
Personality disorder	2	5	0	0	0	0	2
Mental subnormality	0	0	3	14	0	0	3
Total	41		22		25		88

29% had required psychiatric advice, the commonest problems were neurotic, followed by intellectual defects and personality disorders, at least some of which were attributable more to associated brain damage than to epilepsy. In the Isle of Wight study of schoolchildren Graham & Rutter (1968) again found a preponderance of neurotic disorder or antisocial conduct.

In the recent general practice study of epileptic patients over the age of 16 by Edeh & Toone (1987), all patients who were rated as a psychiatric case according to CIS criteria received a clinical diagnosis according to ICD 9. The results are summarised in Table 16.2. Depressive and anxiety neurosis greatly exceeded all other categories, accounting for over three-quarters of all the psychiatric cases. Various forms of psychosis and personality disorder each accounted for less than 10% of the cases.

The very selected view which emerges from the study of epileptic patients admitted to mental hospitals is illustrated by Betts (1981). In two Birmingham mental hospitals in 1967 he found 78 patients with epilepsy in the *chronic* wards. The psychiatric diagnosis when originally admitted is summarised in Table 16.3. Psychoses of various kinds dominate the picture, approximately half the patients having been admitted with some kind of paranoid illness. Betts then surveyed all the *acute* epileptic admissions during one year to the Birmingham mental hospitals and psychiatric

Table 16.3 Chronic mental hospital epileptic population (from Betts 1981)

Diagnosis on admission	
Paranoid psychosis	28
'Furor'	20
Paranoid schizophrenia	15
Confusion/dementia	8
Hebephrenic schizophrenia	4
Other	3
Total	78

Table 16.4 Acute epilepsy admisssions to mental hospitals or psychiatric units in one year (From Betts 1981)

Main reason for admission		Main psychiatric diagnosis	
Acute brain syndrome (delirium,	16	Depressive illness (12 endogenous)	22
confusion, intoxication, etc.)	15	Brain syndrome (dementia,	22
Acute behaviour disturbance		intoxication, twilight state, etc.)	
Attempted/threatened suicide	14	Personality disorder/psychopathy	15
Assessment	12	Social distress	4
Depression	11	Paranoid psychosis	3
Social reasons	4	Phobic anxiety	3
		Psychiatrically normal	2
		Not known*	1
Total	72		72

*Absconded before assessment.

units. The main reasons for admission and the main psychiatric diagnosis in the 72 epileptic subjects are summarised in Table 16.4. In this very different population acute behavioural disturbances, confusion or delirium were mainly responsible for admission, and the commonest psychiatric diagnoses were depression and organic brain syndrome.

In summary the general practice and community studies suggest that much the commonest psychiatric diagnoses are mood disorders, especially depression; and, to a lesser extent conduct/behaviour/personality problems. Depression also contributes to a large extent to acute hospital admissions, as do acute behavioural disturbances or organic brain syndromes, at least some of which are related to an increase in seizure frequency or to drug intoxication. The rather uncommon chronic psychoses tend to accumulate in mental hospitals, from where through the studies and writings of many psychiatrists they have tended to dominate the literature.

AETIOLOGY

Whatever the psychiatric diagnosis, it is notable that similar aetiological factors are frequently discussed, although no doubt they operate in different proportions and to variable degrees in different psychiatric categories or individual patients. These factors affecting mental function in epilepsy are:
1. Seizures
2. Brain damage
3. Heredity
4. Psychosocial
5. Anticonvulsant drugs.

It is worth emphasising at the outset that the high incidence of mental disorder in epileptic patients is not unique to epilepsy but is also seen in patients with other forms of brain disorder (Lishman 1978). It underlines the view that much of the psychopathology does result from a disturbance in cerebral function, a conclusion which was also reached from the careful epidemiological study of Graham & Rutter (1968), in which they compared the psychological consequences of epilepsy and other cerebral disorders with those due to other chronic non-neurological handicaps, such as asthma and diabetes. What might these disturbances in cerebral function be? Two leading candidates for consideration are brain lesions associated with epilepsy, and the seizures themselves.

Cerebral pathology

As is well known, epilepsy is commonly symptomatic of cerebral pathologies of varying type and extent. Probably the more extensive the pathology the greater the risk of epilepsy and the more difficult the seizures are to control. Epilepsy, even of so-called idiopathic type, may also result in brain damage from a variety of mechanisms, such as head injuries or cerebral anoxia, especially the undesirable consequences of status epilepticus. Modern imaging techniques such as CT or MRI have added to earlier neuropathological studies in revealing previously unsuspected brain lesions in patients with epilepsy, but it remains true that such pathology is more likely to be found in patients with partial seizures and in those with adult onset epilepsy. The subject has most recently been reviewed by Marsden & Reynolds (1988). As such pathology can contribute to mental disorders in the absence of epilepsy (Lishman 1978), it is reasonable to suspect that it contributes to the psychopathology of epilepsy. Indeed Graham & Rutter (1968) showed that the combination of brain lesions and epilepsy increased the incidence of psychiatric disorders to 58%, compared to 34% for uncomplicated epilepsy. On the basis of his Icelandic survey Gudmundsson (1966) concluded that the extent of brain pathology was the most important of the various factors which contribute to mental change. Special attention has been focussed on the temporal lobes. But first we must consider the possible influence of the seizures themselves.

Seizure activity

As already emphasised, there is no shortage of speculation about the possible role of seizure activity in generating mental symptoms in epileptic patients. Furthermore, as discussed above, such speculation has extended to mental illness in the absence of overt seizures, either because the mental symptoms are to some extent paroxysmal or because of the discovery of mysterious 'epileptiform' or other abnormalities on the surface EEG. I have previously reviewed possible mechanisms by which seizure activity may contribute to psychopathology (Reynolds 1981). These include: the transient or more prolonged seizure discharges which are detectable on surface EEGs and shown to correlate with mental symptoms, as in psychomotor status; the hypothetical 'subclinical' discharges which are not detectable on the EEG but which are presumed to occur in deeper structures; kindling; the Gowers phenomenon, in which seizures (or mental symptoms?) generate further seizures (or mental symptoms); repeated exposure to the transient disturbance in cognitive function which occur during seizures, or brief EEG 'epileptiform' discharges of either a generalised or focal kind (Aarts et al 1984); and, of course, brain damage due to seizures.

We are, however, also confronted by a paradox. Seizures, especially of a generalised kind, are a powerful therapeutic weapon in the treatment of some forms of mental illness, i.e. ECT for the treatment of depression (and psychoses). And yet depression is the commonest mental disorder associated with epilepsy! It is interesting that in some epileptic patients depression occurs at a time of better seizure control, whether spontaneous or drug induced (Betts 1981). This phenomenon of alternating seizures and mental illness is better known in relation to epilepsy and psychoses, an observation that led to the introduction of convulsive therapy and the concepts of biological antagonism (Meduna 1937, Reynolds 1968, Wolf & Trimble 1985) and 'forced normalisation' (Landolt 1958, Wolf 1986). There is clinical, physiological, pharmacological and biochemical support for the concept of biological antagonism (Reynolds 1968, 1981, Trimble & Meldrum 1979). But there is also evidence that depression, psychoses and behaviour disorders occur commonly at times of exacerbation of epilepsy. No doubt multiple and different mechanisms operate in different subjects, including the influence of psychological, social and genetic factors, as well as anticonvulsant therapy (vide infra).

We remain very ignorant about the pathophysiological mechanisms involved in the psychiatric disorders of epilepsy, mainly because we have relied so long on surface EEG recordings. For ethical reasons, depth electrode studies are mostly confined to chronic epileptic subjects with partial seizures undergoing evaluation for temporal lobe or other forms of surgery. However, these studies have confirmed how unreliable the surface EEG may be, even for localising the site of origin of seizures. Depth electrode studies increase the numbers of patients in whom it is possible to localise accurately the site of origin of seizures by at least a third (Fenwick 1988). They have also confirmed the long-held suspicion that subcortical electrical seizure discharges may not be propagated to the surface, and they are leading to a re-evaluation of long-held views about the localising significance of some of the symptoms of complex partial seizures, especially as it is now apparent, for example, that frontal lobe discharges may be propagated through temporal lobe circuits (Williamson & Spencer 1986, Fenwick 1988). If the ethical difficulties can be overcome, or if magnetoencephalography proves to be a sensitive non-invasive technique for studying deeply placed electrical events on a long-term basis, then similar studies may eventually shed light on the pathophysiology of the psychological disorders associated with epilepsy, as already glimpsed by Heath (1986).

Temporal lobe epilepsy

Since the original report of Gibbs et al in 1948 of an association between anterior temporal EEG abnormalities and personality disorder in patients with psychomotor seizures, an enormous and controversial literature has grown on the alleged special association between temporal lobe epilepsy and a variety of psychiatric disorders, notably personality disorder and certain behavioural traits, schizophrenia-like psychoses and sexual dysfunction. A characteristic temporal lobe behavioural syndrome has been proposed which includes features such as hypergraphia, hyper-religiosity, viscosity in thinking, circumstantiality, anger, labile emotionality, altered sexuality and increased concern with philosophical and cosmic issues (e.g. Geschwind 1979, Bear & Fedio 1977). Despite deeply held convictions about some of these putative associations it is fair to say, after 40 years of controversy, that these matters are far from clarified and considerable doubt must therefore remain about their validity. Reviews of the extensive literature can be found in Lishman (1978), Reynolds & Trimble (1981), Koella and Trimble (1983), Blumer (1984) and Dodrill and Batzel (1986). I have previously discussed some of the reasons for this long-running uncertainty (Reynolds 1981, 1983a). There is frequently clinical imprecision in the diagnosis of 'temporal lobe epilepsy'. This is partly semantic in origin as 'psychomotor seizures' have evolved into 'temporal lobe epilepsy' and more recently 'complex partial seizures', terms which have been, but which should not be, used interchangeably. Imprecision also arises from the variable EEG criteria which have been employed to support the diagnosis and from the unreliability of the surface EEG, especially interictally, and even ictally, to localise the origin of seizures. It is now apparent that complex partial seizures, previously thought to be temporal lobe in origin, may arise in the frontal lobes and may be propagated through temporal/limbic structures (Williamson & Spencer 1986). Another problem is the biased selection of patients for study in hospitals or institutions, whether neurological or psychiatric. Patients with epilepsy of partial onset are more difficult to control and tend to accumulate in hospital clinics, where patients with 'temporal lobe epilepsy' may account for up to 70% of a neurological clinic population (Alving 1978). If psychiatrists find a high incidence of temporal lobe epilepsy amongst their patients with psychiatric disorders this may not be of significance without an appropriate control group.

The study of general practice populations can overcome some of these selection biases, provided the patients have been carefully investigated and characterised, as has recently been attempted by Edeh & Toone (1987). In their south London urban population they were able to compare the psychiatric associations of 41 patients with primary generalised epilepsy (PGE), 25 patients with temporal lobe epilepsy (TLE) and 22 patients with focal non-TLE. As shown in Table 16.2, a greater prevalence of psychiatric morbidity was found in both focal groups compared with the PGE group. Furthermore, the severity of psychiatric disturbance (total CIS score) did not differ between the two focal groups, both being significantly higher than the PGE group. Only on the symptom rating of anxiety and the 'manifest abnormality' of depression did the TLE group score significantly more highly than the focal non-TLE group. This study therefore suggests that higher rates of psychiatric morbidity are found in focal (partial) epilepsies of all types compared to PGE, rather than the older controversial distinction between TLE and other forms of epilepsy. Other differences between the PGE group and the two focal groups were that the latter had more CT scan abnormalities, less well-controlled epilepsy, and more anticonvulsant therapy. Such factors may contribute to the increased psychiatric morbidity (Reynolds 1983a).

Anticonvulsant therapy

Until quite recently the possible contribution of anticonvulsant therapy to the psychological disorders of epilepsy had been much neglected. This was all the more surprising considering the widespread use of prolonged polytherapy in epileptic patients (Reynolds & Shorvon, 1981). Furthermore, it is the most remediable of all the adverse influences on mental function. When Trimble and Reynolds reviewed the literature in 1976 it was clear that there had been very little study of this potentially important area. Since then, however, there has been a considerable growth of interest with increasing study of psychological disorder and psychometric function in relation to different anticonvulsant drugs in adults and children with chronic or newly diagnosed epilepsy, as well as in normal volunteers. The literature has been reviewed by Reynolds (1983b), Trimble & Reynolds (1984), Hirtz & Nelson (1985) and Trimble (1988).

Reduction of unnecessary polytherapy (Shorvon & Reynolds 1979) not only alerted epileptic patients but also alerted physicians to the adverse cognitive, behavioural and emotional effects of such therapy. Such effects had long been known in children treated with phenobarbitone, but had been little studied. The advent of blood level monitoring of anticonvulsant drugs soon revealed similar previously unsuspected cognitive and behavioural effects of other drugs, notably phenytoin, in the absence of the more classical signs of toxicity. An 'encephalopathy' or 'psychosis' has also occasionally been attributed to ethosuximide or valproate.

These clinical observations have stimulated many psychometric studies. Subtle effects of the drugs on attention, concentration, psychomotor performance, memory, motor and mental speed, and problem solving have been observed, especially with phenobarbitone, phenytoin and benzodiazepines and to some extent with valproate, but most of all with polytherapy. A number of studies have compared phenytoin and carbamazepine and have consistently found more adverse effects with the former, whether in normal volunteers, chronic or newly diagnosed epileptic patients (Andrewes et al 1986).

The metabolic mechanisms by which the drugs may exert their influence on mental function has also been explored and include effects on folate, monoamine and hormone metabolism (Reynolds 1983b). In view of the differences between carbamazepine and phenytoin on psychometric performance it is of interest that the former drug elevates plasma levels of free tryptophan whereas the latter (and phenobarbitone) depresses it (Pratt et al 1984). In epileptic subjects carbamazepine has notably fewer adverse behavioural effects than the other drugs, especially in adults. There has also been considerable interest in the therapeutic use of this tricyclic drug in manic-depressive and other non-epileptic psychiatric disorders (Okuma 1983). It seems probable that chronic therapy with most of the anticonvulsant drugs contributes to the high incidence of depression in epilepsy and to the apparently low incidence of mania.

Other factors

Two other important considerations in the genesis of the psychiatric disorders of epilepsy are 1. genetic and 2. psychosocial factors. About the former there is very little to say, about the latter too much! It is remarkable that in the space of a century we have moved from a situation in which Morel's genetic theories have dominated thinking on this subject to one in which little attention is given to genetic factors, despite their importance in other psychiatric disorders and the modern tools available for their investigation. This is probably too great a swing of the pendulum (Reynolds 1981).

The potent influence of psychological and social stress factors, of anxiety, attitudes and stigma, of disturbed relationships in the family and outside, of impaired prospects for employment, marriage, driving and so many aspects of normal living; all of this is sufficiently self-evident not to demand detailed attention here. The emotional impact of epilepsy and its consequences is well described by Williams (1981). The importance of this subject is also emphasised by its long historical roots, summarised at the beginning of this chapter.

CONCLUSIONS

Until near the end of the 19th century epilepsy and mental illness were almost synonomous. The separation of the two was linked in time to the development of neurology as independent discipline, distinct from psychiatry. Although most epileptic patients have normal mental states it is apparent from epidemiological and general practice studies that there is a high incidence of psychiatric disorder in patients with active epilepsy. The distinction between ictal and interictal psychiatric disorders is probably an oversimplification and we remain ignorant of the neurophysiological mechanisms involved, whether the psychological disorder is linked temporally to an increase in seizures, or, as also occurs, at times of better seizure control. The suspicion of a special relationship between temporal lobe epilepsy and psychological disorders of various kinds has not been unequivocally confirmed. Rather it seems that patients with partial (focal) epilepsies of various types are more vulnerable than those with generalised epilepsies. Several factors may contribute to this increased risk. Patients with partial epilepsies have more brain lesions, their seizures are more difficult to control and they receive more anticonvulsant therapy. For all these reasons they also accumulate more psychological and social problems. It is this complex interaction between cerebral pathology, various neurophysiological mechanisms, pharmacological and biochemical factors, genetics and powerful psychological and social influences, which probably is the key to understanding the associated psychopathology.

The psychiatric disorders of epilepsy have long been regarded as valuable models for the study of other forms of mental illness. They also challenge us to understand the paradox of the influence of convulsive therapy in psychiatry. Finally, they continue to illustrate the close links between neurology and psychiatry.

REFERENCES

Aarts J H P, Binnie C D, Smit A M, Wilkins A J 1984 Selective cognitive impairment during focal and generalized epileptiform EEG activity. Brain 107: 293–308

Alving J 1978 Classification of the epilepsies. An investigation of 1508 consecutive adult patients. Acta Neurologica Scandinavica 58: 205–212

Andrewes D G, Bullen J G, Tomlinson L, Elwes R D C, Reynolds E H 1986 A comparative study of the cognitive effects of phenytoin and carbamazepine in new referrals with epilepsy. Epilepsia 27(2): 128–134

Bear D M, Fedio E 1977 Quantitative analysis of interictal behaviour in temporal lobe epilepsy. Archives of Neurology 34: 454–467

Berrios G E 1984 Epilepsy and insanity during the early 19th century. Archives of Neurology 41: 978–981

Betts T A 1981 Epilepsy and the mental hospital. In: Reynolds E H, Trimble M R (eds) Epilepsy and psychiatry. Churchill Livingstone, Edinburgh, p 175–184

Blumer D (ed) 1984 Psychiatric aspects of epilepsy. American Psychiatric Press, Washington

Dodrill C B, Batzel L W 1986 Interictal behavioral features of patients with epilepsy. Epilepsia 27(2): S64–S76

Dongier S 1959 Statistical study of clinical and electroencephalographic manifestations of 536 psychotic episodes occurring in 516 epileptics between clinical seizures. Epilepsia 1: 117–142

Edeh J, Toone B 1987 Relationship between interictal psychopathology and the type of epilepsy. Results of a survey in general practice. British Journal of Psychiatry 151: 95–101

Esquirol J E D 1838 Des maladies mentales. J B Baillière, Paris

Falret J 1860–1861 De l'état mental des épileptiques. Archives of General Medicine 16: 661–679, 17: 461–491, 18: 423–443

Fenton G W 1978 Epilepsy and psychosis. Journal of the Irish Medical Association 71: 315–324

Fenton G W 1981 Psychiatric disorders of epilepsy: classification and phenomenology. In: Reynolds E H, Trimble M R (eds) Epilepsy and psychiatry. Churchill Livingstone, Edinburgh p 12–26

Fenwick P 1988 Seizures, EEG discharges and behaviour. In: Trimble M R, Reynolds E H (eds) Epilepsy, behaviour and cognitive function. Wiley, Chichester, p 55–61

Geschwind N 1979 Behavioural changes in temporal lobe epilepsy. Psychological Medicine 9: 217–219

Gibbs E L, Gibbs F A, Fuster B 1948 Psychomotor epilepsy. Archives of Neurology and Psychiatry 60: 331–339

Goodridge D M G, Shorvon S D 1983 Epilepsy in a population of 6000. 1. Demography, diagnosis and classification, and the role of the hospital services. 2. Treatment and prognosis. British Medical Journal 287: 641–647

Gowers W R 1881 Epilepsy and other chronic convulsive diseases. Churchill, London

Graham P, Rutter M 1968 Organic brain dysfunction and child psychiatric disorder. British Medical Journal 3: 695–700

Gudmundsson G 1966 Epilepsy in Iceland. A clinical and epidemiological investigation. Acta Neurologica Scandinavica Supplement 25

Guerrant J, Anderson W W, Fischer A, Weinstein M R, Jaros R M, Deskins A 1962 Personality in epilepsy. Thomas, Springfield

Heath R G 1986 Studies with deep electrodes in patients intractably ill with epilepsy and other disorders. In: Trimble M R, Reynolds E H (eds) What is epilepsy? Churchill Livingstone, Edinburgh p 126–138

Herpin T 1852 Du pronostic et du traitment curatif de l'epilepsie. J B Baillière, Paris

Hill D 1964 The bridge between neurology and psychiatry. Lancet i: 509–514

Hill D 1981 Historical review. In: Reynolds E H, Trimble M R (eds) Epilepsy and psychiatry. Churchill Livingstone, Edinburgh, p 1–11

Hirtz D G, Nelson K B 1985 Cognitive effects of antiepileptic drugs. In: Pedley T A, Meldrum B S (eds) Recent advances in epilepsy (2) Churchill Livingstone, Edinburgh, p 161–181

Jackson J H 1873 On the anatomical, physiological, and pathological investigation of epilepsies. Reports of the West Riding Lunatic Asylum 3: 315–339

Jackson J H 1890 On convulsive seizures. British Medical Journal i: 703–707

Koella W P, Trimble M R (eds) 1982 Temporal lobe epilepsy, mania and schizophrenia and the limbic system. Advances in Biological Psychiatry, vol 8. Karger, Basle

Landolt H 1958 Serial electroencephalographic investigations during psychotic episodes in epileptic patients and during schizophrenic attacks. In: Lorentz de Haas A M (ed) Lectures on epilepsy. Elsevier, Amsterdam, p 91–133

Lennox W G, Lennox M A 1960 Epilepsy and related disorders. Little Brown, Boston

Lishman W A 1978 Organic psychiatry: the psychological consequences of cerebral disorder. Blackwell Scientific Publications, Oxford

Marsden C D, Reynolds E H 1988 Neurology. In: Laidlaw J, Richens A, Oxley J (eds) A textbook of epilepsy. Churchill Livingstone, Edinburgh p 144–182

Meduna L von 1937 Die Konvulsionstherapie der Schizophrenie. Marhold, Halle

Morel B A 1857 Traité des Dégenerescences Physiques, Intellectuelles et Morales de L'Espèce Humain et des Causes qui Produisent ses Variétés Maladaptives, vol 1. Ballière, Paris

Morel B A 1860 D'une forme délire, suite d'une sur excitation nervous se rattachant a une variéte non encore decrite d'épilepsie (épilepsie larvee). Gaz. Hebdomad Med. Chir. 3: 773–775, 819–821, 836–841

Okuma T 1983 Therapeutic and prophylactic effects of carbamazepine in bipolar disorders. In: Diagnosis and treatment of affective disorders. Psychiatric Clinics of North America, vol 6, p 157–174

Pond D 1981 Epidemiology of the psychiatric disorders of epilepsy. In: Reynolds E H, Trimble M R (eds) Epilepsy and psychiatry. Churchill Livingstone, Edinburgh, p 27–32

Pond D A, Bidwell B H 1960 A survey of epilepsy in 14 general practices. 2. Social and psychological aspects. Epilepsia 1: 285–299

Pratt J A, Jenner P, Johnson A L, Shorvon S D, Reynolds E H 1984 Anticonvulsant drugs alter plasma trytophan concentrations in epileptic patients: implications for antiepileptic action and mental function. Journal of Neurology, Neurosurgery and Psychiatry 47: 1131–1133

Reynolds E H 1968 Epilepsy and schizophrenia. Relationship and biochemistry. Lancet i: 398–401

Reynolds E H 1981 Biological factors in psychological disorders associated with epilepsy. In: Reynolds E H, Trimble M R (eds) Epilepsy and psychiatry Churchill Livingstone, Edinburgh, p 264–290

Reynolds E H 1983a Interictal behaviour in temporal lobe epilepsy. British Medical Journal 286: 918–919

Reynolds E H 1983b Mental effects of antiepileptic medication; a review. Epilepsia 24 (suppl 2): S85–S95

Reynolds E H 1986 The clinical concept of epilepsy: an historical perspective. In: Trimble M R, Reynolds E H (eds) What is epilepsy? Churchill Livingstone, Edinburgh, p 1–7

Reynolds E H 1987 Early treatment and prognosis of epilepsy. Epilepsia 28 (2): 97–106

Reynolds E H, Shorvon S D 1981 Monotherapy or polytherapy for epilepsy? Epilepsia 22: 1–10

Reynolds E H, Trimble M R 1981 (eds) Epilepsy and psychiatry. Churchill Livingstone, Edinburgh

Reynolds E H, Elwes R D C, Shorvon S D 1983 Why does epilepsy become intractable? Prevention of chronic epilepsy. Lancet ii: 952–954

Reynolds J R 1861 Epilepsy: its symptoms, treatment and relation to other chronic convulsive disorders. John Churchill, London

Shorvon S D, Reynolds E H 1979 Reduction of polypharmacy for epilepsy. British Medical Journal ii: 1023–1025

Temkin O 1945 The falling sickness. The John Hopkins Press, Baltimore

Toone B 1981 Psychoses of epilepsy. In: Reynolds E H, Trimble M R (eds) Epilepsy and psychiatry. Churchill Livingstone, Edinburgh p 113–137

Trimble M R 1988 Anticonvulsant drugs, mood and cognitive function. In: Trimble M R, Reynolds E H (eds) Epilepsy, behaviour and cognitive function. John Wiley, Chichester, p 135–143

Trimble M R, Meldrum B S 1979 Monoamines, epilepsy and schizophrenia. In: Obiols J, Ballus E, Gonzales M, Pujol J (eds) Biological psychiatry today. Elsevier, Amsterdam, p 470–475

Trimble M R, Reynolds E H 1976 Anticonvulsant drugs and mental symptoms. A review. Psychological Medicine 6: 169–178

Trimble M R, Reynolds E H 1984 Neuropsychiatric toxicity of anticonvulsant drugs. In: Matthews W B, Glaser G H (eds) Recent advances in clinical neurology. Churchill Livingstone, Edinburgh p 261–280

Trimble M R, Reynolds E H 1986 (eds) What is epilepsy? Churchill Livingstone, Edinburgh

Williams D 1981 The emotions and epilepsy. In: Reynolds E H, Trimble M R (eds) Epilepsy and psychiatry. Churchill Livingstone, Edinburgh p 49–59

Williamson P D, Spencer S S 1986 Clinical and EEG features of complex partial seizures of extratemporal origin. Epilepsia 27 (suppl 2): S46–S63

Wolf P 1986 Forced normalization. In: Trimble M R, Bolwig T G (eds) Aspects of epilepsy and psychiatry. John Wiley, Chichester, p 101–115

Wolf P, Trimble M R 1985 Biological antagonism and epileptic psychosis. British Journal of Psychiatry 146: 272–276

The significance of a seizure

For many years it has been customary to teach each new generation of medical students that epilepsy is a medical condition. Seizures arise as a result of abnormal brain discharges, usually caused by a damaged area of brain tissue. Abnormal electrical activity arising from this area leads to the genesis of a seizure, either by a change in the physiology of the brain or for some other unspecified reason. Although it is becoming recognised that this model of seizure genesis is too simple, it is not generally appreciated that there must, of necessity, be a close relationship between ongoing cerebral activity, and the capacity of those cells involved in that activity to be diverted into a seizure process. This article examines in some detail the relationship between brain activity, the psychic life of the individual, and the genesis of seizure activity.

THE BRIDGE BETWEEN PSYCHIATRY AND NEUROLOGY

Psychiatry is the study of the diseased mind. Neurology studies the diseased brain. From the point of view of reductionist science, these two words — mind and brain — are synonyms. Reductionist science sees every aspect of mind as determined entirely by alterations in brain states. With the abolition of brain function there is an abolition of mind. It matters not whether we wish to describe the subjective experience of our perceived worlds in terms of the alteration of the flow of neural impulses in different cerebral circuits or whether we wish to describe it in terms of emotion, intellect and volition. Reductionist science, by definition, is unable to draw a distinction between these two. Thus, from the point of view of the reductionist, the psychiatrist with his emphasis on mind, or the neurologist with his emphasis on brain, must be discussing a similar structure, albeit from different viewpoints.

Because the reductionist viewpoint is not properly understood, the sciences of psychiatry and neurology are seen as fundamentally different. This has led to a division within the clinic. For the neurologist seeks to define pathological brain states and rectify these with his physical and physiological treatments (usually drugs), whereas the psychiatrist seeks to define pathological states of mind, and often attempts to rectify these by manipulating the patient's mind (counselling, analysis, behavioural treatment) as well as by physical treatments (drugs).

A study of epilepsy is a study of the bridge between these two disciplines. The pathological seizure discharge can be seen by the neurologist as arising in a particular structure and spreading through distinct brain areas. For the psychiatrist, the aura which is the beginning of the seizure discharge is an experience which is followed by an alteration in the subjective world of the sufferer as the epileptic discharge sweeps through his brain. Within the seizure discharge is the synthesis of neurology and psychiatry. The discharge is a pure demonstration of the precise linking of mind and brain. It also emphasises the point that a true understanding of an epileptic patient and his seizures requires both the neurological and the psychiatric points of view.

The chasm between neurologists and psychiatrists which is the result of the alienation of mind by the 19th century neurologists is bridged in the epilepsy clinic. It is as wrong for the neurologist in his clinic to say, 'Take these drugs and you will be seizure free', as it is for the psychiatrist to say, 'Mend your relationships and you will be seizure free'. For each of these viewpoints gives only half the answer. The neurologist needs to disentangle the psyche of the individual in order to assist the effects of his drugs, while the psychiatrist needs to investigate abnormalities of brain function to make his psychological treatments effective. Perhaps the true balance is to be found in neuropsychiatry, which bestrides both brain and mind.

SEIZURE GENESIS

The most elegant model of seizure genesis is that of focal epilepsy, proposed by the Seattle group. Lockard (1980a), using aluminium hydroxide paste, produced focal epileptogenic lesions in the cortex of monkeys. This epileptogenic area was then implanted with microelectrodes and two populations of epileptogenic cells defined which were called group 1 and group 2. Group 1 neurones were situated at the centre of the focus, were partially damaged, and always fired in an epileptic, bursting mode. These cells were pacemaker cells, and fired abnormally all the time. Their activity was not modified to any significant extent by surrounding brain activity.

Group 2 cells were partially damaged neurones surrounding the focus. They could fire in both the bursting, epileptic mode, and in a normal mode. Thus the activity of these cells could be modified by surrounding brain activity. When a seizure occurred, group 1 cells, which were continually discharging, managed to recruit group 2 cells into the process of the seizure discharge. The spreading out of abnormal discharges within the group 2 cells was a focal seizure. If group 2 cells were able to recruit cells in the normal brain surrounding the abnormal discharges, then the focal seizure would become secondarily generalised, and spread throughout the brain.

What this model clearly shows is that there are two points in the evolution of a seizure where ongoing brain activity can either increase or decrease the likelihood of a seizure. The first is between group 1 and group 2 neurones, and the second between group 2 and normal brain neurones. If this model is correct, then it would indicate that the activity of the background populations of cells would be of crucial importance in determining whether or not a seizure is likely to occur, and whether or not it is likely to spread. When it is recognised that behaviour can alternatively be described in terms of excitation and inhibition of populations of neurones, then it must follow that behaviour should be extremely important in the genesis of seizure activity.

SPIKE AND WAVE SEIZURES

New information has recently become available concerning the likely mechanism of spike and wave seizures. The model which has been proposed by Gloor and co-workers (1980) and Avoli & Gloor (1982) at the Montreal Neurological Institute, is based on the effect of penicillin on the cortex of the cat. Penicillin injected into the cat causes the appearance of generalised spike and wave activity. The underlying mechanism is thought to be the inhibition of the inhibitory processes within the cell by penicillin, leading to hyperexcitability of cortical neurones. The above workers have convincingly shown that spike and wave generation is predominately cortical and that the thalamus plays only a secondary role. He has suggested that the generators of spike and wave activity are cortical, but they can be modifed by reticular formation stimulation. Thus, a complete description of the generator is probably reticulocortical. If this model is correct for man, and there is sufficient indirect evidence that this may be so (Fenwick 1981), then it would be expected that overall changes in reticular activity would be likely to lead either to the genesis or inhibition of seizure discharges. Reticular activity also, like cortical activity, varies as a function of behaviour and, thus again, behaviour could be expected to have a direct effect on seizure frequency.

Spike activity

Lockard (1980b) has suggested that spike activity is caused by the synchronisation of populations of group 1 neurones. The exact reason for this synchronisation is not clear, but on their model, spikes are seen as excitatory. An alternative significance for epileptic spikes has been suggested by Engel et al (1981), who have postulated that epileptic spikes may be inhibitory in nature. He points to, amongst other evidence, the commonly observed fact that spike activity usually slows and then ceases before the development of a grand mal seizure. Whichever model is used, it is likely that changes in spike frequency can be related to seizure frequency.

Lockard (1980b) has also shown that the numbers of spikes occurring at any one time can be modified by, amongst other things, psychosocial processes. In an elegant experiment, she carried out spike counts on her epileptic monkeys before, during and after the exposure of an epileptic monkey low down on the social hierarchy to a more dominant monkey. This exposure significantly increased spike firing, and presumably the likelihood of seizures.

Cortical excitation and behaviour

The contingent negative variation (CNV) is a slow negative potential shift which arises on the surface of the cortex in a forewarned reaction time task. This potential has been called the 'readiness' potential, as it is thought to indicate cortical priming which occurs before the onset of a piece of behaviour. It is only one of a number of negative potential shifts which occur prior to activity. For example, the breitschaftspotential occurs over the motor cortex, just prior to a movement. It is argued that these potentials increase the likelihood of neuronal firing and thus facilitate the expected action. More recent work has shown that the CNV can be activated asymmetrically over the right or left cortex, and this activation is related to specific tasks (Brown et al 1988, Anderson & Fenwick 1988). For example, right temporal tasks, e.g. the classifications of line diagrams, activate the right temporal region more than the left, whereas the classification of line drawn pictures by a verbal category activates the left temporal region more than the right. Additional evidence suggests that there are differences in CNV amplitude related to personality factors (Howard et al 1982). Other studies have shown evoked potential differences for personality factors and for intelligence (Gasser et al 1983). All these studies point to an interaction between behaviour, personality, intelligence and cerebral excitability.

Recent measurement of scalp DC (or very low frequency waves) potentials carried out at the University of Tubingham Department of Psychology has shown that in the seconds before a seizure occurs there is a rapid increase in the scalp negativity. This could be due to the onset of the seizure discharge in the depths, or to a generalised recruitment process which just antedates the seizure.

It would thus be surprising if the facilitatory negative shifts, which are the normal accompaniment of cerebral activity, did not also increase the likelihood of abnormal cerebral discharges. These negative shifts may recruit populations of cells whose activity is being enhanced by alterations of behaviour.

Synchronisation of cell populations

Photosensitive epilepsy is a good example of the way that external stimuli can trigger a seizure. The precise mechanism has been studied in detail by many workers. The clearest account and model is that of Wilkins et al (1980, 1981) and Binnie et al (1985). What they suggest is that rhythmic driving of the retina produces rhythmic stimulation of cells in the visual cortex. Providing a sufficient number of cells are stimulated, then the discharges will spread from the cells which are being driven to normal cells surrounding them, and a generalised seizure may occur. Their hypothesis suggests that both spatial and temporal summation of a stimulated population of cells is required before a critical mass of excited cells is reached. They have shown, as have other workers (Jeavons & Harding 1975, Newmark & Penry 1979) that a simple way of preventing photic seizures is to close one eye. The effect of this is to reduce the population of cells within the visual cortex which are being directly stimulated by the light flashes, and thus the critical mass of excited cells is never reached.

Photosensitive epilepsy is only one example in which rhythmic stimulation of the sensory input to the body may lead to an evoked seizure. It is a general property of the central nervous system that, in susceptible individuals, any form of appropriate (usually rhythmic) peripheral stimulation may evoke a seizure.

Evoked seizures are said to occur in about 5% of people with epilepsy (Symonds 1959). However, rather higher rates are given, particularly in hospital populations, and Fenwick (1981) has suggested in those epileptics attending the Maudsley Hospital that the rate may be nearer 25%. Reading, eating, stimulation of the skin, movement, sounds, smells, can all trigger seizures (Merliss 1974, Fenwick 1981). Although the mechanism has not been established in every case, it is presumed to be similar to that of photic stimulation. The current concept is that peripheral stimulation raises the level of activity within a damaged area of the cortex by rhythmic driving of the cells, and so allows seizure discharges to spread within this area. Alternatively, using the model of Lockard mentioned above, peripheral activity would so increase the level of excitation within a population of neurones that group 1 neurones would be able to recruit group 2 neurones and thus allow a focal seizure discharge to develop. This second hypothesis has the consequence that the opposite can also occur, i.e. that a reduction (or alteration) in the level of excitation in that area of damaged cortex where the epileptic focus is will *prevent* seizure activity from arising and spreading. This point will be discussed further below.

THE THINKING EPILEPSIES

In exactly the same way that stimulation of the brain by a peripheral input will, in certain cases, cause seizures, so will activity within the brain caused by thinking. These have been called the thinking epilepsies by Ingvar & Nyman (1962), Fenwick (1981) and Merliss (1974). Mental activity, such as multiplication or addition, can precipitate seizure activity (Bingel 1957, Symonds 1959, Gomez & Escueta 1977, Ch'en et al 1965, Forster et al

1975, Forster 1977a, Cirignotta et al 1980). Wilkins et al (1980) have documented a case of a patient with a parietal lobe lesion who, whenever he carried out a mathematical calculation, would have an absence attack. The subject was given the WAIS intelligence test while measuring his EEG. Some subtests on the WAIS produced excessive amounts of spike and wave activity. These subtests were testing predominately spatial abilities: the one that produced the greatest increase was block design. It was shown that specific tests which activated the parietal region were the most effective in producing spike and wave activity. Thus, there is little doubt that some specific stimuli, either mental, or physical, can produce epileptic seizures.

Psychogenic seizures

In 1981 Fenwick proposed a classification of seizures generated by an action of mind. These seizures he called psychogenic seizures, indicating that they arose as a consequence of mental activity. He divided psychogenic seizures into primary and secondary. Primary psychogenic seizures are those produced by the direct action of will — the patient deliberately attempts to induce a seizure. Secondary psychogenic seizures are those which occur when the subject is thinking, but not trying to induce a seizure. Clearly, secondary psychogenic seizures are the same as the thinking epilepsies, as they are caused by ongoing activity of the mind.

Primary psychogenic seizures are those seizures which the patient attempts to precipitate deliberately by an act of will. He has usually learned by experience that, by thinking specific thoughts or feelings, he is able to generate a seizure at will. Thus, by a willed action the patient alters neuronal activity in brain areas surrounding his epileptogenic focus and allows a seizure to arise. Psychogenic seizures are common; some examples may be helpful.

Case 1: A young man aged 36 had suffered from partial complex seizures since the age of 4 years, following an attack of meningitis. His seizures commenced in his left temporal lobe and were accompanied by an epigastric aura and a feeling of sadness. He had discovered, when an adolescent, that thinking sad thoughts could cause an aura which would then go on to trigger a secondary generalised seizure. At the time of his father's death, when in his late teens, he would frequently use his seizures to blot out his miseries and unhappiness. He could generate his own seizures by encouraging feelings of unhappiness to arise within him.

Case 2: A 40-year-old woman suffered from brain damage at birth and focal adversive seizures arising in her right frontal lobe. These seizures would start with her head and eyes turning slowly to the left, followed by secondary generalisation and a tonic-clonic grand mal seizure. She discovered, again in her teens, that she could generate these seizures herself, by slowly moving her head in the direction that it was moved by the aura, at the same time deliberately looking out of the left hand corner of her eyes. She found the seizures were even more likely to occur if this procedure was accompanied by chomping movements of her jaws. She too, as an adolescent, would carry out this manoeuvre to produce seizures when her mother had upset her.

It is not only patients with focal epilepsy who can generate their own seizures. Patients with either absence attacks or primary grand mal seizures are also able to do this.

Case 3: A 19-year-old boy had suffered from petit mal epilepsy since the age of 7. His mother had suspected for many years that, when she was cross and scolding him, he would have a shower of absence attacks. However, he had always denied it. In the clinic he told me how he achieved it. He did this by an alteration of his attention. While listening to his mother scolding him, he would suddenly swing his attention to the periphery of his visual attentional field, so as in some way to produce a split in his concentration. This would automatically induce a small absence seizure. He retained this ability right up to the age at which he finally lost his absence attacks.

Case 4: A 22-year-old man with a strong family history of epilepsy had had tonic clonic seizures from the age of 9. There was no evidence of any brain damage either in his history or in his investigations. His seizures commenced with his losing consciousness without a warning and had no focal features. He discovered that he could generate his seizures by lying on the bed and deliberately holding his mind empty and blank for a number of minutes. This would lead to a grand mal seizure and he would then awake in a postictal state, confused and disorientated, a sensation that he quite enjoyed. Not infrequently he would do this when bored and fed up at the weekends.

Both these patients with generalised seizures were able to generate their attacks by manipulating their processes of attention. It thus seems clear that primary psychogenic seizures may be produced either by activating specific brain areas, as in the case of focal seizures, or by using the mechanism of attention and thus altering arousal levels throughout the brain in the case of generalised seizures.

In a recent survey of 76 patients attending the epilepsy clinic at the Maudsley hospital, 22.4% (Fig. 17.1) answered yes to the question, 'This may seem a strange question, but some people with epilepsy have at some time, by a conscious wish, caused a seizure to occur. Have you ever done this?'

In answer to the question, 'Have you ever, when feeling upset in some way, encouraged a seizure to come?' 15.6% said that they had. However, when asked, 'Can you describe what you need to do to make a seizure occur,' 28.6% were able to do so. These figures suggest that between a quarter and a third of patients attending a psychiatric epilepsy clinic are able at will to generate their own seizures. It is well known that patients describe having more seizures in certain situations. In the above survey, over 50% of the patients said that they had seizures when they were tense, depressed, or tired, and over 30% had them when they were angry, excited, or bored. There is thus a very fine line between deliberate induction of seizures and allowing oneself the luxury of a mental state that you know is likely to induce a seizure (Fig. 17.2).

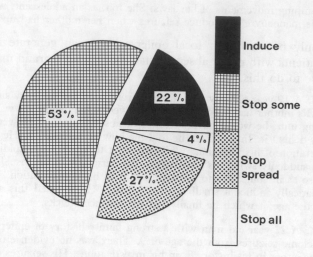

Fig. 17.1 In a recent study of 76 patients at the Maudsley Hospital Epilepsy Clinic, carried out by Dr Loza, 22% could voluntarily induce their seizures; 53% could sometimes stop their seizures; 27% were able to stop their seizures from spreading; only 4% were always able to inhibit their seizures once they had started.

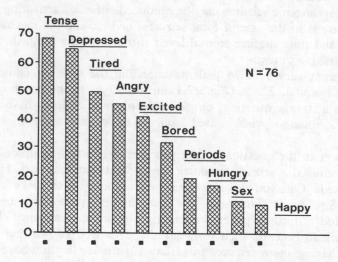

Fig. 17.2 In a recent survey at the Maudsley Hospital, patients were asked which mental states tended to precipitate seizures. The above graph shows the most important factors. It is interesting that nearly 70% of patients had more seizures when they were tense or depressed and only 7% when they were happy. It would seem that happiness is a powerful anticonvulsant.

SEIZURE INHIBITION

Seizure inhibition, like seizure generation, consists of both primary and secondary components. Primary seizure inhibition is the direct inhibition of seizures by an act of will, whereas secondary seizure inhibition is the stopping of seizures by an action of mind or behaviour which interferes with the generation of the seizure process, but is not deliberately intended to do so.

Primary inhibition

The use of external stimulation to inhibit seizure occurrence is already well reported (Efron 1956, Forster et al 1969, Forster 1977b, de Weerdt and van Rijn 1975). Most patients, when asked, have a mental mechanism by which they attempt to inhibit their seizures. A study at the Maudsley Hospital cf 76 patients in the outpatient clinic showed that 53% of these patients claimed that they could sometimes stop their seizures. In answer to the question 'Do you sometimes make yourself have fewer seizures?' 33.8% said yes; 'Can you sometimes stop your seizures from happening?' 36.4% said yes; 'Can you stop your seizures from spreading?' 27.3% said yes (Fig. 17.1).

Thus about a third of patients, when asked, state that they have a mental mechanism by which they stop or inhibit their seizures. These mechanisms do not always succeed, as clearly patients do have seizures which they wish did not occur. To the question, 'Can you always stop seizures if you try?' 3.9% said yes. However, the removal of specific precipitants can be very valuable.

> *Case 5:* A 42-year-old woman had her first grand mal seizure at the age of 16, when she then came to medical attention. She also mentioned that since the age of 6 or 7 she had had feelings of deja vu which had at times been associated with feelings of guilt. She also mentioned an occasion when her vicar called and she had not done her typing for the church magazine. She felt very guilty and immediately had a seizure. Her therapy, in part, consisted of helping her deal with her guilt. She relates that the most powerful anticonvulsant that she has ever been given was, firstly, the recognition that guilt brought on her seizures and secondly, to be taught a method of dealing with this guilt.

When seizures arise from a different area of cortex, different inhibitory strategies will be needed.

> *Case 6:* A 28-year-old man had been suffering from focal motor seizures for two years. These seizures were confined to his left leg and consisted of rhythmical jerking of the leg lasting from a few seconds to a minute, with practically no impairment of consciousness. He found that walking down an incline, or walking into a large room were both likely to precipitate an attack. In both cases, it was the feeling of unsteadiness which he felt was the trigger. In the case of the incline, it was due to poor balance, and in the case of the

room, to a sudden change in visual cues. His seizures were considerably helped by telling him to keep his gaze fixed on a point both when walking down an incline or entering a wide open space. He reported that after doing this there was a significant reduction in his seizure frequency in those situations.

Although it is not possible to be certain why this strategy succeeded, it is known that with routine low-key movements, such as stepping and possibly ordinary, habitual walking, task-related fusimotor drive — or 'set' — is operated at a low level and is static in type. However, when behaviour is difficult or unpredictable, then dynamic gamma-motor neuronal drive is turned hard on, and there is enhanced feedback from the muscle spindles (Prochazka et al 1985). It is possible that this change in feedback in some way alters the excitability of the cortex and, thus, the ability of cells to be recruited into the seizure discharge. Further evidence for this comes from magnetic stimulation of the brain. It is known that the threshold of the motor cortex controlling a limb is considerably reduced if the limb is either taking part in or is about to be used in a voluntary movement. Again, this suggests that the excitability level of motor neurone pools is susceptible to the anticipation of conscious movement. It is possible that by getting this patient to fix his gaze on a specific point, and thus stabilise his walking, he did not have to bring into action his dynamic fusimotor drive, and the motor cortex threshold was not significantly changed as no complex movements were required.

Efron (1956), described a patient with temporal lobe epilepsy who experienced an unusually prolonged and stereotyped aura, beginning with depersonalisation and proceeding through phases of forced thinking, olfactory hallucinations and auditory hallucinations, to adversive head movement and a tonic-clonic seizure. Application of an unpleasant odour prior to the phase of forced thinking, aborted a seizure, but this method alone was not sufficient to reduce the overall frequency of auras. Presumably the stimulus altered the excitability of cells surrounding the focus in some non-specific way, thus preventing further spread of the seizure discharge. Later, it was possible to condition the patient to a visual stimulus; a bracelet which was present at the same time as the smell, so that seizures could be aborted by looking at the bracelet alone. It was fortuitously discovered that a similar effect occurred if the patient thought about the bracelet instead of actually looking at it. Following this there was a decline in seizure frequency until the patient eventually considered herself cured. On the model that is being put forward, it would have to be argued that thinking about the conditioned stimulus changed neuronal excitability in the area of the brain from which seizures were arising. Some support for this is provided by blood-flow studies, which show that blood flow is increased in the expected cortical areas when thinking takes place, and recent EEG brain mapping work which indicates a change in EEG frequencies over the active area of cortex.

Indirect primary inhibition

Indirect primary inhibition of seizures occurs when the patient carries out a set of actions, either physical or mental, which are designed to stop the seizure occurring or generalising, but which act in a non-specific way.

Although it is convenient to think of both seizure induction and inhibition as capable of altering the level of cortical excitability surrounding an epileptic focus, and thus either facilitating or inhibiting the spread of seizure discharges, there are cases where this model does not seem to fit so well. Penn & Wada (1986) described the case of a woman with a right temporal lesion and an aura of deja vu who was able to inhibit her partial complex seizures by singing. She was being assessed for temporal lobec-tomy, so from the intracarotid sodium amytal test results her cerebral dominance for speech was known to be located in the left hemisphere and music in the right hemisphere. Humming was found not to inhibit seizure activity, although singing did so. Unfortunately, she misunderstood instruc-tions to try words or writing, so it is not known if verbal activity on its own would be as effective as singing. What this case showed was that left hemisphere involvement was essential (the words of the song and not just the tune) if her seizures were to be inhibited. It is not known what mech-anism was involved.

Because the excitability of the brain can be altered in a global fashion by changes in reticular formation activity, many non-specific strategies make use of this mechanism to inhibit seizures. For example, Mostofsky & Balaschack (1977) give examples of different strategies which have been found to be effective in stopping seizures. The main mechanism of action is the alerting of the patient, so altering the level of cortical excitability in a non-specific way. This may be accomplished in different ways. Patients whose seizures have focal onsets will commonly either say 'no' to them-selves, or try to attend to something different at the onset of the aura.

A 35-year-old woman with focal motor seizures starting in the arm would, immediately they started, walk about the room or in some other way alert herself. By doing this she was sometimes able to stop the seizures from spreading.

Another patient would hit his arm at the seizure onset, and this would sometimes prevent the seizure from generalising. Whether this functioned by non-specific arousal, or by local stimulation of the arm, so indirectly changing cortical motor excitability, is debatable. The modification of focal cortical epileptogenic discharges by afferent impulses has been described by Prince (1966) and Tassinari (1969).

Deliberate alerting in boring situations has been known to produce a reduction in petit mal seizures. Jung (1962) showed that seizure frequency fell in a patient with petit mal epilepsy when he was kept interested. In another single case study, Ounsted et al (1966) described the case of a girl with petit mal absences who was subjected to a burst of photic stimulation, described by her as mildly unpleasant, whenever a spike-wave paroxysm occurred on her EEG during the experimental sessions. From being severely incapacitated by frequent absence seizures, the patient improved and had only occasional seizures. The authors speculated that repeated photic bombardment raised the total level of physiological arousal, and analysis of background EEG data supported this by showing a decrease in slow wave components.

Secondary inhibition

Secondary inhibition is caused by the activity which occurs when a patient either behaves or thinks in such a way as to produce a reduction in seizure frequency, without deliberately intending to do so. Maintaining interest or not becoming drowsy are such measures. A recent study in an epilepsy centre (Brown, personal communication, 1988) measured the number of seizures, that children had during an art class when soothing music was played and when they were kept interested in painting and modelling. Their seizure frequency was compared with that in ordinary classes and other activities elsewhere in the centre. During the interesting and relaxed art classes significantly fewer seizures occurred.

It is usual for patients to state that there are situations in which they seldom, if ever, have seizures. This varies from patient to patient and with the type of epilepsy. Some patients will have a greatly reduced seizure frequency, or even no seizures, when they are on holiday. Others say they are unlikely to have seizures at the theatre, or in situations in which their interest is held. Yet other patients report that a low key lifestyle, with regular and habitual activity, is the one way in which they can keep themselves seizure free. For them, overstimulation or excess novelty is likely to precipitate seizures. In the Maudsley hospital questionnaire study referred to above, 40.8% of patients said excitement increased their seizures, 45.3% anger, and 58.4% tension and anxiety.

It is not possible to be certain in general why these particular strategies work for particular people, but what can be said is that certain types of activity are likely to enhance the possibility of seizure occurrence, while others will prevent it. The final common pathway for all such activity in those patients who have focal seizures is the stimulation of group 2 neurones, so that they become sufficiently excited to take part in the seizure discharges. A reduction in the excitability levels of this pool of neurones will, of course, directly lead to seizure inhibition. Changes in reticular formation activity, which result from either interest or boredom in the task that the epileptic is carrying out, will also lead to modification and excitability in pools of group 2 neurones and thus alter the likelihood of seizure discharges.

Seizure behaviour

Patients who have generalised grand mal tonic clonic seizures show stereo-typed behaviour consisting of loss of consciousness, falling to the ground, followed by tonic-clonic jerking movements and a postictal confusional state. Because of the complete and total disruption of brain activity, there is no integration between the seizure behaviour and the patient's environment. But those patients who have focal seizures, particularly those whose seizures are followed by complex automatisms, will show a very wide range of behaviour during the seizure itself, and during the period of automatic activity.

The time course of an automatism can be divided into three parts:

1. The initial phase, which lasts only seconds and usually consists of staring or simple mouthing and chewing movements.

2. More complex behaviour, which is still stereotyped and repetitive, such as fumbling with objects, picking at clothes or standing up and turning. This lasts a further few seconds or minutes.

3. In the final phase, behaviour is most complex and may range from the sterotyped into the normal. Complex movements of turning and standing may progress to searching, handling and walking, and then merge imper-ceptibly into normal behaviour (Fenton 1972).

Memory is always impaired during an automatism because, for the automatism to arise, there must have been a bilateral spread of the seizure discharge into both periamygdaloid-hippocampal structures. Jasper (1964) has shown that in stimulation experiments at operation, automatisms arise when the bilateral involvement of the amygdaloid hippocampal structures spreads to the mesial diencephalon and temperoparietal cortex. Automa-tisms usually arise from temporal lobe lesions, but are also seen in discharging lesions of the frontal lobe and orbitofrontal and parietal regions of the mesial surface of the hemisphere (Geier et al 1976, 1977). Conscious-ness is also interfered with during an automatism, so that actions are poorly directed and executed. The patient behaves as if confused, is dazed and disorientated. Aggressive acts are very rare. Most automatisms are brief. Knox (1968) found that 80% last less than 5 minutes, 12% less than 15 minutes and the remaining 8% less than an hour. In a study of 40 patients with 163 partial complex seizures, 14% lasted less than 30 seconds, with the ictal phase ranging from 3 to 343 seconds (mean 54 seconds) and the postictal phase ranging from 3 to 767 seconds (mean 89 seconds) (Theodore et al 1983).

There is always an interaction between the patient and his environment during a seizure: the form the automatism takes is at least partly determined by the patient's thought content and surroundings before a seizure begins. Forster & Liske (1963) quote the case of an organist who had a seizure while playing a hymn. He stopped during the aura and then played a few bars of jazz before recommencing the hymn again. Thus, if a crime is committed during an epileptic automatism, it is possible that some elements of the action may appear purposive.

Because the seizure discharges activate structures which are already involved in ongoing behaviour, the later phases of the automatism contain activity which is relevant to the patient. Thus, patients who have partial complex seizures on the pavement seldom walk into the road, and patients who have seizures on station platforms seldom fall onto the track. Although both these do happen, they happen less frequently than might be expected.

CONCLUSION

Significance of a seizure

Epileptic seizures should not be thought of as arising randomly. They occur, in the case of focal seizures, when the pools of group 2 neurones are sufficiently excitable for seizure activity to spread. Generalised seizures occur when the level of cortical excitability, or corticoreticular excitation, has reached a point at which thalamic recruiting volleys generalise and start to spread.

In the case of the focal epilepsies, a detailed clinical history should be taken as to the nature and characteristics of the aura, and the form that seizure generalisation or spread may take. This information allows the accurate location of the seizure focus and a knowledge of the cerebral structures through which the seizure discharge passes. The position of the focus will determine the relationship between the individual and his epilepsy. It will define those aspects of the psychic life or behaviour of a patient which will both trigger and inhibit seizure activity.

Detailed discussion of this information with the patient will allow the patient to understand that his seizures are not part of a random process, but are intimately related to how he feels, what he is doing and what he is thinking. A complete treatment of epilepsy is not just the giving of drugs, but includes the teaching of the patient about his brain and its functioning, and how his feelings, thinking and behaviour can all be used in the control of his epilepsy.

REFERENCES

Anderson E, Fenwick P 1988 CNV used as an indicator of temporal lobe damage in patients with TLE. (in preparation)
Avoli M, Gloor P 1982 Role of the thalamus in generalised penicillin epilepsy; observations on decorticate cats. Experimental Neurology 77 (2): 386–402
Bingel A 1957 Reading epilepsy. Neurology 7: 752–756
Binnie C, Findlay J, Wilkins A 1985 Mechanisms of epileptogenesis in photosensitive epilepsy implied by the effects of moving patterns. Electroencephalography and Clinical Neurophysiology 61: 1–6
Brown D, Fenwick P, Howard R 1988 CNV asymmetries in response to a task of right or left temporal lobe activation. (in preparation)
Brown S 1988 Personal communication.

Ch'en H, Ch'in C, Ch'u C 1965 Chess epilepsy and card epilepsy. Chinese Medical Journal 84: 470–474

Cirignotta F, Cicogna P, Lugaresi E 1980 Epileptic seizures during card games and draughts. Epilepsia 21: 137–140

de Weerdt C J, van Rijn A J 1975 Conditioning therapy in reading epilepsy. Electroencephalography and Clinical Neurophysiology 39: 417–420

Efron R 1956 The effect of olfactory stimuli in arresting uncinate fits. Brain 79: 267–281

Engel J, Alzerman R, Caldecott-Hazard F, Kuhl D 1981 Epileptic activation of antagonistic systems may explain paradoxical features of experimental and human epilepsy: a review. In: Wada J (ed) Kindling, vol 2. Raven Press, New York

Fenton G W 1972 Epilepsy and automatism. British Journal of Hospital Medicine 7: 57–64

Fenwick P 1981 Precipitation and inhibition of seizures. In: Reynolds E H, Trimble M R (eds) Epilepsy and psychiatry. Churchill Livingstone, Edinburgh, p 306–321

Forster F M 1977a Epilepsy evoked by higher cognitive functions; decision-making epilepsy. In: Reflex epilepsy, behaviour therapy and conditioned reflexes. Charles C Thomas, Springfield, p 124–134

Forster F M 1977b Behavioral therapy of reflex epilepsy: maintenance or reinforcement of therapy. In: Reflex epilepsy, behaviour therapy and conditioned reflexes. Charles C Thomas, Springfield, p 242–255

Forster F M, Liske E 1963 Role of environmental clues in temporal lobe epilepsy. Neurology (Minneap) 13: 310–305

Forster F M, Paulsen W, Baughman F 1969 Clinical therapeutic conditioning in reading epilepsy. Neurology 19: 71–77

Forster F M, Richards J F, Panitch H S, Huisman R E, Paulsen R E 1975 Reflex epilepsy evoked by decision making. Archives of Neurology 32: 54–56

Gasser T, von Lucadou-Müller I, Verleger R, Bächer P 1983 Correlating EEG and IQ: a new look at an old problem using computerised EEG parameters. Electroencephalography and Clinical Neurophysiology 55: 493–504

Geier S, Bancaud J, Talairach J, Bonis A, Szikla G, Enjelvin M 1976 Automatisms during frontal lobe epileptic seizures. Brain 99: 447–458

Geier S, Bancaud J, Talairach J, Bonis A, Szilkla G, Emjelvin M 1977 The seizures of frontal lobe epilepsy. Neurology 27: 951–958

Gomez G L, Escueta A V 1977 In: Forster F M (ed) Reflex epilepsy, behavioural therapy and conditional reflexes. Charles C Thomas, Springfield

Howard R, Fenton G, Fenwick P 1982 Event-related brain potentials and personality in psychopathology: a Pavlovian approach. Research Studies Press. John Wiley, Chichester

Ingvar D H, Nyman G E 1962 Epilepsia arithmetices. Neurology 12: 282–287

Jeavons P, Harding G 1975 Photosensitive epilepsy. A review of the literature and a study of 460 patients. Heinemann, London

Jung R 1962 Blocking of petit mal attacks by sensory arousal and inhibition of attacks by an active change in attention during the epileptic aura. Epilepsia 3: 435

Knox S 1968 Epileptic automatisms and violence. Medicine, science and the law 8: 96–104

Lockard J S 1980a A primate model of clinical epilepsy: mechanisms of action through quantification of therapeutic effects. In: Lockhard J S, Ward A A (eds) Epilepsy: a window to brain mechanisms. Raven Press, New York, p 11–50

Lockard J S 1980b Social primate model of epilepsy. In: Lockhard J S, Ward A A (eds) Epilepsy: a window to brain mechanisms. Raven Press, New York, p 165–190

Merliss J K 1974 Reflex epilepsy. In: Vinken P J, Bruyn G W (eds) Handbook of clinical neurology, vol 15. North Holland Publishing Company, Amsterdam, p 440–456

Mostofsky D I, Balaschak B A 1977 Psychobiological control of seizures. Psychological Bulletin 84: 723–759

Musgrave J, Gloor P 1980 The role of the corpus callosum in bilateral interhemisphereic synchorny of spike and wave discharge in feline penicillin epilepsy. Epilepsia 21: 369–378

Newmark M E, Penry A K 1979 Photosensitivity and epilepsy. A review. Raven Press, New York

Ounsted C, Lee D, Hut S J 1966 Electroencephalographic and clinical changes in an epileptic child during repeated photic stimulation. Electroencephalography and Clinical Neurophysiology 21: 388–391

Penn A, Wada J 1986 Differential effects of singing and dressing/undressing on complex partial seizures originating in the speech non-dominant hemisphere. (AES Proceedings, p 629) Epilepsia 27: 590–650

Prince D A 1966 Modification of focal cortical epileptogenic discharges by afferent impulses. Epilepsia 7: 181–201

Prochazka A, Hulliger M, Zangger P, Appenteng K 1985 'Fusimotor set': new evidence for alpha-independent control of gamma-motor neurones during movement in the awake cat. Brain Research. 339 (1): 136–140

Symonds C 1959 Excitation and inhibition in epilepsy. Brain 82 (2): 133–146

Tassinari C A 1969 Suppression of focal spikes by somato-sensory stimuli. Electroencephalography and Clinical Neurophysiology 25: 574–578

Theodore W, Porter R, Penry K 1983 Complex partial seizures: clinical characteristics and differential diagnosis. Neurology 33: 1115–1121

Wilkins A, Binnie C, Darby C 1980 Visually-induced seizures. Progress in Neurobiology 15: 85–117

Wilkins A J, Binnie C D, Darby C E 1981 Interhemispheric differences in photosensitive epilepsy 1: pattern sensitivity thresholds. Electroencephalography and Clinical Neurophysiology 52: 461–468

Dyscontrol

INTRODUCTION

A relationship between brain pathology and aggressive behaviour was recognised as early as 1715, when Boerhaave noted the relationship between aggression and a rabid infection of the central nervous system. He describes patients as 'gnashing their teeth and snarling like a dog.' Gowers (1892) described his patients as being 'exhausted by attacks of fury.' The relationship of rabies to aggression was explored further by Gastaut et al (1955) who found that the limbic system is heavily involved in the pathological process. This finding was widely recognised as indicating a possible relationship between cerebral damage, but specifically limbic damage, and aggression. These early findings have been amply confirmed by recent brain studies, which have shown a clear relationship between brain damage and aggressive behaviour.

The questions that remain to be answered are where brain lesions have to occur for aggressive behaviour to develop and whether specific behavioural syndromes can arise from specific brain lesions. This article will explore the possibility that abnormal paroxysmal discharges occurring deep in the brain can lead to paroxysmal disorders of behaviour.

Kaplan (1899), gave this description of sudden paroxysmal violent behaviour:

> Following the most trivial and most impersonal causes, there is the effect of rage with its motor accompaniments. There may be the most grotesque gesticulations, excessive movements of the face, and a quick, sharp explosiveness of speech; there may be cursing and outbreaks of violence which are often directed towards things; there may or may not be amnesia for these events afterwards. These outbursts may terminate in an epileptic fit. There is an excess in the reaction with inadequate adaptation to the situation which is so remote from a well considered and purposeful act that it approaches a pure psychic reflex.

This concept of a psychic reflex or a sudden massive outpouring of rage in response to a trivial stimulus is the basis of the modern dyscontrol syndrome.

With the discovery of the EEG, it was hoped that the question of the nature of paroxysmal rage attacks would be solved. Indeed, when it was demonstrated that epilepsy showed distinctive patterns, a search was made for paroxysmal discharges from the cortex which would be the electrical equivalent of an episode of rage. Unfortunately, this was not found, although occasionally minor paroxysmal discharges were noted. This led to the conclusion that rage attacks and paroxysmal cortical discharges (epilepsy) were different. However, the recent information from those laboratories with electrodes implanted in the limbic structures is that limbic discharges can occur without generalising to the cortex. It is this finding that prompts a re-examination of the relationship between dyscontrol and epilepsy.

THE DYSCONTROL SYNDROME

Early EEG studies showed a relationship between paroxysmal discharges in the EEG during a seizure and alterations of behaviour. It was also established that similar discharges could occur in the EEGs of patients who were not having a seizure but who were liable to show paroxysmal disorders of aggressive behaviour. It was therefore postulated that paroxysmal disorders of behaviour could be due to 'covert epilepsy' (sometimes called epileptic equivalent) — an abnormality of brain function which, although not epileptic in the clinical sense, was dependent on abnormal cerebral discharges.

Heath & Mickle (1960) and Sem-Jacobson (1968), using neurosurgical implantation of electrodes, showed a correlation between deep-seated limbic discharges and disorders of behaviour in patients whose cortical rhythms were unaffected by the subcortical discharges. These findings led Monroe (1970) to suggest that paroxysmal disorders of behaviour arising from paroxysmal discharges of subcortical structures were not necessarily recorded by the EEG on the surface of the cortex. He proposed a specific behavioural syndrome, episodic dyscontrol, which he defined (Monroe 1974) as:

> an interruption in the lifestyle and life flow of the individual, involving either a single act or short series of acts with a single intention . . . the common features . . . are precipitous onset of symptoms, equally abrupt remissions, as well as the tendency of frequent recurrences.

Monroe was careful to point out that this syndrome could only occur in patients who did not have a long-standing disorder of personality. He was also careful to distinguish between cases in which these episodes of behaviour were out of character and atypical for the individual and those in which there is a chronic and persistent disorder of behaviour, with waxing and waning, as occurs in habitually violent individuals.

Mark & Ervin (1970) were more specific in the behavioural characteristics that they attributed to this syndrome, and suggested the following features:

1. A history of physical assault, especially wife and child beating.

2. The symptoms of pathological intoxication — i.e. drinking even a small amount of alcohol triggers acts of senseless brutality.

3. A history of impulsive sexual behaviour, including at times sexual assaults.

4. A history in car drivers of many traffic violations and serious automobile accidents.

Maletsky (1973) described 22 patients with episodic dyscontrol who fitted the criteria of Monroe and Mark & Ervin.

> The subjects demonstrated violent loss of control upon minimal provocation, aurae [sic] and postictal states following such episodes, a history of alcoholism and increased aggression after alcohol, a childhood history of hypokinesis and truancy, and a family background of alcoholism, sociopathy and violence in the males, and depression in the females. Such patients have frequently been in trouble with the law and were especially prone to use their automobiles aggressively.

This group of patients clearly had heterogeneous cerebral pathology and there is little clinical evidence to suggest that their violent behaviour is part of a clinical syndrome. However, this study did demonstrate that a large proportion of these people responded in a dramatic way to medication with phenytoin and, together with the previous work of Mark & Ervin, and Monroe, reinforced the idea of an epileptic diathesis in these patients.

Studies of 130 violent patients and 62 habitually violent men (Bach-y-Rita et al 1971, Bach-y-Rita & Veno 1974), again stress the significance of non-specific brain pathology, especially that related to the limbic system. Their sample contained many patients with multiple pathology similar to that described by Maletsky. However, they again concluded that the dyscontrol syndrome is a specific entity.

A case report of a 24-year-old single female who had episodes of violent behaviour, was deaf, borderline mentally defective and in long-term institutional care led Tunks & Dermer (1977) to suggest that carbamazepine is an effective treatment of the dyscontrol syndrome. However, although this case has been quoted by others as an example of the beneficial effects of carbamazepine in the dyscontrol syndrome, medication was unlikely to have been the sole cause of her improvement, as many other non-specific factors were clearly involved.

Carbamazepine is now widely used in the treatment of episodes of violence, whether or not they have an ictal basis, and other authors have studied the possibility that other anticonvulsant drugs may be effective. Andrulonis et al (1980) studied the effect of ethosuximide in patients described as suffering from:

> . . . acts of violence, drug or alcohol abuse, traffic violations, arrests, job or school failures, suicide attempts, and resistance to conventional psychiatric interventions. As children these patients often suffered from head trauma, hyperactivity and learning disabilities. They had a family history of sociopathy, alcoholism and violence.

The authors conclude, 'that ethosuximide, when used in the treatment of patients exhibiting episodic dyscontrol, has the potential for producing an excellent clinical response with few side effects'. Again it should be noted that the heterogenous nature of this population of patients makes it impossible to be certain either that a specific pathological entity is being treated or that these results are not due to non-specific factors.

Two studies by Elliott (1976, 1982) examined the relationship of aggressive and violent behaviour with both organic brain disease and minimal brain dysfunction. In the first study of 70 patients with organic cerebral pathology from numerous different causes, symptoms of emotional dyscontrol or violence were elicited in half the patients only after careful questioning. In a second retrospective study he reports:

> . . . the neurological findings in 286 patients with a history of recurrent attacks of uncontrollable rage occurring with little or no provocation and dating from early childhood or from a physical brain insult at a later date. Objective evidence of developmental or acquired brain defects was found in 94%. The most common abnormality was found in minimal brain dysfunction, which was found in 41%. The diagnosis was not made on behavioural symptoms alone; there had to be positive neurological and/or laboratory evidence. The most common symptom, apart from episodic dyscontrol, was complex partial seizures which had occurred at some time in the life of 30% of the patients. In many, the seizures had not been recognised as epileptic because of their subtle form and rare occurrence. Convulsions and dramatic attacks with unconsciousness were rare. One-third of the patients presented a variety of psychiatric disorders, persisting for days, weeks or months, in addition to episodic rage.

A review of the literature relating to the dyscontrol syndrome by Ratner & Shapiro (1979) includes a report of a case of paroxysmal and violent behaviour in a usually placid man which led to him killing. The neurological, neuropsychological and neuroradiological investigations showed some evidence of organic brain dysfunction. The authors stress the significance of a response which is out of proportion to the stimulus and which lacks a reflective component — the epileptic equivalent (epileptoid response) of Monroe. They are the first authors, as far as I know, to have taken the concept of dyscontrol to its logical conclusion, by acknowledging that if organic pathology is involved and a defect in impulse control results from it, then offenders with this defect should not have to accept complete responsibility for their acts. They said:

> Though still 'experimental', the concepts we presented were persuasive to the authors, although the concept and precise criteria for the organic or epileptoid dyscontrol syndrome are still evolving. We do not feel we would be more correct to have ignored this material and insisted, with the government psychiatrist, that in spite of the substantial evidence of brain dysfunction in our patient, and despite the classic similarity of his history and behaviour pattern to that of individuals with known neurological disease, our patient was merely suffering from a 'personality disorder'. We therefore concluded in our letter to the court that (the patient) was, in our opinion, not guilty by reason

of insanity at the time of the offence, by virtue of a mental defect, namely, episodic dyscontrol syndrome, epileptoid type.

Statistical clustering has been used to differentiate patients with episodic dyscontrol from other patients who are diagnosed as having a borderline personality (Andrulonis et al 1982). A group of patients with the episodic dyscontrol syndrome was distinguished by means of cluster analysis from a patient population diagnosed as borderline personality, using the criteria of the DSM-III. Of interest is the high degree of organic brain pathology shown by patients within this subgroup, who not only had the episodic dyscontrol syndrome as defined by Monroe, but also showed minimal brain damage or limbic system disorders.

THE NEUROPHYSIOLOGICAL BASIS OF AGGRESSION

It has been suggested that aggression is not a simple unitary emotion and that it may have several components. Moyer (1971) has suggested a neural basis of aggression based on a survey of research in this area. He has shown that aggression falls into a number of different categories, which he has defined as predatory, territorial, inter-male, maternal, defensive fear-induced, irritable and instrumental. Each category has either a specific outward behaviour or a definite stimulus which determines it. The dyscontrol syndrome is based on the hypothesis that there are specific brain structures which are related to the mediation of aggression: studies of aggression in animals indicate that several sites within the limbic system and hypothalamus can potentially enhance, modify or reduce aggression.

Some neurophysiological evidence that the different aggression circuits are situated in the lateral and medial hypothalamus and the ventromedial nucleus of the hypothalamus is given by Moyer (1971). There is some evidence that these circuits are cholinergic (Smith et al 1970). Yasukochi (1960) has suggested that fear-induced aggression arises from the anterior hypothalamus and the dorsal hypothalamus (Romaniuk 1965).

The amygdala may play both an inhibitory and an excitatory role in aggression (Gloor et al 1981). Moyer has suggested that there are eight identifiable nuclei in the amygdala, each of which is involved in the localisation of aggression. Irritable aggression in animals is facilitated from the medial nuclei and inhibited from the central nuclei. The rhinencephalic structures, hippocampus and cingulate gyrus (limbic system, Papez circuit) are also involved. Hippocampal lesions appear to increase irritable aggression in cats (Green et al 1957), and cholinergic stimulation of the hippocampus has confirmed this (Maclean & Delgado (1953). Destruction of the cingulate gyrus in both dogs (Brutkowski et al 1961), and cats (Kennard 1955), has been shown to lead to an increase in irritable aggression. However, this is clearly species specific as cingulectomy in monkeys (Kennard 1955) and in man (Le Beau 1952, Tow & Whitty 1953) has been shown to make monkeys tamer and more docile and lead to the calming of violence in man.

Kindling and neuroresponsiveness

Adamek & Stark-Adamek (1983) suggest that cats with higher discharge rates of the basal amygdala showed most defensive and least aggressive behaviour when activity of their amygdala was directed towards the medial hypothalamus. They found that more aggressive cats showed higher discharge rates of the ventral hippocampus. Prekindling of the amygdala in cats led to an increase in discharge rates to the medial hypothalamus and inhibition of amygdala discharges to the ventral hippocampus, and to behaviour which was more defensive and less aggressive (Fig. 18.1).

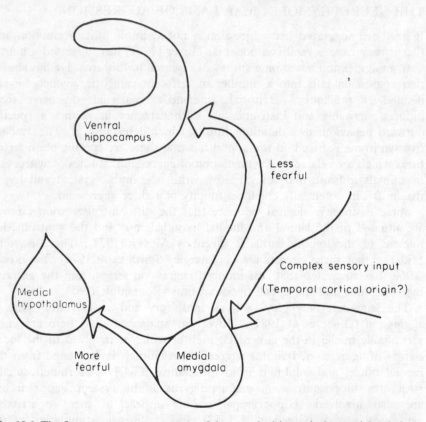

Fig. 18.1 The figure represents a summary of data acquired by evoked potential techniques which indicate different preferential routes of conduction of evoked excitatory neural activity from the amygdala to the ventromedial hypothalamus (VMH-or medial hypothalamus in the figure), and from the amygdala to the ventral hippocampus. More fearful cats display enhanced conduction from amygdala to the VMH. Less fearful cats show the strongest conduction from the amygdala to the ventral hippocampus. (Reproduced with kind permission from Adamek & Stark-Adamek 1983).

These authors support the current idea that kindling, leading to a permanent change in the neurotransmission characteristics of the structures already mentioned, may make the animal permanently either more or less aggressive and argue that this could apply to man, although they admit that in this case the evidence is less secure. In support of this view they quote the evidence, amongst others, of Hermann (1982) who showed different MMPI profiles for patients with complex partial seizures, depending on whether or not the seizure started with an aura of fear, showing limbic system involvement. Halgren et al (1978) and Gloor et al (1982) have shown that human emotions can be altered by direct electrical limbic system stimulation, which again suggests a change in limbic system functioning in patients with epilepsy.

If further evidence is found that kindling is not species specific, but is applicable to man, then it could be argued that discharging lesions or brain injury situated in the limbic system but specifically involving the amygdala, ventral hippocampus and medial hypothalamus, would modify the functioning of these structures. Individuals would become more or less aggressive; more aggressive if the functioning of the amygdala towards the ventral hippocampus was enhanced, less aggressive and more fearful if the activity of the amygdala towards the medial hypothalamus was enhanced. The idea of 'periods' in development may also be relevant to this theory. Taylor (1981) has consistently emphasised that the effect of brain damage will depend on when during development the damage occurs. The timing of the onset of the brain injury may thus be crucial in its effect on limbic functioning.

NEUROPHYSIOLOGICAL AND SURGICAL STUDIES IN MAN

The mediation of aggression

Intracranial stimulation in man has provided some evidence that there are specific brain areas which are involved with the mediation of aggression and others which, when stimulated, will tranquillize. Electrodes implanted in the centromedian thalamus have been shown to lead to very high self-stimulation rates, and repeated stimulation rapidly led to an aroused angry state (Heath 1963). The behaviour of a second patient, stimulated in the septral region while he was in an agitated, violent and psychotic state, almost instantly changed to behaviour that was happy and mildly euphoric. Mark & Ervin (1970) report the case of a patient who became aggressive and violent during a partial complex seizure. Electrodes implanted in the amygdala showed that abnormal behaviour coincided with an amygdala-ictal discharge. Hitchcock & Cairns (1973) induced both rage and escape attempts in a patient by stimulation of the amygdala. Heath & Mickle (1960) found a wide range of responses, including aggressive behaviour, following stimulation.

However the idea that aggression arises when specific neural pathways in man are stimulated or invaded by seizure discharges has now fallen out of fashion. Amygdala stimulation in man has very rarely been shown to lead to the expression of violence (Gloor 1972); Higgins et al (1956) and Chapman (1958) were unable to evoke aggressive behaviour with peri-amygdaloid and temporal lobe stimulation. Amygdala stimulation may have a paradoxical effect; direct stimulation and ictal discharges normally lead to the sensation of fear, whereas the abnormally facilitated response to an external stimulus is seldom fear but a outburst of fighting (Gloor 1978). Wieser (1983) reports two patients in whom there is a clear relationship between aggressive behaviour and ictal activity in the deep limbic structures. Cortical detection of these deep seizures was not always possible.

In summary, it seems probable that the amygdala, hippocampus and the hypothalamus are all involved in the mediation of aggression in man. It is thus logical to assume that either damage to or seizure discharges traversing these structures and interfering with their function may well lead to aggressive behaviour.

Amygdalectomies in man

Although animal experiments do not make clear the precise role of the amygdala in man, there is nevertheless sufficient evidence to suggest that neurosurgical intervention in man could lessen aggressive behaviour.

Narabayashi et al (1963) and Hitchcock & Cairns (1973) reported significant improvements in the majority of subjects in whom they carried out amygdalectomies. Mark et al (1975) described six patients who had received bilateral amygdala lesions. In three of these the rage attacks ceased; in one attacks decreased, while two patients experienced no relief from their aggressive episodes. Unfortunately again, quantifiable data was not presented.

Not all studies have been as successful. Kim & Umbach (1973) found no decrease in aggressive behaviour after amygdala lesions. Although this may, in part, have been due to the rather different patient populations that they used, Nádvorník et al (1973) have confirmed these negative results using a population similar to that of the more successful studies.

Sano et al (1970), building on the observation in animal work that the posterior hypothalamus is involved with the mediation of aggression, induced lesions in the posterior hypothalamus in 44 patients. They were successful in reducing aggression, as 12 patients had excellent results.

It may be remembered that in Heath's (1963) study, stimulation of the central median nucleus of the thalamus led rapidly to an aroused, angry state. Andy (1970) argued that destruction of this area by thalamotomy, was likely to reduce aggressive behaviour. Five patients had surgical lesions in this area and he reports an attenuation of aggressive behaviour in all these patients.

Although amygdalectomy has been found to be helpful only in some studies, many of the populations which were treated had large numbers of brain damaged and mentally subnormal patients. Neurosurgery may still prove to have a place in the treatment of aggressive behaviour, but it is clear that the criteria needed to choose those patients who can be helped by amygdalectomy are not yet sufficiently understood.

AGGRESSIVE BEHAVIOUR IN EPILEPSY AND THE DYSCONTROL SYNDROME

It has often been suggested that, if there is a connection between epilepsy, aggression and the dyscontrol syndrome, then populations of patients with epilepsy should show a higher prevalence of aggressive behaviour. Unfortunately, in many of these studies aggressive behaviour is not precisely defined and therefore comparison between studies is difficult. An additional difficulty is the difference in reported incidence between different populations; higher rates of aggression are to be expected in those populations whose epilepsy is more intractable. These patients are likely to be on higher doses of anticonvulsant medication and to have more severe brain damage (Stevens 1975). It is well known that brain damage, poor impulse control and aggression are all related.

Violent behaviour may be the result of cultural, situational, or pathological factors, and is usually a combination of all three factors. A higher proportion of violence is found in social class III and IV than in I and II (Whitman et al 1980). Socioeconomic factors, such as poor housing and education, are generally accepted as contributory to these higher levels of violence. Situational violence is determined by specific factors at the time of the violent behaviour. Most murders, for example, are committed within the family and many acts of violence take place in the context of crime. Severe injury is more likely to result from an act of violence if the victim is elderly or young.

The prevalence of paroxysmal rage

Gastaut et al (1955) reported an unusually high incidence of paroxysmal rages (50%) in his group of patients with temporal lobe epilepsy. Currie and coworkers (1971), in a survey of 666 patients with temporal lobe epilepsy of mixed aetiology and type at the London Hospital found aggression reported in 7%. Pathological aggression was reported in only 4.8% of a population of 700 cases from the Michigan Epilepsy Centre (Rodin 1973). The majority of the aggressive group were young men with below-average intelligence. When compared to a control group without aggressive outbursts and matched for age, sex and IQ, those with aggression had a higher rate of psychiatric problems and showed more evidence of organic damage in the central nervous system. Bingley (1958), looking at 90 patients from both neurological and neurosurgical clinics of a general hospital in Sweden, found that 17% of patients with temporal lobe epilepsy showed aggressive behaviour. However, patients attending neurology clinics have been shown to be selected by the presence of psychiatric disorder (Pond & Bidwell 1960) and the true prevalence of aggressive behaviour in Bingley's study may have been masked by this factor.

A study of patients with severe epilepsy who were assessed for temporal lobectomy at the Maudsley Neurosurgical Unit showed a high prevalence of aggressive behaviour (Falconer 1973). In those patients who had a predominately unilateral spike focus (mainly left sided), pathological outbursts of aggressive behaviour occurred in 38% of 50 cases. Many of these individuals were well adjusted. A further 14% showed milder or more persistent aggresiveness associated with a paranoid outlook. These patients had been originally described by James (1960), Serafetinides (1965) and Taylor (1969). This was a patient population with a high rate of psychiatric disorder and severe drug-resistant epilepsy. In many of these patients there was evidence of brain damage and an early onset of epilepsy, both of which could be expected to lead to aggressive behaviour due to poor impulse control and disordered social development.

An increased prevalence of patients with epilepsy in prison populations has been found in many different studies (Whitman et al 1984, King & Young 1978, Derro 1978, Norvik et al 1977, Gunn & Fenton 1969, 1971). This increased prevalence is, however, likely to be due to many non-specific factors:

1. Prisoners are selected from populations of socioeconomic class III and IV, in which there is already a higher prevalence of epilepsy.

2. Some studies have found a higher prevalence of post-traumatic epilepsy in prison populations, which again suggests that these prisoners came from a violent subculture.

3. There is a weak link between aggressive behaviour and committal to prison.

4. There is no difference in the number or nature of violent crimes committed by prisoners with epilepsy and those without.

5. Those studies which have specifically compared violent with non-violent prisoners (Gunn & Bonn 1971) found no differences in the prevalence of epilepsy.

EVIDENCE FOR SEIZURE DISCHARGES IN LIMBIC STRUCTURES LEADING TO AGGRESSIVE BEHAVIOUR

Although there is a clear relationship between brain damage, poor impulse control and aggression, it is not clear whether, in the absence of brain damage, seizure discharges within the limbic system can lead to violent and aggressive behaviour. It has been suggested that aggressiveness is more frequently reported in patients with seizures and especially those with temporal lobe seizures. Aggressive behaviour may conveniently be classified into that occurring during the seizure and postictally and that which is interictal, occurring between seizures in a setting of clear consciousness.

Ictal aggression

Aggressive episodes of disordered behaviour, which have as their basis an ictal discharge, have already been mentioned. There is evidence that temporal lobe discharges, which involve the hippocampus, amygdala and hypothalamus, are particularly likely to lead to episodes of violent behaviour. These episodes have the characteristics that would be expected if they were due to seizure activity: there is a disorder of consciousness, and the aggressive activity is usually carried out in a disordered, uncoordinated and non-directed way. However, the number of cases of ictal aggression published in the literature is small. One reason for this is the difficulty in being certain that the event described is ictal in origin, as it has not previously been possible to monitor patients continuously in the community (Lewis & Pincus 1983 — letter).

Delgado-Escueta et al (1981), in a comprehensive study, rated 5400 videotaped seizures collected from different units throughout the world according to the degree of ictal violence. They concluded that frank ictal violence is very rare — only 13 cases of violent behaviour were found (most of which were postictal and occurred in a confusional setting), and only 3 patients had attacked people.

This study is methodologically sound, but the authors did not, unfortunately, take into account that the form an epileptic seizure takes is dependent, not only on the spread of the discharge through the brain, but also on the thought content of the patient at the time of the seizure. The literature provides many examples of the interraction between the patient's intended action and the modification of this by the seizure. It is thus not surprising that Delgado-Escueta and co-workers should find so few cases of ictal aggression in the clinical situation of a videotape recording laboratory.

Aggression occurs to a much lesser extent in hospital than it does in the community — a point amply demonstrated in a study by King & Ajmone Marsan (1977) who studied 270 epileptic patients with temporal lobe foci and observed complex partial seizures in 199 of these. Twenty of these patients had a history of interictal violent behaviour, but none displayed interictal violence in hospital. However, 9 of the 199 patients for whom well-observed seizures had been recorded had periictal behaviour that could be defined as violent. In most cases this was postictal and confusional in nature. Rodin (1973), who recorded 150 patients with seizures in hospital between 1959 and 1964, also found that with one possible exception, none at any time showed clear evidence of ictal aggression. Rodin and subsequent workers interpreted this finding as suggesting that ictal violence is rare, but it could in part be due to the recording situation in hospital. Further evidence can only be obtained by portable recording devices used at home.

Other examples of ictal aggression have already been mentioned (Heath, Mark, Ervin, Gloor and Wieser). Knox (1968), in a systematic study of the relationship between epileptic automatism and violence in 434 epileptic outpatients, found only 1 patient who had acted in an aggressive and violent fashion. Gunn (1979) and Gunn & Fenton (1969, 1971), in a survey of epileptic offenders in prisons and borstals in England and Wales found only 2 persons out of a total of 158 whose crime was probably committed during or following a seizure, 1 in a possible postictal automatism, the other in a postictal phase. A survey of the 29 male epileptic offenders in Broadmoor hospital, a special hospital for violent psychiatric offenders, found a definite relationship between crime and seizures in only 2 cases, both of which had behaved violently in a postictal confusional state. Fenwick (1984) describes the case of a brain-damaged man with complex partial seizures who attacked and severely injured a neighbour during a witnessed automatism. Another case to come before the British courts was a man who also suffered from TLE and, during a presumed automatism, killed a woman with a chisel. Further cases of ictal aggression have been described by Stevenson (1963), Brewer (1971) Gunn (1978), Milne (1979), Cope & Donovan (1979) and Simon & de Silva (1981).

Not all of these studies provide clear evidence that direct ictal behaviour was the sole responsible cause for the aggressive acts mentioned, but there is certainly evidence to support the conclusion that ictal violence, though rare, does occasionally occur. (For a fuller review see Treiman & Delgado-Escueta 1983 and Fenwick 1986.)

Lewis et al (1982), in a study of children in a reform school, found 5 of the 78 violent boys had committed violent acts during an ictus. Lewis & Pincus (1983) state: 'Clearly, most violence in this group was not caused by epilepsy, but neither was the association (with ictal discharge) exceedingly rare'.

Not every authority concurs with the view that ictal violence does occur, despite the positive evidence. Penfield and Jasper (1954) state, regarding anger: 'So far as our experience goes, neither localised epileptic discharge, nor electrical stimulation, is capable of awakening any such emotion'. Gloor (1967) reports never having seen a case of ictal rage. Later evidence suggests that this may be due to selection of cases rather than to a lack of association between ictal violence and epilepsy.

Interictal aggression

The literature on interictal aggression is confused. The definition of aggression is unclear in many studies and most fail to describe the relationship of the aggressive behaviour to the underlying personality. Mungus (1983) using cluster analysis, was able to define five homogenous subgroups derived from 138 neuropsychiatric outpatients who attended UCLA Neurobehavioural Clinic. Seizure disorders were related to only two of these categories, and these showed a high frequency of impulsive, violent acts. Specific seizure type was not investigated, owing to sample size, and no relationship was found between temporal lobe abnormalities and any of the five categories. He concluded that violent behaviour was not a unitary measure and that seizures were not related to all types of violence.

Violent individuals tend to come from the lower socioeconomic groups where there are higher levels of perinatal mortality, infections and trauma. Many come from violent families and have a history of violent behaviour since childhood. Most are males under the age of 40 and a large number show 'soft' neurological signs and abnormal EEGs. They often show cognitive impairment, a high proportion are left handers and many show poor attention span and occasionally focal cognitive deficits. When all these factors are taken into account, many of the associations of aggression and violence with epilepsy become weaker (Stevens & Hermann 1981).

Despite all the evidence that temporal lobe epilepsy may have a special relationship to violence (Nuffield 1961, Currie et al 1971, Lindsay et al 1979, Fenwick & Fenwick 1985), methodological difficulties and patient selection weaken the correlations found between interictal aggression and temporal lobe epilepsy. The commonest fault in all these studies is a lack of adequate control groups. When they are used, many of the differences which were apparently significant disappear. It is clear that there is a relationship between aggressive behaviour and epilepsy, but two recent reviews of the literature conclude that this is probably due to non-specific factors which are common in both violent populations and patients with epilepsy, most significantly the associated brain damage (Kligman & Goldberg 1975, Stevens & Hermann 1981).

Relationship of EEG abnormalities to aggressive behaviour and dyscontrol

Both Stafford-Clarke & Taylor (1949) and Hill & Pond (1952) studied the EEGs of alleged murderers. Only a third of those patients who had claimed epilepsy as a defence had specific abnormalities which were thought to be epileptic in nature. Non-specific abnormalities were common, but no more so than in other studies of prison populations. Williams (1969) found that 65% of 333 habitually aggressive prisoners showed abnormal EEGs, compared to 12% of the normal population. Although these patients did not necessarily have temporal lobe epilepsy, he felt there was a relationship between temporal lobe epilepsy, pathology and aggression. However, many of these patients had other weak indicators of associated brain damage and these other variables tend to confound the suggested relationship between temporal lobe epilepsy and aggression.

Numerous studies in the 1960s showed that, in many psychiatric conditions, e.g. schizophrenia and psychopathy, cortical excitability was increased and thus seizure threshold was reduced (Hill & Parr 1963).

Monroe believed that specific EEG patterns occurring during cortical activation were indicative of an epileptic tendency and poor impulse control, and that they might therefore be directly related to the dyscontrol syndrome. However, this was not found to be so, as many studies also showed that the EEGs of patients with different types of psychiatric disorder showed paroxysmal activity which could be produced by activation techniques (Monroe et al 1956).

Some of the EEG abnormalities found in these populations have been clearly shown to be the results of perinatal cerebral insults or later acquired damage (Volavka & Matousek 1969). But these early studies did show definite evidence that an increase in cortical excitability was frequently found in groups of patients with behaviour disorders. Small showed the presence of spikes correlated with a significant increase in suicide attempts and psychotic depressive episodes (Small 1970, Small et al 1975), a finding enlarged by Struve et al (1977) to include suicidal ideation. However, an increase in cortical excitation even without spiking is significant. Small (1971) found that raised cortical excitability, shown by the presence of photoconvulsive responses correlated with attempts of suicide in a psychiatric population. Impulsive suicide attempts are significantly increased in patients with schizophrenia who show phenothiazine evoked EEG abnormalities. Davies et al (1975) have demonstrated a lowered seizure threshold in these patients.

It seems probable that the EEG changes found in patients with the dyscontrol syndrome are non-specific and are more likely to relate to underlying cerebral pathology than to a specific epileptic mechanism. Riley & Niedermeyer (1978) found slightly abnormal EEGs in 6.6% of 212 patients who were referred for acts of violence and outbursts of aggression without provocation, although none of these abnormalities was characteristic of epilepsy. They suggested that there was no definite relationship between aggressive behaviour as such and EEG abnormalities and certainly there was nothing to suggest that epilepsy was involved.

BRAIN DAMAGE, EPILEPSY AND DYSCONTROL

The previous section reviewed the literature relating to aggression arising interictally in clear consciousness in patients with epilepsy, and concluded that although there is an association between epilepsy and violence, this is not on a one-to-one basis, and many non-specific factors are involved. There is a very wide literature relating to brain damage and poor impulse control; this section is not an exhaustive review but will extract some of the main points for consideration.

Rutter (1982), in a review paper on concepts, issues and prospects in developmental psychiatry, examines the behavioural sequelae of head injuries in childhood, and the relationship between the severity of the injury and the type of neurological deficit and psychiatric morbidity which follows.

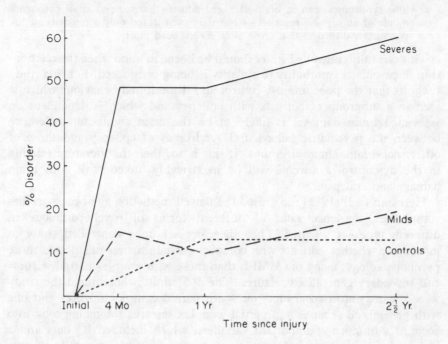

Fig. 18.2 Rates of new psychiatric disorders in children with closed head injuries. (Reproduced with kind permission from Rutter 1982.)

In a 2½-year prospective study of children suffering closed head injuries they looked at the relationship between those with severe head injuries (post-traumatic amnesia greater than 7 days), mild head injuries (PTA greater than 1 hour but less than 7 days), and a group of control children who were admitted to hospital with non-cephalic, mainly orthopaedic injuries. The patients' behaviour *before* the injury was assessed by interview with parents, teachers, etc. Following the injury the patients' psychiatric and neurological status were examined at 4 months, 1 year and 2½ years. The results of this study are shown in Figure 18.2.

It can be seen that it is only severe brain damage that leads to a high incidence of psychiatric morbidity. In comparing the controls and the brain damaged groups, they conclude:

> According to the psychiatric diagnoses, detailed parental interview ratings of individual behaviours, observations during psychological testings, and teacher questionnaire ratings: all of these separate comparisons were in agreement in showing that, with the sole (but important) exception of socially inappropriate and disinhibited behaviour, the emotional and behavioural problems attributable to head injury were closely similar to those known *not* to be due to brain damage. The great majority of the 'organic' psychiatric reactions were *not* recognisably different from functional disorders . . . It was only the disinhibited patterns of behaviour (of a type rather comparable to so-called frontal

lobe syndromes seen in brain-damaged adults) that seemed at all pathognomonic of an organic reaction — but they constituted only a minority of the
psychiatric disorders that arose after severe head injury.

This carefully controlled study should be borne in mind when the relationship of psychiatric morbidity to epilepsy is being considered. For this study
suggests that the poor impulse control and disinhibited behaviour which is
seen in a subgroup of patients with epilepsy and which is dependent on
associated brain damage, is likely to be the main significant difference
between the psychiatric behavioural syndromes of epilepsy and those of
other, non-brain-damaged groups. If this is so, then the literature relating
to the dyscontrol syndrome will be inextricably linked with both brain
damage and epilepsy.

Hermann et al (1982) recognised the flawed methodology of most studies
comparing prevalence rates of different forms of psychopathology in
different types of seizures. They therefore set up a controlled study to
investigate whether patients with complex partial seizures manifested more
psychopathology, using the MMPI, than those with complex partial seizures
and secondary generalised seizures. The 165 adults who entered the study
were divided into two groups, one with partial complex seizures and one
with generalised seizures and partial complex seizures. Matching took into
account a number of important variables, which included IQ data and a
Halstead Impairment Index (test of brain damage), as well as age,
education, age of onset of seizures and duration of seizures.

Hermann et al found that the group with multiple seizure types scored
higher in the increased psychopathological direction than the single seizure
group on every measure used in the study. This finding is important as it
could have been argued that multiple seizure types correlated with higher
degrees of brain damage and it was the brain damage which led to the
increased rates of psychiatric morbidity. It is of interest that the psychopathic deviance scale of the MMPI was one of the scales to show the
greatest difference between the groups. This scale is known to be associated
with poor impulse control and thus this study can be interpreted as indicating that patients with multiple seizure types show increased aggression.
Hermann has interpreted this study as supportive of the theory put forward
by Stevens & Hermann in 1981 that 'there are a number of factors which
increase the risk of psychopathology in individuals with TLE. The most
powerful factors identified are clinical, EEG, and radiological evidence of
bilateral, deep, or diffuse cerebral pathology'. Added to these, they suggest,
are the possible changes in cerebral functioning produced by the presence
of generalised seizures.

The hypothesis that specific brain damage may lead to unopposed
aggressive responses has been suggested by Bear (1983). This theory is of
interest because it links many of the empirical findings of the literature
related to episodic dyscontrol and impulsive and aggressive behaviour, with
damage to the orbital frontal surface of the cortex, and limbic system

dysfunction. It reinforces the view that patients with epilepsy and brain damage to specific cerebral systems which mediate impulse control are likely to suffer aggressive outbursts. Seizure activity may also interfere with the functioning of these impulse control systems.

Pontius (1984) has suggested that a syndrome of sudden outbursts of violence which are inappropriate to the situation and which are released by specific triggers can be explained by a neurological system intimately related to memory and impulse control. He describes eight cases in which sudden acts of motiveless violence, triggered by an apparently irrelevant stimulus, erupted from a non-aroused state. He suggests that poor impulse control and inappropriate response to a specific stimulus could be explained by frontal lobe dysfunction. This author makes no suggestion that an epileptic process is involved, but they do question whether hippocampal, amygdala and hypothalamic function are involved, and quotes Nauta & Domesick (1982) in postulating that limbic system dysfunction was also involved: 'That the functional set of the limbic system affects not only, as generally acknowledged, the organism's visceral and endocrine functions and its motivational state, but also the sensory and associated mechanisms involved in its perceptions and ideational processes'.

The link between epilepsy and dyscontrol is a close one (Elliott 1976, Monroe 1970). Patients who are thought to have episodic dyscontrol often show similar characteristics to populations of patients with epilepsy, and non-specific factors such as brain damage, violent backgrounds, low socioeconomic status, trauma and infections are common in both groups. Lewis et al (1982), as we have seen, found that 5 of the 78 violent boys in a study of children in a reform school had committed violent acts during an ictus. However, the high prevalence of minimal brain damage, soft neurological signs, and abnormal EEGs, suggested that the violence was more related to organic factors than to epilepsy. Acts of violence in epileptic populations are not necessarily all the result of epilepsy. Leicester (1982), in a review of the literature, points out that in many of the studies which have already been quoted, violence could be due to a disorder of behaviour (temper tantrums) rather than to epilepsy.

Patients who are diagnosed as showing episodic dyscontrol therefore probably form a heterogenous population. The common factors are minimal trauma to the central nervous system in conjunction with socioeconomic factors, both of which can lead to a violent behaviour.

Cortical excitability and abnormal behaviour

The relationship of poor impulse control to brain mechanisms and brain damage has already been described. Drugs which change neurohumoral transmission within the brain are frequently used to modify episodes of violent and abnormal behaviour. Fenwick et al (1983) suggested a relationship between poor impulse control and changes in brain catecholamines.

This hypothesis is based on the behaviour inhibitory system (BIS) of Gray (1979), which controls activity in the hippocampus and projects to the frontal and septal regions of the forebrain. It has been shown to be enervated by the dorsal noradrenergic tracts originating in the nucleus coeruleus. This system mediates the passive avoidance behaviour which Gray suggests is equated with anxiety. We suggest that lack of passive avoidance in an animal model can also be equated with behavioural impulsiveness, and that

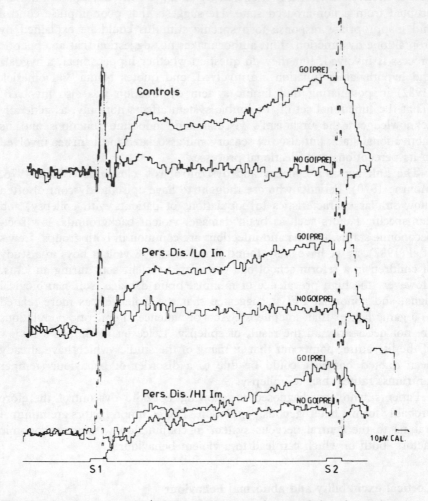

Fig. 18.3 This figure show GO/NO GO CNV averages in a population of controls and patients from Broadmoor Special Hospital. Sixteen trials are averaged in each condition. It can be seen that those with personality disorders who were highly impulsive show poor differentiation of the GO/NO GO response, whereas those who showed low impulsiveness showed a greater differentiation. (Reproduced with kind permission from Howard et al 1982.)

in man this system mediates not only anxiety but also impulse control. In several experiments in various populations of patients we have shown that changes in cortical excitabilities (represented by differentiation of the CNV GO/NO GO amplitudes) correlates with poor impulse control. We have also shown that drugs which modify the action of the BIS by decreasing passive avoidance also decrease the CNV differentiation (Fenwick et al 1983, Howard et al 1982) (Figs 18.3, 18.4).

On the basis of these observations we suggest that poor impulse control and episodic violent behaviour in man is mediated by a noradrenergic system, the BIS of Gray. Episodes of disordered behaviour which characterise the dyscontrol system can arise either from a modification of activity

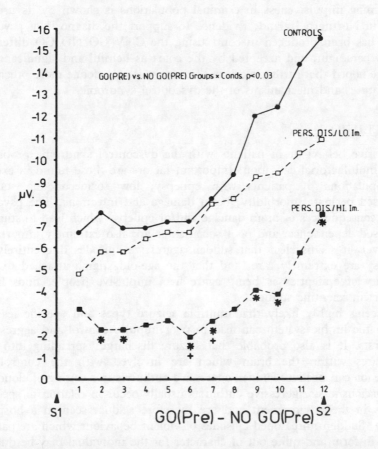

Fig. 18.4 This figure shows the difference of the 12 CNV points between GO/NO GO responses in the patient groups shown in Figure 18.3. Highly significant differences can be seen between the differentiations of the personality disorders that were highly impulsive, and the controls, whereas there are no significant differences between the low impulsive personality disorders and the controls. $\star$ $p < 0.05$, $+$ $p < 0.01$. (Reproduced with kind permission from Howard et al 1982).

in the mesolimbic or septal regions, or from a change in impulse control by the frontal cortex. Depletion of norepinephrine will lead to an increase in cortical excitability, an increase in impulsiveness and a decrease in CNV differentiation. This hypothesis contains many similar features to those of both Stevens and Bear, which have been mentioned above.

We have also shown that the activity of this system can be measured by using the CNV. Further information confirming these results has recently been found in a population of normal subjects. Poor GO/NO GO differentiation was found to correlate with impulsiveness on Eysenck's 15 questionaire. This suggests that our findings are not limited only to pathological populations, but do reflect quite generally a system which underpins the mechanism of impulsiveness (Brown et al 1988). The success of this system in defining impulsiveness in criminal populations is shown by its use in court in Northern Ireland. Evidence to support the diagnosis of psychopathy has been produced in court using the CNV GO/NO GO differentiation paradigm, and accepted by the court as helpful and significant. It is to be hoped that further work in this area will help define more precisely the features and mechanisms of the dyscontrol syndrome.

CONCLUSION

Aggressive behaviour in patients with the dyscontrol syndrome probably has a multifactorial causation. Important factors are those found in excess in populations of patients with epilepsy; low socioeconomic status, increased perinatal morbidity, brain damage and infections. The psychosocial consequences of brain damage and/or epilepsy which lead to stigma, increased dependence, and poor social skills are also extremely important. However, it seems clear that sudden aggressive episodes due entirely to epilepsy are extremely rare, and that the age-old stigma attached to the majority of epileptics as being aggressive, impulsive people, finds little support in scientific studies.

It seems highly likely that multiple seizure types and specific lesions within the limbic system can lead to poor impulse control and aggressive outbursts. It is also probable that seizure discharges spreading into the structures within the brain which are involved with the control of aggression can produce sudden aggressive outbursts in a setting of clouding of consciousness. Aggressive outbursts usually occur in relation to specific factors in the environment and are therefore seldom seen in a hospital setting. Sudden unreasoned episodes of violent behaviour which are paroxysmal in form and quite out of character for the individual may be due to brain damage to both the orbital surface of the frontal lobe and to the limbic system. The significant association shown by the dyscontrol syndrome is between poor impulse control and brain damage; brain damage and not epilepsy seems likely to be the main common factor.

The bridge between psychiatry and neurology

Paroxysmal outbursts of aggressive behaviour are the final common pathway of both psychiatric and neurological disease processes. For aggressive behaviour can arise in many different circumstances and need not even be related to brain pathology. It is not uncommon for adolescents to display sudden outbursts of aggressive behaviour which have no apparent trigger and which are — to the parents — socially inappropriate. Young children when frustrated may respond to a trivial stimulus by an outburst of destructive and violent aggression. In adults, temper outbursts are more likely to be a function of personality than the result of a brain lesion.

Aggressive behaviour also occurs in a large number of neurological illnesses. Here, the aggressive behaviour arises from a disorder of brain function which is dependent on structural brain damage. The brain damage can be confined to those structures which are thought to underpin aggressive behaviour (the hypothalamus and limbic system), but lesions in other parts of the brain which affect behaviour can also lead to aggression. For example, damage to left hemisphere structures can lead to sudden and violent outbursts of frustration — the catastrophic syndrome.

Psychiatric disorders — the functional illnesses such as the schizophrenias and affective disorders — are commonly associated with violent aggressive outbursts. Here the aggression is a result of the misinterpretation of environmental cues by the patient. Paranoid or depressive reactions can both lead to sudden outbursts of aggresive behaviour. Psychopathic disorder, drug addiction, alcoholism and stress within the patient's life, are all potent generators of aggressive behaviour. Indeed, few of us, when under stress, would consider that we are immune to aggressive outbursts.

Implantation of depth electrodes in the amygdala and hippocampal structures, has created a new synthesis between neurology and psychiatry. Previously neurology had been regarded as relating entirely to the disorders of brain function, and psychiatry as relating to disorders of mind. This simple distinction is now no longer possible. Paroxysmal discharges within the amygdala can arise from pathology within these structures, but it is also possible for normal activity within these structures to trigger a paroxysmal discharge. Paradoxically, normal brain functioning may itself be an effective stimulus of abnormal discharges and outbursts of aggressive behaviour. It is perfectly possible that many unexplained aggressive outbursts result from covert limbic system discharges in patients who may not even be epileptic. These deep limbic discharges can lead to violent behaviour even though they are confined to the limbic system and produce no change in cortical rhythms. The neurological touchstone that no paroxysmal disorder of behaviour is epileptic unless disorders of scalp rhythms are associated with it is now no longer true. These findings bring the neurologist closer to the psychiatrist.

REFERENCES

Adamek R E, Stark-Adamek C 1983 Limbic kindling and animal behaviour: implications for human psychopathology associated with complex partial seizures. Biological Psychiatry 18: 269–273

Andrulonis P A, Donelly J, Blueck B C et al 1980 Preliminary data on ethosuximide and the episodic dyscontrol syndrome. American Journal of Psychiatry 137: 1455–1456

Andrulonis P A, Glueck B C, Strobel C F, Vogel N G 1982 Borderline personality subcategories. Journal of Nervous Disorder and Mental Disease 170: 670–679

Andy D J 1970 Thalamotomy in hyperactive and aggressive behaviour. Confinia Neurologica 32: 322–325

Bach-y-Rita G, Lion J R, Climent C F, Ervin F R 1971 Episodic dyscontrol: a study of 130 violent patients. American Journal of Psychiatry 127: 1473–1478

Bach-y-Rita G, Veno A 1974 Habitual violence: a profile of 62 men. American Journal of Psychiatry 131: 1015–1017

Bear D 1983 Hemispheric specialization and the neurology of emotion. Archives of Neurology 40: 195–202

Bingley T 1958 Mental symptoms in temporal lobe epilepsy and temporal lobe gliomas with special reference to laterality of lesion and the relationship between handedness and brainedness. Acta Psychiatrica Scandanavica 33(suppl 120): 1–151

Boerhaave H 1715 Aphorisms concerning the knowledge and cure of disease, translated by G Delacoste, London

Brewer C 1971 Homicide during a psychomotor seizure. Medical Journal of Australia i: 857–859

Brown D, Fenwick P, Howard R 1988 The contingent negative variation (CNV) in a GO/NO GO avoidance task: relationship with personality, subjective state and cognitive function. Psychophysiology (in press)

Brutkowski S, Fonberg E, Mempel E 1961 Angry behaviour in dogs following bilateral lesions in the genual portion of the rostral cingulate gyrus. Acta Biologici Experimentalis 21: 199–205

Chapman W P 1958 Studies of the periamygdaloid area in relation to human behaviour. Association of Research in Nervous and Mental Disease 36: 258–277

Cope R, Donovan W 1979 A case of insane automatism? British Journal of Psychiatry 135: 574–575

Currie S, Heathfield W, Henson R, Scott D 1971 Clinical course and prognosis of temporal lobe epilepsy: a survey of 666 patients. Brain 94: 173–190

Davies R, Neil K, Himmelhoch J 1975 Clinical Electroencephalography 6: 103–115

Delgado-Escueta A, Mattson R, King L 1981 The nature of aggression during epileptic seizures. New England Journal of Medicine 305: 711–716

Derro R 1978 Admission health evaluation of a city-county workhouse. Minnesota Medicine 61: 333–337

Elliott F 1976 The neurology of explosive rage. Practitioner 217: 51–60

Elliott F 1982 Neurological findings in adult minimal brain dysfunction and the dyscontrol syndrome. Journal of Nervous and Mental Desease 170: 680–687

Falconer M 1973 Reversibility by temporal lobe resection of the behavioural abnormalities of temporal lobe epilepsy. New England Journal of Medicine 289: 451–455

Fenwick P 1984 Epilepsy and the law. British Medical Journal 288: 1938–1939

Fenwick P 1986 Aggression and epilepsy. In: Bolwig H, Trimble M (eds) Aspects of epilepsy and psychiatry. John Wiley, Chichester, p 62–98

Fenwick P, Fenwick E 1985 (eds) Epilepsy and the law — a medical symposium on the current law. International Congress and Symposium Series, no 81. The Royal Society of Medicine, London, p 3–8

Fenwick P, Howard R, Fenton G 1983 Review of cortical excitability, neurohumeral transmission and the dyscontrol syndrome. In: Parsonage M et al (eds) Advances in epileptology: XIVth epilepsy international symposium. Raven Press, New York, p 181–191

Gastaut H, Morrin G, Lesevre N 1955 Etudes du compartment des epileptiques psychomoteur dans l'interval de leurs crises. Annals of Medical Psychology 113: 1–29

Gloor P 1967 Discussion of 'Brain mechanisms related to aggressive behaviour', by B Kaada. In: Clemente C, Lindsay D (eds) Aggression and defence: neural mechanisms and social patterns, vol 5: Brain Function, p 116–127

Gloor P 1972 Temporal lobe epilepsy: its possible contribution to the understanding of the functional significance of the amygdala and of its interaction with neocortical-temporal mechanisms. In: Eletheriou B (ed) The neurobiology of the amygdala Plenum Press, New York, p 423–458

Gloor P 1978 Inputs and outputs of the amygdala: what the amygdala is trying to tell the rest of the brain. In: Livingstone and Hornykiewicz (eds) Limbic mechanisms: the continuing evolution of the limbic system concept. Plenum Press, New York, p 189–209

Gloor P, Olivier A, Quesney L F 1981 The role of the amygdala in the expression of psychic phenomena in temporal lobe seizures. In: Ben-Azi Y (ed) The amygdaloid complex. Elsevier/North Holland Biomedical Press, Amsterdam, p 489–498

Gloor P Olivier A, Quesney L F, Andermann F, Horowitz S 1982 The role of the limbic system in experimental phenomena of temporal lobe epilepsy. Annals of Neurology 12/2: 129–144

Gowers W R 1892 Diseases of the nervous system, vol 2, p 928

Gray J 1979 Anxiety. In: Izard C (ed) 1979 Emotions in personality and psychopathology, vol 10. Plenum Press, New York, p 303–331

Green J D, Clement C D, De Groot J 1957 Rhinencephalic lesions and behaviour in cats. Journal of Comparative Neurology 108: 505–536

Gunn J 1978 Epileptic homicide: a case report. British Journal of Psychiatry 132: 510–513

Gunn J 1979 Forensic psychiatry. In: Granville-Grossman K (ed) Recent advances in clinical psychiatry. Churchill Livingstone, Edinburgh, p 271–295

Gunn J, Bonn J 1971 Criminality and violence in epileptic prisoners. British Journal of Psychiatry 118: 337–343

Gunn J, Fenton G 1969 Epilepsy in prisons: a diagnostic survey. British Medical Journal iv: 326–328

Gunn J, Fenton G 1971 Epilepsy, automatism and crime. Lancet i: 1173–1176

Halgren E, Walter R D, Cherlow D G, Crandall P G 1978 Mental phenomena evoked by electrical stimulation of the human hippocampal formation and amygdala. Brain 101: 83–117

Heath R G 1963 Electrical self stimulation of the brain in man. American Journal of Psychiatry 120: 571–577

Heath R G, Mickle W A 1960 Evaluation of seven years experience with depth electrode studies in human patients. In: Ramey E R, O'Doherty D (eds) Electrical studies of the unanaesthetised brain. Paul B Hober, New York, p 214–247

Hermann B P 1982 Interictal psychopathology in patients with ictal fear. A quantitative investigation. Neurology 32: 7–11

Hermann B P, Dikmen S, Schwartz M S, Karnes W E 1982 Interictal psychopathology in patients with ictal fear: a quantitative investigation. Neurology 32: 7–11

Higgins J W, Mahl G F, Delgado J, Hamlin H 1956 Behavioural changes during intracerebral electrical stimulation. Archives of Neurology and Psychiatry 76: 399–419

Hill D, Parr G 1963 The EEG in psychiatry. In: Electroencephalography: a Symposium of its Various Aspects, 2nd edn. Macdonald, London, p 360–428

Hill D, Pond D 1952 Reflections on a hundred capital cases submitted to EEG. Journal of Mental Science 98: 23–43

Hitchcock E, Cairns V 1973 Amygdalotomy. Postgraduate Medical Journal 49: 894–904

Howard R, Fenton G, Fenwick P 1982 Conclusions and directions for future research. In: Event-related brain potentials in personality and psychopathology: a Pavlovian approach, Research Studies Press, London, p 81–89

James I 1960 Temporal lobectomy for psychomotor epilepsy. Journal of Mental Science 106: 543–558

Kaplan J 1899 Kopftrauma unt psychosen. Allgemeine Zeitschrift für Psychiatrie 56: 292–296

Kennard M A 1955 Effects of bilateral ablation of cingulate area on behaviour of cats. Journal of Neurophysiology 18: 159–169

Kim Y, Umbach W 1973 Combined stereotactic lesions for treatment of behavioural disorders and severe pain. In: Laitinen L, Livingstone K (eds) Surgical approaches in psychiatry. University Park, Baltimore, p 182–188

King D, Ajmone Marsan C 1977 Clinical features and ictal patterns in epileptic patients with EEG temporal lobe foci. Annals of Neurology 2: 138–147

King D, Young Q 1978 Increased prevalence of seizure disorders among prisoners. Journal of the American Medical Association 239: 2674–2675

Kligman D, Goldberg D T 1975 Temporal lobe epilepsy and aggression. Journal of Nervous and Mental Disease 160: 324–341

Knox S 1968 Epileptic automatisms and violence. Medicine, Science and the Law 8: 96–104

Le Beau J 1952 The cingular and precingular areas in psychosurgery (agitated behaviour, obsessive compulsive states, epilepsy). Acta Psychiatrica et Neurologica, Copenhagen 27: 305–316

Leicester J 1982 Temper tantrums, epilepsy and episodic dyscontrol. British Journal of Psychiatry 141: 262–266

Lewis D, Pincus J, Shanok S, Glaser G 1982 Psychomotor epilepsy and violence in a group of incarcerated adolescent boys. American Journal of Psychiatry 139: 882–887

Lewis D, Pincus J 1983 Psychomotor epilepsy and violence. American Journal of Psychiatry 140: 646–648

Lindsay J, Ounstead C, Richards P 1979 Long-term outcome in children with temporal lobe seizures. (3) Psychiatric aspects in childhood and adult life. Developmental Medicine and Child Neurology 21: 630–636

Maclean P D, Delgado J 1953 Electrical and chemical stimulation of front temporal portion of limbic system in waking animal. Electroencephalography and Clinical Neurophysiology 5: 91–100

Maletsky B M 1973 The episodic dyscontrol syndrome. Diseases of the Nervous System 36: 178–185

Mark V H, Ervin F 1970 Violence and the brain. Harper and Rowe, New York

Mark V H, Sweet W, Ervin F 1975 Deep temporal lobe stimulation and destructive lesions in episodically violent temporal lobe epileptics. In: Fields W, Sweet W (eds) Neural bases of violence and aggression, Warren H Greem, St Louis, p 379–391

Milne H 1979 Epileptic homicide: drug induced. British Journal of Psychiatry 134: 547–548

Monroe R 1970 Episodic behavioural disorders. Harvard University Press

Monroe R 1974 Episodic behavioral disorders: An unclassified syndrome. In: Arieti (ed) American handbook of psychiatry Vol 3, 2nd edn. Basic Books, New York, p 237–254

Monroe R, Jacobson G, Ervin F 1956 Activation of psychosis by a combination of scopolamine and alpha-chloralose. Archives of Neurology and Psychiatry 76: 536–548

Moyer K E 1971 The physiology of hostility. Markham, Chicago

Mungus D 1983 An empirical analysis of specific syndromes of violent behaviour. Journal of Nervous and Mental Disease 171: 354–361

Nádvorník P, Pogady J, Sramka M 1973 The result of stereotactic treatment of the aggressive syndrome. In: Laitinen L, Livingstone K (eds) Surgical approaches in psychiatry. University Park, Baltimore, p 125–128

Narabayashi H, Nagao T, Yosluda M, Nagahata M 1963 Stereotaxic amygdalotomy for behaviour disorders. Archives of Neurology 9: 1–16

Nauta W J B, Domesick V B 1982 Neurological association of the limbic system. In: Beckman A (ed) Neurological basis of behaviour. Spectrum, New York, p 175–206

Norvik L, Dellapenna R, Schwartz M et al 1977 Health status of the New York city prison population. Medical Care 15: 205–217

Nuffield E 1961 Neurophysiology and behaviour disorders in epileptic children. Journal of Mental Science 107: 438–458

Penfield W, Jasper H H 1954 Epilepsy and the functional anatomy of the human brain. Little, Brown, Boston, p 113–143

Pond D, Bidwell B 1960 A survey of epilepsy in 14 general practices. II Social and psychological aspects. Epilepsia 1: 285–299

Pontius A 1984 Specific stimulus evoked violent action in psychotic trigger reaction: a seizure-like imbalance between frontal lobe and limbic systems. Perceptual and Motor Skills 59 (1): 299–333

Ratner R R, Shapiro D 1979 The episodic dyscontrol syndrome and criminal responsibility. Bulletin of the American Academy of Psychiatry and the Law 7: 422–431

Riley T, Niedermeyer E 1978 Rage attacks and episodic violent behaviour electroencephalographic findings and general consideration. Journal of Clinical Elecroencephalography 9: 113–139

Rodin E 1973 Psychomotor epilepsy and aggressive behaviour. Archives of General Psychiatry 28: 210–213

Romaniuk A 1965 Representation of aggression and flight reactions in the hypothalamus of the cat. Acta Biologicae Experimentalis Sinica, Warsaw 25: 177–186

Rutter M 1982 Concepts, issues and prospects in development psychiatry. Journal of Clinical Neuropsychology 4: 91–115

Sano K, Mayanagi Y, Sekino H E, Ajashiwa M, Ishyima B 1970 Results of stimulation and destruction of the posterior hypothalamus in man. Journal of Neurosurgery 33: 689–707

Sem-Jacobson C W 1968 Vegetative changes in response to electrical brain stimulation. Electroencephalography and Clinical Neurophysiology 24: 88

Serafetinides E 1965 Aggressiveness in temporal lobe epilepsy and its relation to cerebral dysfunction and environmental factors. Epilepsia 6: 33–47

Simon R, de Silva M 1981 Intercranial tumour coexistant with uncinate seizures in violent behaviour. Journal of the American Medical Association 245: 1247–1248

Small J 1970 Small sharp spikes in a psychiatric population. Archives of General Psychiatry 22: 277–484

Small J 1971 Photoconvulsive and photomyoclonic responses in psychiatric patients. Clinical Electroencephalography 2: 78–88

Small J, Small I, Milstein V, Moore D 1975 Familial associations with eeg variants in manic-depressive disease. Archives of General Psychiatry 32: 43–48

Smith D E, King M D, Hoebelb G 1970 Lateral hypothalamic controls of killing: evidence for a cholinergic mechanism. Science 167: 900–901

Stafford-Clarke D, Taylor F 1949 Clinical and electroencephalographic studies of prisoners charged with murder. Journal of Neurology, Neurosurgery and Psychiatry 12: 325–329

Stevens J R 1975 Interictal clinical manifestations of complex partial seizures. Advances in Neurology 11: 85–107

Stevens J R, Hermann B 1981 Temporal lobe epilepsy, psychopathology and violence: the state of the evidence. Neurology (New York) 31: 1127–1132

Stevenson H 1963 Psychomotor epilepsy associated with criminal behaviour. Medical Journal of Australia 50: 784–785

Struve F, Kishore R, Arco R, Klein D, Becker D 1977 Relationship between paroxysmal electroencephalographic dysrhythmia and suicide ideation and attempts in psychiatric patients. In: Shagass G, Gershon S, Friedhoff A (eds) Psychopathology and brain dysfunction. Raven Press, New York, p 199–221

Taylor D 1969 Aggression and epilepsy. Journal of Psychosomatic Research 13: 229–236

Taylor D 1981 Brain lesions, surgery, seizures, and mental symptoms. In: Reynolds E, Trimble M (eds) Epilepsy and psychiatry. Churchill Livingstone, Edinburgh, p 227–241

Tow P M, Whitty C W 1953 Personality changes after operations in the cingulate gyrus in man. Journal of Neurology, Neurosurgery and Psychiatry 16: 186–193

Treiman D, Delgado-Escueta A 1983 Violence and epilepsy: a critical review. In: Pedley T, Meldrum B (eds) Recent Advances in Epilepsy 1. Churchill Livingstone, Edinburgh, p 179–209

Tunks E R, Dermer S W 1977 Carbamazepine in the dyscontrol syndrome associated with limbic system dysfunction. Journal of Nervous and Mental Disease 164: 56–63

Volavka T, Matousek M 1969 The relation of pre- and perinatal pathology to the adult EEG. Electroencephalography and Clinical Neurophysiology 27: 667

Wieser H G 1983 Depth recorded limbic seizures and psychopathology. Neuroscience and Behavioural Reviews 7 (3): 427–440

Whitman S, Colman T, Borg B et al 1980 Epidemiological insights into the socioeconomic correlates of epilepsy. In: Hermann B P (ed) A Multidisciplinary Handbook of Epilepsy. Charles C Thomas, Springfield III, p 243–271

Whitman S, Coonley-Hoganson R, Desai B 1984 Comparative head trauma experiences in two socioeconomically different Chicago-area communities: a population study. American Journal of Epidemiology 119: 570–580

Williams D 1969 Neural factors related to habitual aggression. Brain 92: 503–520

Yasukochi 1960 Emotional responses elicited by electrical stimulation of the hypothalamus in cats. Folia Psychiatrica et Neurologica Japanica 14: 260–267

Laterality in neuropsychiatry

In this chapter I will review the evidence for lateralised disturbances of hemisphere function or structure in the chronic interictal psychoses of epilepsy and discuss their implications for the major psychoses.

THE CHRONIC INTERICTAL PSYCHOSES OF EPILEPSY

This term, for all its questionable aetiological assumptions, has stood the test of time and will be used here. It describes those chronic psychotic disorders that develop in association with epilepsy, but which pursue a fluctuating course largely uninfluenced by seizure activity, and which resemble in many aspects the so-called functional psychoses. Schizophrenia-like states in particular have attracted considerable attention, but uncertainties about the exact nature of the relationship with epilepsy remain unresolved (Stevens 1966, Toone 1981) and fresh doubts about their nosological status have recently been expressed (Murray et al 1985, Toone 1986).

These uncertainties have always existed. Early studies (e.g. Kraepelin 1910) supported the notion of an affinity between the two disorders. Later writers (e.g. Muller 1931) were more impressed by the beneficial effect of seizure activity on the psychotic process; observations that gave rise to the 'antagonism' hypothesis and to the introduction of artificially induced convulsion therapy by Meduna.

More recent developments, in particular the increasing diagnostic precision within epilepsy due to electrocephalography, have led to further revision and to a return to the original 'affinity' hypothesis, albeit an affinity that permits symptomatic antagonism to occur between the two conditions. Psychoses develop in the wake of epilepsy, and the epilepsy is more usually expressed in the form of complex partial seizures arising in the temporal lobes, though this latter view is still disputed (Stevens 1966).

DISTURBANCE OF FUNCTION AND LATERALITY

In 1969 Pierre Flor-Henry's study of temporal lobe epileptic patients with psychoses was published. Many aspects of the complex relationship between epilepsy and psychosis were considered, but one set of observations commanded immediate attention: the association between laterality of epileptic foci and form of psychosis. This seminal paper was highly influential and its impact extended well beyond the relatively narrow diagnostic confines of the clinical material studied. Cerebral dominance and hemisphere specialisation had already received considerable attention. The risk of major psychiatric disorder (Lishman 1968, 1973), or of psychosis (Hillbom 1951) had been shown to increase following injury to the dominant hemisphere; damage or disease to that hemisphere may be associated with psychotic phenomena (Davison & Bagley 1969). Hitherto, little attempt had been made to relate lateralised disturbances in hemisphere function (as opposed to structural damage) to vulnerability to psychosis. Flor-Henry's findings gave fresh impetus to the study of the epileptic psychoses. Of far greater importance, it stimulated a novel approach to the study of the aetiology of the functional psychoses: one that sought to relate symptom and syndrome pattern to lateralised hemisphere dysfunction. For these reasons this work will be described in some detail.

Flor-Henry identified retrospectively from among those patients attending the Maudsley Hospital between 1950 and 1965, 50 in whom a diagnosis of temporal lobe epilepsy (TLE) was combined with a psychosis. A control group was formed from temporal lobe epileptic patients attending the hospital with some form of psychiatric disorder other than psychosis and from epileptic patients awaiting temporal lobe surgery.

The principle findings that relate to laterality of focus and psychosis are as follows. Among the psychotic patients, bilateral foci occur more commonly than among the controls: if unilateral cases alone are considered, twice as many psychotic patients have left-sided foci as right. The reverse is the case in the control group. In the psychotic group, 'the highest incidence of right-sided unilateral (non-dominant) foci is found in the manic-depressive and in the schizoaffective psychoses. In schizophrenic psychoses the dominant temporal lobe is predominantly involved'. Group differences are said to be significant in each case.

The large proportion, almost half, of psychotic patients with bilateral pathology is consistent with previous Maudsley studies (Slater et al 1963, Toone et al 1982b) but not with some from other centres (Gregoriadis et al 1971, Hara et al 1980, Ounsted & Lindsay 1981). This could be due to a methodological bias. The Maudsley has a long-standing interest in this group of patients and they have often been intensively investigated over a lengthy period of contact with the hospital. According to the methodology used (and this is not always clearly stated) the probability of bilaterality would increase in step with the number of EEGs carried out. Also a referral bias against bilaterality would operate in the TL surgery patients.

The interpretation of the finding of a relative excess of left-sided foci in the psychotic group is also rendered more difficult. The possibility exists of referral bias in the control group (patients with dominant hemisphere foci are less likely to be referred for surgery). Again this may best be approached by reference to large unselected TLE series. In Currie et al's (1971) series of 666 patients treated at the London Hospital, unilateral foci were on the left in 60% of cases. The distribution in Flor-Henry's psychotic group (19L;9R) does not differ significantly, whereas the control group (13L;25R) very clearly does. The differences reported here seem more likely to be due to the use of a control group that is highly atypical in this respect.

It is in his observation of the relationship between form of psychosis and laterality of focus that Flor-Henry's work has been most influential (Table 19.1). The subset numbers, perhaps inevitably given the size of the group, are small. Subset differences are not analysed in terms of Chi squared distribution (this does not approach significance) but as a trend, and this is stated to be significant at the 5% level. However, it is not permissible to use trend tests on data that lack any natural order of progression (e.g. a comparison of patient groups that differ in terms of age, height, or any other quantifiable dimension). It is not possible to discern any comparative progression in the series mania/depression-mixed-confusional-schizophrenia, nor is this claim made by the author. The use of this test is therefore open to question.

Table 19.1 Laterality of focus and form of psychosis (Flor-Henry 1969)

Epileptic foci	Manic-depressive	Mixed	Confusional	Schizophrenic
Right	4	2	1	2
Left	2	4	4	9
Bilateral	3	5	4	10

This work contains one of the more comprehensive studies of the chronic interictal psychoses of epilepsy; it is also one of the first to use a reference group for comparative purposes. Its findings must, however, due to the unrepresentative nature of the control group, be interpreted with caution.

Since 1969 a number of studies have addressed the issue of lateralisation of pathology in patients with epilepsy and chronic psychoses. A few have reported on structural abnormalities (Toone et al 1982a, Sherwin 1984), but the majority have been concerned with disturbance of function. The widespread adoption of internationally agreed criteria for psychiatric diagnosis and classification has been a relatively recent development and in some early studies in particular the amount of clinical information provided leaves room for diagnostic uncertainty. Other studies (e.g. Shukla & Katiyar 1980) failed to distinguish between schizophrenia and manic depressive psychosis, thus invalidating any attempt to further explore Flor-Henry's central hypothesis. An excess of sinistral patients may make interpretation difficult e.g. Taylor 1975). First to be considered are those studies in which diagnostic criteria approach present day standards.

Flor-Henry's study introduced the concept of psychosis and laterality: it has therefore been considered first. It was preceded by a work that was equally influential in its delineation of the salient features of the schizophrenia-like psychosis of epilepsy. Slater and his associates (Slater et al 1963) reported on 69 patients in whom a diagnosis of epilepsy was combined with one of schizophrenia. Temporal lobe foci were recorded in 48. In 16 the focus was in the dominant lobe, in 12 the non-dominant lobe, and in 20 there were bilateral foci. The authors had previously further subdivided the schizophrenia-like illness into chronic psychosis proceeded by repeated short-lived confusional episodes, chronic paranoid states and hebephrenic states. No obvious lateralisation pattern is described which may distinguish between any of these subcategories.

Data from two major neurosurgical series were published in 1979. Jensen & Larsen (1979) reported on 74 patients who underwent temporal lobe surgery for epilepsy. Eleven were psychotic prior to surgery (though none prior to epilepsy), and a further 9 became psychotic subsequently. Six were said to have a 'manic depressive or schizoaffective psychosis and were treated with ECT or tricyclic antidepressants'. Thirteen had a schizophrenia-like psychosis. Three were 'simple schizophrenics while the remaining 10 patients showed the picture of the chronic paranoid state'. A quantitative analysis of laterality of foci is not provided, but 'operations on the right or on the non-dominant side were more frequent in psychotic patients but no segregation by handedness or by dominance was found when the various psychotic groups were compared with each other'.

Kristensen & Sindrup (1978) compared 96 patients with complex partial seizures and a history of paranoid/hallucinatory states with a same size group with complex partial seizures only. Psychosis was documented in a hospital setting and was said to be present when 'one or more psychotic episodes (duration several weeks) or permanent psychosis characterised by paranoid ideas and/or hallucinations in a state of clear consciousness' were present.

Among the psychotic groups, successfully performed waking, sleep and sphenoidal EEG's showed unilateral spike activity on the left in 24, on the right in 30 and bilaterally in 33. Respective figures for the control group were 34, 19 and 15. Even when allowances are made for a further 6 psychotic patients with a slow wave focus only (the direction of the unilaterality is not disclosed), the excess of sinistrality within the psychotic group (16 against 5 controls), and the possibility that some of the patients with 'paranoid ideas' were not psychotic, the laterality ratios are in the opposite direction to that which Flor-Henry's findings would have predicted. The psychotic group also showed more diffuse slow wave activity, multiple spike foci and fewer normal recordings. These observations, taken in conjunction with the greater proportion of psychotic patients with bilateral foci, might suggest more extensive brain damage in this group. Lumbar air encephalography, however, did not distinguish psychotic patients from controls.

In a more recent study (Perez et al 1985), a subgroup of 17 patients with TLE and psychosis was analysed with respect to laterality. Using the PSE (Wing et al 1974) and CATEGO diagnostic criteria, patients were divided into either nuclear schizophrenia, or into some other CATEGO subclass of psychosis. In the first group, 7 had unilateral left-sided foci, 2 unilateral right-sided foci (but 1 of these was left handed), and 2 had bilateral foci. Six patients had some other form of psychosis. One had a unilateral focus on the left, 2 on the right, and 2 bilaterally (in 1 no focus could be demonstrated). The association between left-sided focal discharge and schizophrenia was significant at the 5% level.

Other studies have given little or no indication of the criteria used for diagnosis of psychosis, or have employed descriptive terms or included case studies that call into question the validity of diagnosis. Taylor (1972) studied a consecutive series of 100 patients undergoing temporal lobectomy. Sixteen had a history of psychosis or were shown to be psychotic prior to surgery; 4 developed psychosis postoperatively. In the first group EEG provided evidence of foci (and this was later confirmed by surgery) on the left in 7, on the right in 5, and bilaterally in the remainder. The psychoses are not further differentiated, but individual case reports suggest that 4 may have been schizophrenic (2 had left unilateral foci, 2 right), 2 depressive (1 left, 1 right). These findings regarding the relationship between laterality and psychosis subtype are therefore inconclusive.

In a further study Taylor (1975) identified 13 cases of psychosis from two carefully selected groups of postlobectomy patients with either 'alien tissue' lesions or mesial temporal sclerosis. The criteria introduced by Slater et al (1963) were used to diagnose 'a schizophrenia-like psychosis'. Seven of the patients were left handed. Side of surgery did not distinguish between schizophrenic and non-schizophrenic patients in terms of cerebral dominance. Interpretation would, in any case, have been difficult due to the unusually high proportion of sinistrals among the psychotics.

Sherwin (1977, 1981, 1984) has written at length on the relationship between epilepsy, laterality and psychosis in patients referred for temporal lobe surgery. In one early paper (1977) he identified 36 patients with 'intractable epilepsy' who showed a 'psychotic-like reaction with aggressivity'. Thirty-four had surface EEG recordings only and half of these displayed localising abnormalities in the temporal lobes. In 11 cases these were left sided, 3 right sided and in 3 they were bilateral. However, in a later paper (1984) Sherwin states that only 6 of the 17 showed definite EEG evidence of epilepsy. The remainder showed monophasic sharp waves or runs of rhythmic activity coming from the temporal lobe. In a further series 63 patients with unilateral temporal lobe epileptic foci undergoing investigation for temporal lobe surgery (Sherwin 1981) were thought to be psychotic. Six were diagnosed as having a paranoid or schizophrenic type of psychosis, 1 a schizoaffective psychosis with marked depressive features. The ratio for left- to right-sided foci for the psychotic and non-psychotic groups respectively were 5:2 (and the 2 patients with right-sided foci included the 1 with a schizoaffective illness) and 10:44. The psychotic patients may have been atypical in certain respects. In discussing the reasons for the predominance of right-sided lesions (in the first study the majority were left sided), the author explains that the cases were selected to exclude patients with a severe behaviour disorder or active psychosis at the time of investigation. Elsewhere, Sherwin states that the psychotic disorders differ from schizophrenia in that 'the psychosis often was more periodic and that frequently it did not require the use of major tranquillisers'. In a similar study (Sherwin et al 1982), absolute or relative freedom from seizures after temporal lobe surgery was used as a criterion for unilaterality of focus. Seven schizophrenics, atypical in the same respects as the previous cohort, received surgery, 5 on the left, 2 on the right. Among the non-psychotic patients the corresponding figures were 15 and 58. However, 5 of the psychotics were left handed and, using the Wada test as a criterion, the groups did not differ in terms of cerebral dominance.

The remaining studies may be more briefly described. Gregoriadis et al (1971) reported on 52 hospitalised psychotic epileptic patients. In 43, a history of schizophrenia and paranoid symptoms could be obtained and in this group evidence of left temporal involvement was invariably present. The remaining 9 patients, who had predominantly affective symptoms, showed right temporal lobe involvement. Lindsay and her coworkers, in an important series of papers, reported on the adult outcome of a cohort of 100 patients with 'limbic epilepsy' referred to a special centre during childhood. Nine of 87 patients had developed 'schizophreniform psychosis'; 9 had an epileptic focus on the left, 2 bilateral foci (Lindsay et al 1979). Pritchard et al (1980) identified from among 56 TL epileptics, 3 schizophrenics (2 left, 1 right-sided foci) and 2 depressives (1 left-sided, 1 bilateral foci).

Finally, Hara et al (1980) described 40 episodes of psychiatric disturbance in 32 epileptic patients. In one subgroup, referred to as 'paranoid state or disturbances of thought or comprehension, so called schizophrenia-like state', 6 of 10 cases showed a left temporal focus. In another group characterised by dysphoric or depressive mood swings, generalised epilepsy or 'right lateralisation' predominated.

LATERALITY AND STRUCTURAL BRAIN DAMAGE

This has received less detailed study. Evidence comes mainly from neuroradiological data, particularly from lumbar air encephalography (LAEG) and computerised tomography (CT) studies. LAEG was carried out in 56 of Beard's 69 cases (Slater et al 1963) and was reported to be abnormal in 39. Abnormalities were found on the left in 15, on the right in 11, and bilaterally in 13. If abnormalities in the temporal lobes alone are considered (and these patients were all TL epileptics) left-sided abnormalities were present in 3, right-sided in 5. Gregoriadis et al (1971) reported LAEG findings consistent with EEG abnormalities described in the same paper. Sherwin (1977) reported LAEG abnormalities in 18 out of 25 cases; in 14 TL abnormalities were noted, 13 left-sided, 1 bilateral.

Toone et al (1982a) carried out CT scanning on 57 patients at the Maudsley Hospital with a combined diagnosis of epilepsy and psychosis. Psychiatric diagnosis had originally been established by the responsible clinician, but was further determined by the use of the syndrome check list, a schedule derived from the PSE (Wing et al 1974) and adapted to the needs of retrospective case history evaluation. A control group of 78 patients with epilepsy and some form of psychiatric illness other than psychosis was used for the purpose of radiological comparison. The groups did not differ in terms of the prevalence of abnormality (44% in the index group, 50% in the control group) nor in the distribution. Within the psychotic group, unilateral abnormalities were present in 7 cases. Four patients with a schizophrenic, and 1 with a paranoid psychosis, had left-sided abnormalities; 2 patients with affective psychoses had right-sided abnormalities. An absence of right-sided involvement in patients who were hallucinated was noted, but this just failed to achieve significance.

A Maudsley Hospital cohort of psychotic epileptic patients has been studied with respect to radiological abnormalities (Toone et al 1982a) and clinical characteristics (Toone et al 1982b). The EEG characteristics have not previously been reported and their contribution to the issue will now be considered.

The Maudsley hospital has acted as a tertiary referral centre for epilepsy with psychiatric disorders for over three decades. A computer search for the years 1967–79 identified 90 patients in whom the diagnosis of epilepsy (using the criteria suggested by Gunn & Fenton 1969) and psychosis were combined. Following upon a careful examination of the case notes, 21 cases were excluded (because of inadequately recorded information regarding epilepsy — 10, psychosis — 8, or doubtful diagnosis — 3). All but 1 of the remainder were traced. Two had died, 2 emigrated, and 7 refused to co-operate. A final total of 58 patients entered the study. Routine EEGs have been carried out in every case and in the majority multiple recordings including sleep and specialised electrode placements had been performed. Psychiatric diagnosis was based on recorded information using the Syndrome Check List and the CATEGO Diagnostic System.

Twenty-five patients received a diagnosis of schizophrenia (CATEGO subclass diagnosis S). Many had more than one discreet episode and in 5 cases an episode received some diagnosis other than schizophrenia. Temporal lobe epilepsy was diagnosed in 12, some other form of focal epilepsy (FE) in 5, primary generalised epilepsy (PGE) in 6, and secondary generalised epilepsy in 1 case. In 1 patient PGE and FE were combined, and in 1 no diagnosis was possible. The lateral distribution of significant EEG abnormalities is shown in Table 19.2. The majority of patients with focal abnormalities showed spike or sharp wave discharges, but in 1 subject

Table 19.2 The distribution with respect to laterality of EEG discharges indicative of epilepsy in different CATEGO subclasses

	Unilateral Left or bilateral (L > R)	Unilateral right or bilateral (R > L)	Bilateral	General	Normal	Unclassified
A *CATEGO subclass (S) diagnosis of schizophrenia*						
All forms of epilepsy	9(3)	7(3)	3	2	3	1
Temporal lobe epilepsy	3(0)	6(3)	2	0	1	0
B *CATEGO subclass (N,R,D,M) diagnoses of affective disorder*						
All forms of epilepsy	9(2)	6(3)	5	1	4	0
Temporal lobe epilepsy	8(2)	4(2)	1	0	0	0

who experienced clonic seizures without focal onset, a right-sided slow wave focus was the only abnormality.

The EEG distribution for the affective disorders (CATEGO subclass diagnoses N,D,R,M) are shown in the same table. Temporal lobe epilepsy was diagnosed in 13 of the 25 cases. The remaining 8 patients either received a diagnosis of paranoid psychosis or showed evidence of a post ictal psychosis.

Each of the patients answered questions relating to handedness (Annett 1979). The preferred hand for writing was known in 49 out of the 50 patients and in 10 was on the left. If these patients are then excluded (Table 19.3) an excess of unilateral left or bilateral left predominant foci becomes apparent in both schizophrenic and affective groups. This finding, based on limited data, is consistent with the distribution of unilateral foci in an unselective series of epileptic patients reported by Currie et al (1971), but differs from that study in the observation that almost half of the patients

Table 19.3 The distribution as in Table 19.2 after removal of sinistral patients

	Unilateral left or bilateral (L > R)	Unilateral right or bilateral (R > L)	Bilateral	General	Normal	Unclassified
A *(S)*						
All forms of epilepsy	7(2)	5(3)	2	2	1	1
Temporal lobe epilepsy	2(0)	5(3)	1	0	1	0
B *(N,R,S,M)*						
All forms of epilepsy	8(1)	5(2)	4	1	4	0
Temporal lobe epilepsy	7(1)	4(2)	1	0	0	0

with focal lesions show bilateral involvement. These data might also support the speculation that psychotic illness was associated with disturbance in the dominant hemisphere; they do not provide any evidence for an association between affective disturbance and non dominant hemisphere foci.

CONCLUSION

The difficulties inherent in this area of research cannot be overstressed. These disorders are relatively uncommon and in order to collect a series of sufficient size most researchers have resorted to retrospective case identification, with all the limitations implicit in that methodology. The proportion of subjects with this diagnosis who will have an unusual or complicated pattern of cerebral dominance is increased and this will render interpretation more difficult. The longer the period of observation and the more thoroughly it is conducted, the more difficult it becomes confidently to assign the patient to one or other categories. This applies equally to psychiatric and to epileptic classification. The probability that a patient may on different occasions receive a diagnosis of schizophrenia and affective disorder increases with the length of the illness and the number of relapses. A similar relationship exists between the demonstration of bilateral EEG abnormality and the number of EEG recordings.

These caveats notwithstanding, an attempt should be made to reach some form of conclusion. Table 19.4 summarises findings derived from those studies in which a distinction has been made between schizophrenia and affective psychosis and in which problems of cerebral dominance appear to be not insuperable. There is an obvious excess of left-sided foci among the schizophrenic group and of right-sided foci among the affective group. In this approach equal weight is given to each case and no account is taken

Table 19.4 Epilepsy discharge, lateralisation and type of psychosis: a summary*

	Schizophrenia			Affective disorder		
	L	R	Bilateral	L	R	Bilateral
Slater et al (1963)	16	12	20			
Flor-Henry (1969)	9	2	10	2	4	3
Kristensen & Sindrup (1969)	24	30	33			
Taylor (1972)	2	2	0	1	1	0
Gregoriadis et al (1973)	43	0	0	0	9	0
Lindsay et al (1979)	9	0	2			
Pritchard et al (1980)	2	1	0	1	0	1
Hara et al (1980)	6	4	0			
Sherwin (1981)	5	1	0			
Perez et al (1985)	7	2	2			
Toone (this chapter)	6	4	11	7	3	11
Totals	129	58	78	11	17	15

* The study by Jensen & Larson (1979) is not included as these authors did not refer to any numerical data relating to laterality.

of the differences in reporting of diagnostic categories. There is a persisting excess of patients with bilateral involvement among both psychotic categories.

In 1969 Flor-Henry introduced the possibility of an association between psychosis subtype and lateralisation of epileptic discharge. This concept has attracted, due in part perhaps to its misleading simplicity, considerable attention and there have been numerous attempts to replicate. The lack of agreement is a reflection, not only of the inadequacies of an evolving methodology, but also of the unavoidable problems facing any investigator into such a complex and ill-understood condition. Epilepsy and psychosis are each dynamic processes, shifting and changing pattern in response to environmental stresses, treatment programmes and, where they coexist, in relation to each other. Functional lateralisation, whether normal or pathological, is often incomplete and may be highly unstable. It follows that 'snapshot' cross-sectional observations that have as their purpose the formation of categories that are stable, enduring and non-interactive, may be inaccurate and misleading. A prospective, closely observed longitudinal study would be time-consuming and costly, but it may be the only means by which reliable and conclusive data can be obtained.

There is, however, one remaining methodological difficulty that may prove insuperable. Any attempt to relate laterality of focus to form of psychosis depends on the prior assumption that the two disorders are causally linked. But epilepsy and psychosis are both common disorders and chance association accounts for a substantial proportion of those patients who have chronic interictal psychosis (including those with temporal lobe foci). Nor is it easy, in individual cases, to determine if the association is chance or causal. Given this amount of random variability, it may not be possible to confirm or to refute Flor-Henry's findings. The enduring significance of this study may then come to lie in the body of research it has generated: the investigation of a laterality effect in the aetiology of the psychoses.

Implications for the major psychoses

The next decade after Flor-Henry's paper saw the introduction of computerised tomography (CT) and, prompted by the results of neuroimaging studies, a rekindling of interest in cerebral structure and neuropathology. It was also a period that witnessed rapid advances in psychophysiology technology. How does the laterality effect stand now?

Inquiries into the causes of schizophrenia lie somewhat becalmed. The dopamine hypothesis remains intact, but seemingly incapable of further immediate development. The effectiveness of dopamine postsynaptic receptor blockade and the close association between blocking capability and therapeutic efficacy constitute the two inescapable facts in the pharmacological treatment of schizophrenia. But convincing evidence of disturbance in dopamine synthesis, metabolism or transmission in the untreated state is entirely lacking and it seems probable that dopamine 'overactivity' is relative and a consequence of an imbalance created by a defect elsewhere in a complex counterpoised neurotransmitter/neuromodulator system. An association between cerebral atrophy (as demonstrated by CT), cognitive impairment and 'soft' neurological involvement has suggested a new approach to classification (Crow 1980). A familial/sporadic dichotomy may also provide a useful heuristic model (Lewis et al 1987).

Neuropathological studies (Bogerts et al 1985, Brown et al 1986, Jakob & Beckmann 1986) have emphasised the significance of temporal lobe (and, in particular, the hippocampus and its cortex) malfunction, but neuroimaging techniques, using cerebral blood flow (CBF) and glucose utilisation, have demonstrated frontal hypofunction, at rest but particularly during conditions of mental stress (Weinberger et al 1986). Increasing attention is paid to prenatal and perinatal risk factors (season of birth effect; obstetric accidents) and the concept of schizophrenia as a neurodevelopmental rather than a neurodegenerative disorder has gained support.

The affective psychoses are, in clinical terms, less clearly delineated and less homogenous; but the same biological risk factors and interventions are of a similar order of importance here. Thus genetic loading, season of birth, cerebral atrophy, and the antipsychotic specificity of dopamine blockade appear relevant to an understanding of both forms of psychosis. Affective psychosis secondary to organic brain disease, e.g. secondary mania (Krauthammer & Klerman 1978) has recently achieved more prominence.

The importance of laterality in these more recent developments has been fairly limited. With each technological advance, psychophysiological methodology has grown increasingly sophisticated, but as experimental paradigms increase in complexity, so interpretation becomes more uncertain and results of investigations (in skin conductance, EEG power spectral analysis, sensory processing, abnormalities of lateral gaze, and handiness, to name only a few of the more prominent lines of enquiry) cannot readily be integrated into any simple or consistant laterality theory for either of the major psychoses (Gruzelier 1981). CT has confirmed the earlier air encephalography findings of generalised cerebral atrophy (lateral ventricular dilatation, sulcal atrophy, cerebellar vermis atrophy) in schizophrenia, and also in the affective psychoses. In general, asymmetry of atrophy has not been a feature, but CT imaging of the temporal lobe is relatively limited. Measures of hemispheric density, though prone to artifact, may have more discriminatory power. Golden et al (1981) have shown that schizophrenics have lower mean brain density than controls in the left anterior hemisphere and Reveley et al (1987) have found that in monozygotic twins discordant for schizophrenia, the affected twin has a lower left hemisphere density (see page 220).

The more recent neuroimaging techniques, magnetic resonance imaging (MRI), single photon emission computerised tomography (SPECT) and positron emission tomography (PET), are at a developmental stage and their contribution to the laterality debate is limited. Abnormalities of regional CBF (left frontal and right posterior hemisphere) in unipolar depressives have been described (Uytdenhoef et al 1983, Gur et al 1984), but not always in the same direction. A reduction in left hemisphere CBF in major depressive disorder has also been reported (Mathew et al 1980) but not replicated (Gustafson et al 1981).

Final confirmation of a laterality effect may rest with autopsy studies. But, for logistic reasons, few recent investigations have been carried out. Reynolds (1987) has reported an increase in dopamine and its major metabolite, HVA, in the left but not the right amygdala, but this has not been confirmed. Enlargement of the temporal horns and thinning of the parahippocampal cortex, more marked on the left, have also been described (Brown et al 1986).

It would be quite premature at this moment to make any pronouncement on the significance of cerebral lateralisation in the aetiology of the major psychoses. Cerebral function is far more complex than could have been envisaged even 20 years ago. New techniques are being introduced that have a penetrance and precision that must inevitably yield a great increase in our understanding; but these techniques are in their infancy and the findings that derive from them are of the most preliminary kind. The one prediction that may be made with some confidence is that the pathological mechanisms that underlie the major psychoses are complex and diffuse and unlikely to be confined solely to one or other hemisphere or part of the brain.

REFERENCES

Annett M 1979 A Classification of hand preferences by association analysis. British Journal of Psychology 61: 303–21
Bogerts B, Meertz E, Schonfeldt-Bausch R 1985 Basal ganglia and limbic system pathology in schizophrenia. A morphometric study of brain volume and shrinkage. Archives of General Psychiatry 42: 784–791
Brown R, Colter N, Corsellis J A N et al 1986 Postmortem evidence of structural brain changes in schizophrenia. Differences in brain weight in temporal horn area and parahippocampal gyrus compared with affective disorder. Archives of General Psychiatry 43: 36–42
Crow T J 1980 Molecular pathology of schizophrenia; more than one disease process? British Medical Journal ii: 66–68
Currie S, Heathfield K W G, Henson R A, Scott D F 1971 Clinical course and prognosis of temporal lobe epilepsy. Brain 94: 173–190
Davison K, Bagley C R 1969 Schizophrenia-like psychoses associated with organic disorders of the central nervous system: a review of the literature. In: Herrington R N (ed) Current problems in neuropsychiatry. British Journal of Psychiatry Special Publication no 4. Headley Brothers, Ashford, Kent, p 150–152
Flor-Henry P 1969 Psychosis and temporal lobe epilepsy: a controlled investigation. Epilepsia 10: 363–395
Golden C J, Graber B, Coffman J, Berg R A, Newlin D B, Block S 1981 Structural brain deficits in schizophrenia: identification by computed tomographic scan density measurements. Archives of General Psychiatry 38: 1014–1017

Gregoriadis A, Fragos E, Kapslakis Z, Mandouvalos B 1971 A correlation between mental disorders and EEG and AEG findings in temporal lobe epilepsy. Abstracts from the first world congress of psychiatry 1971, Mexico. La Prensa Medica Mexicana, Mexico, p 325

Gruzelier J H 1981 Cerebral laterality and psychopathology: fact and fiction. Psychological Medicine 11: 219–227

Gunn J, Fenton G W 1969 Epilepsy in prisons: a diagnostic survey. British Medical Journal iv: 326–328

Gur R E, Skolnick B E, Gur R C et al 1984 Brain function in psychiatric disorders II Regional cerebral blood flow in medicated unipolar depressives. Archives of General Psychiatry 41: 695–699

Gustafson L, Risberg J, Silferskiold P 1981 Cerebral blood flow in dementia and depression. Lancet i: 275

Hara T, Hoshi A, Takase N, Saito S 1980 Factors related to psychiatric episodes in epileptics. Folia Psychiatrica et Neurologica Japonica 34: 329–330

Hillbom E 1951 Schizophrenia like psychoses after brain trauma. Acta Psychiatrica et Neurologica Scandinavica, supplement 60: 36–47

Jakob H, Beckmann H 1986 Prenatal developmental disturbance in the limbic allocortex in schizophrenics. Journal of Neural Transmission 65: 303–326

Jensen I, Larsen J K 1979 Mental aspects of temporal lobe epilepsy. Journal of Neurology, Neurosurgery and Psychiatry 42: 256–265

Kraepelin E 1910 Psychiatrie, 8th edn. Barth, Leipzig

Krauthammer C, Klerman G L 1978 Secondary mania: manic syndromes associated with antecedent physical illness or drugs. Archives of General Psychiatry 35: 1333–1339

Kristensen O, Sindrup E H 1978 Psychomotor epilepsy and psychosis II Electroencephalographic findings. Acta Neurologica Scandinavica 57: 370–379

Lewis S W, Reveley A M, Reveley M A, Chitkara B, Murray R M 1987 The familial-sporadic distinction as a strategy in schizophrenia research. British Journal of Psychiatry 151: 306–313

Lindsay J, Ounsted C, Richards P 1979 Long-term outcome in children with temporal lobe seizures III Psychiatric aspects in childhood and adult life. Developmental Medicine and Child Neurology 21: 630–636

Lishman W A 1968 Brain damage in relation to psychiatric disability after head injury. British Journal of Psychiatry 114: 373–410

Lishman W A 1973 The psychiatric sequelae of head injury: a review. Psychological Medicine 3: 304–318

Mathew R J Meyer J S, Francis D J et al 1980 Cerebral blood flow in depression. American Journal of Psychiatry 137: 1449–1450

Muller G 1931 Anfalle bei schizophrenen erkrankungen. Allgemeine Zeitschrift fur Psychiatrie 93: 235–240

Murray R M, Lewis S W, Reveley A M 1985 Towards an aetiological classification of schizophrenia. Lancet i: 1023–1027

Ounsted C, Lindsay J 1981 The longterm outcome of temporal lobe epilepsy in childhood. In: Reynolds E H, Trimble M R (eds) Epilepsy and psychiatry. Churchill Livingstone, Edinburgh, p 185–215

Perez M, Trimble M R, Murray N M F, Reider I 1985 Epileptic psychosis: an evaluation of present state examination profiles. British Journal of Psychiatry 146: 155–163

Pritchard III P B, Lombroso C T, McIntyre M 1980 Psychological complications of temporal lobe epilepsy. Neurology 30: 227–232

Reveley M A, Reveley A M, Baldry R 1987 Left cerebral hemisphere hypodensity in discordant schizophrenic twins. Archives of General Psychiatry 44: 625–632

Reynolds G P 1987 Postmortem neurochemical studies in schizophrenia. In: Hafner H, Gattaz W F, Janzarik W (eds) Search for the causes of schizophrenia. Springer Verlag, Berlin, p 236–240

Sherwin I 1977 Clinical and EEG aspects of temporal lobe epilepsy with behaviour disorder: the role of cerebral dominance. In: Blumer D, Levin K (eds) McLean Hospital Journal, special issue, p 40–50

Sherwin I 1981 Psychosis associated with epilepsy: significance of the laterality of the epileptogenic lesions. Journal of Neurology, Neurosurgery and Psychiatry 4: 83–85

Sherwin I 1984 Differential psychiatric features in epilepsy: relationship to lesion laterality. Acta Psychiatrica Scandinavica, supplement 313: 92–103

Sherwin I, Peron-Magnan P, Bancaud J, Bonis A, Talairach J 1982 Prevalence of psychosis in epilepsy as a function of the laterality of the epileptogenic lesion. Archives of Neurology 39: 621–625

Shukla G D, Katiyar B C 1980 Psychiatric disorders in temporal lobe epilepsy: the laterality effect. British Journal of Psychiatry 137: 181–182

Slater E, Beard A W, Glitheroe E 1963 The schizophrenia-like psychoses of epilepsy. British Journal of Psychiatry 109: 95–150

Stevens J R 1966 Psychiatric Implications of Psychomotor Epilepsy. Archives of General Psychiatry 14: 461–471

Taylor D 1972 Mental state and temporal lobe epilepsy. Epilepsia 13: 727–765

Taylor D 1975 Factors influencing the occurrence of schizophrenia-like psychoses in patients with temporal lobe epilepsy. Psychological Medicine 5: 245–254

Toone B K 1981 Psychoses of epilepsy. In: Reynolds E H, Trimble M R (eds) Epilepsy and psychiatry. Churchill Livingstone, Edinburgh, p 113–137

Toone B K 1986 Epilepsy with mental illness: interrelationships. In: Trimble M R, Reynolds E H (eds) What is epilepsy? Churchill Livingstone, Edinburgh, p 206–216

Toone B K, Dawson J, Driver M V 1982a Psychoses of epilepsy, a radiological evaluation. British Journal of Psychiatry 140: 244–248

Toone B K, Garralda M E, Ron M A 1982b The psychoses of epilepsy and the functional psychoses: a clinical and phenomenological comparison. British Journal of Psychiatry 141: 256–261

Uytdenhoef P, Portelange P, Jacquy J et al 1983 Regional cerebral blood flow and lateralized hemispheric dysfunction in depression. British Journal of Psychiatry 143: 128–132

Weinberger D R, Berman K F, Zec R F 1986 Physiologic dysfunction of dorsolateral prefrontal cortex in schizophrenia 1 Regional cerebral blood flow evidence. Archives of General Psychiatry 43: 114–124

Wing J K, Cooper J E, Sartorius N 1974 The measurement and classification of psychiatric symptoms. Cambridge University Press, Cambridge

The EEG in neuropsychiatry

To contribute to this volume which honours the memory of Sir Denis Hill gives me great pleasure. This feeling is mixed with sadness, as he is no longer with us to share and discuss its contents. I had the privilege of working in his departments at the Middlesex Hospital Medical School and later at the Institute of Psychiatry for just over 13 years. Amongst his many interests were two that we had in common; the behavioural aspects of epilepsy and the neurophysiology of behaviour.

He made very significant contributions to knowledge and clinical practice in both these fields. He pioneered the EEG study of psychopathic behaviour and schizophrenia and set up the first epilepsy unit in the UK dedicated to the investigation and management of the behavioural problems of epilepsy. In the late 1940s and early 1950s he wrote about the new syndrome of psychomotor/temporal lobe epilepsy and encouraged Murray Falconer, recently arrived at the Maudsley from New Zealand, to develop an interest in its surgical treatment. He was a joint author with Murray Falconer of the early Maudsley publications on the outcome of temporal lobectomy and its effect on behaviour, thus initiating a period of sustained research productivity that has established the Maudsley's international reputation in the field of temporal lobe epilepsy surgery. He drew attention to the relation between temporal lobe epilepsy and a schizophrenia-like psychosis 10 years before Eliot Slater and colleagues published their classic study of epilepsy and schizophrenia in 1963.

Sir Denis was a gifted clinician and a superb clinical teacher in neuro-psychiatry as well as in general psychiatry. His psychiatric interviewing skills were of a very high order and his clinical and EEG assessments a model of clarity and commonsense. His interests spanned the interface between brain and mind, and in his case formulations he had an unparalleled ability to integrate the biological and psychodynamic aspects of the clinical problem under consideration.

WHAT IS THE ELECTROENCEPHALOGRAM?

In order to appreciate the contribution of electroencephalography to the practice of neuropsychiatry, a basic understanding of the neural basis of the EEG and the general principles of EEG interpretation is required. The cerebral cortex is a complex structure consisting of six layers of cells with complex fibre interconnections between them. Many are arranged in a mosaic of vertical columns. Each column consists of apical dendrites running vertically towards the surface of the cortex from the cell body with the axon radiating from the soma in the opposite direction towards the deeper layers of the cortex.

Potentials arising near one or other pole of the vertically arranged columns of neurones cause currents to flow either towards or away from the surface of the cortex due to the summation effect of thousands of excitatory and inhibitory postsynaptic potentials. Such current flow involving the mosaic of neurone columns, when summated, creates a sufficiently strong electrical field to generate the EEG. The original hypothesis of the EEG being due to summated axon action potentials has now been rejected since such potentials have been shown to set up very localised electrical fields that are not evident at the cortical surface (Goldensohn 1979, Driver & McGillivray 1982).

Although the actual potential fields are created by the superficial layers of the cortex, the synchronisation of this cortical activity is controlled by the thalamus via the non-specific thalamic nuclei and the thalamic projection areas of the cortex (Andersen & Andersson 1968). Thus the EEG generators are thalamocortical in nature. In turn the thalamic activity is modulated by tonic bombardment from the midbrain and brainstem reticular activating system. Depression of reticular tone leads to synchronisation of the thalamic rhythms and hence to synchronisation and slowing of cortical EEG activity. An increase in reticular tone leads to EEG desynchronisation due to breaking up of thalamic spindle activity (Andersen & Andersson 1968). The interested reader is referred to the review by Creutzfeldt (1974).

The cranium and soft tissues of the scalp have an attenuating effect on the EEG generated by the cerebral cortex. This attenuation factor varies from 5000 : 1 to 2 : 1 and is determined largely by the extent of cortex involved. The amplitude of the signal generated by the cortex is less important. Hence, cortical activity will only appear prominently in the scalp EEG when there is synchronous involvement of at least 6 cm^2 of cortex. Thus the alpha rhythm arising widely from the postcentral cortex of both hemispheres is only attenuated three-fold while strictly localised cortical spikes can be attenuated 40 times by transmission through the cranial vault to the scalp (Cooper et al 1965).

FACTORS THAT INFLUENCE EEG INTERPRETATION

Location and extent of lesion

From the above observations it can be inferred that disorders of brain function will only produce scalp EEG change when there is synchronous electrical involvement of a relatively large area of cortex. Such a process will be caused by either relatively extensive local cortical lesions or diffuse and synchronous involvement of the cortex due to transmission of diencephalic electrical abnormalities via the diffuse thalamocortical projection systems. These observations lead to an important principle of interpretation: namely, that lesions or dysfunction of the cerebral cortex are much more likely to cause EEG abnormality than those located deep in the brain. For example, posterior fossa tumours produce little EEG change unless secondary pressure effects result in brain stem compression and diencephalic electrical abnormality.

Diencephalic dysfunction causes projected rhythms to arise synchronously from the cortex of both cerebral hemispheres via the diffuse thalamocortical pathways. These disturbances take the form of bilateral high voltage episodes of monorhythmic delta/theta waves, usually most prominent in the frontal areas. The underlying midbrain and brainstem malfunction is a consequence of structural changes due to compression caused by increased intracranial pressure and/or disturbed functioning of the arousal system brought about by pressure effects or metabolic disorder. Diencephalic structures are also probably involved in the process of generalisation of epileptic seizures.

Physiological origins of the EEG

EEG changes caused by cerebral dysfunction result from an alteration in the electrical activity of cortical neurones. However, such abnormal activity can be the final expression of a wide variety of disease processes involving either damage to nerve cells or potentially reversible disturbances in cell metabolism due to such metabolic insults as liver failure, hypothyroidism, hypoglycaemia and acute hypoxia. Therefore, another important principle is that the electrical patterns accompanying brain dysfunction can not be used to predict the precise nature of the underlying pathological process. Their value is limited to assessing the location and extent of the dysfunction, the cause of which can only be determined by consideration of other factors, in addition to the EEG, such as the evolution and course of the illness, the physical signs and the results of other investigations.

Acute and progressive nature of the pathology

The extent and intensity of the EEG changes depend on the acuteness of the lesion as well as its location. The more rapid its progression the greater is the probability of EEG abnormality. For example, a slowly growing tumour such as a meningioma may expand to massive size without affecting the EEG while an acute cerebral abscess will produce a marked local or lateralised slow wave disturbance. Further, the EEG abnormalities are at their peak when the brain dysfunction is most severe and subsequently may resolve almost completely despite residual brain damage. Hence EEG abnormality tends to reflect active disease processes. When the disorder has resolved or ceased to progress, the EEG will show little or no abnormality. For example, cortical cell loss due to brain damage acquired early in life may show little or no EEG change after an interval of time has elapsed following the initial brain insult. An exception to this rule occurs when the lesion develops epileptogenic properties with the generation of spikes, sharp waves, etc.

Epileptogenic lesions

Cerebral neurones involved in the epileptic process produce EEG paroxysmal or epileptiform abnormalities. These appear on the scalp EEG as transient electrical events suddenly arising from the EEG background with a characteristic, sharply contoured waveform, lasting milliseconds to seconds only and then disappearing completely. Those known as sharp waves or spikes (short duration sharp waves; less than 80 ms) are associated with epilepsy due to local cortical damage (partial epilepsy). Hence, they tend to be confined to the site of the diseased cortex causing the fits. In contrast, the so-called generalised spike and wave complexes arise simultaneously from all areas of the cortex of both hemispheres (generalised onset). They consist of a complex of activity: a spike followed by a slow wave, this complex of spike-wave activity often being repeated at a fairly constant repetition rate of around 3 Hz. Such generalised spike-wave activity is commonly a consequence of epilepsy of genetic origin with no underlying brain damage (primary generalised epilepsy). Occasionally, they may be secondary to diffuse cortical damage acquired early in life, when the frequency of the spike-wave complexes tends to be slower (less than 3 Hz). Epilepsy associated with generalised spike-wave discharges due to diffuse acquired pathology is known as secondary generalised epilepsy. Rarely, a local cortical lesion may trigger generalised spike-wave discharges. The location of such lesions tends to be in the mesial surface of the hemisphere, orbitofrontal cortex or in the mesial temporal lobe structures.

These paroxysmal electrical events occur between, as well as during, clinical seizures, though between fits their occurrence is usually relatively transient. The appearance of such paroxysmal abnormalities is a variable and unpredictable phenomenon; sometimes related to level of alertness and time of day, seizure frequency and amount of medication, but often being apparently a random event. From the clinical point of view it is important to bear in mind that such paroxysmal/epileptiform abnormalities can be recorded in the absence of clinical epileptic fits; in a small number of apparently healthy people, during alcohol and drug withdrawal states, as a consequence of antidepressant and neuroleptic medication, or as part of the EEG disturbances accompanying diffuse or focal brain disease without manifest epilepsy. Therefore epilepsy must always be a clinical diagnosis; the EEG being used as confirmatory evidence only.

PATHOLOGICAL EEG CHANGES: SOME GENERAL OBSERVATIONS

Despite these limitations the EEG is a useful non-invasive tool to investigate organic brain disease and epilepsy. Local cortical damage causes a localised reduction or absence of normal EEG background activity from the affected cortex with a resultant amplitude asymmetry compared to the activity generated by the equivalent part of the contralateral hemisphere. An asymmetry in dominant background activity frequency may also develop with frequency slowing over the affected side. If the disease process causing the cortical damage is acute or actively progressing, e.g. acute ischaemia due to a vascular lesion, a cerebral abscess or a malignant tumour, irregular slow waves (less than 4 Hz; local delta activity) will be prominent around the affected area.

In the case of a tumour the slow waves will tend to be most marked around the advancing boundaries of the growth, being generated by tissue that is damaged by infiltration or compression but is still capable of some function. Dead brain tissue is electrically silent. Therefore, the location of the relative amplitude reduction often gives more accurate localisation of the tumour site.

Extracerebral lesions, e.g. subdural haematomas, do not change the spontaneous activity of the cortex unless the mass of the lesion intervenes between the recording scalp electrodes and the brain and so constitutes a low resistance pathway between adjacent pairs of electrodes with consequent electrical 'silence' over the lesion. This can often be misleading in the case of a subdural haematoma since the activity recorded from the contralateral hemisphere may be dominated by high voltage delta activity due to a generalised disturbance of the arousal system or pressure effects. The contralateral side may therefore appear more 'abnormal' than the 'silent' ipsilateral hemisphere. The localisation problems of space-occupying pathology can be further complicated by the not infrequent development of cortical rhythms at a distance from the lesion; bifrontal monorhythmic delta wave episodes due to brainstem malfunction.

In the case of widespread dysfunction involving all or most of the cerebral cortex, the background changes mirror in generalised distribution those observed with local pathology; namely bilateral reduction of normal rhythms and progressive frequency slowing. The main alteration is initial slowing of alpha frequency over both hemispheres; slowing of as little as

1 Hz is significant, since the (alpha) dominant activity frequency in any individual is remarkably consistent over time. It should be noted that although the alpha frequency range is 8–13 Hz, most individuals have 9–10 Hz alpha rhythms. Therefore, a pathological reduction of 1 Hz may still leave alpha frequency with the normal 8–13 Hz range. For this reason, serial EEG recordings are very useful in the investigation of organic brain syndromes (Pro & Wells 1977).

The bilateral alpha rhythm slowing is accompanied by the appearance of diffuse slower frequencies (less than 7 Hz), that replace the alpha rhythm completely as the disorder progresses. Superimposed upon this diffuse slow background, episodic higher voltage runs of rhythmic bifrontal delta activity occur. With severe impairment of cortical functioning the EEG becomes dominated with generalised irregular delta waves. These widespread EEG changes characterised by progressive diffuse slowing are a stereotyped response to the cerebral insult regardless of its nature and occur in the following two main groups of clinical state: acute and chronic brain failure.

ACUTE BRAIN FAILURE

This develops as a consequence of a sudden disturbance of the metabolism of the cortical neurones caused by poisoning with exogenous toxins, toxic products circulating in the blood stream as the result of failure of other bodily organs such as liver or kidney, disruption of the delivery of essential nutrients to the brain, such as oxygen, glucose or the various vitamin B complexes or structural damage due to trauma or diffuse inflammatory processes involving the cortical cells. The EEG changes closely reflect the extent and severity of the disturbance of cortical function caused by such events. Indeed, the EEG slowing may be the first herald of incipient brain failure and of value in the early detection of recurrent episodes of such disorder, e.g. in hepatic encephalopathy (Parsons-Smith et al 1957). These changes are potentially reversible and the EEG will revert towards normality if and when the underlying brain dysfunction resolves or remits. However, should residual damage remain, some degree of diffuse slowing may be permanent.

Electrolyte disturbances

Calcium metabolism upsets are associated with the most marked changes. Hypocalcaemia causes diffuse slowing along with epileptiform activity and seizures, while hypercalcaemia is known to produce generalised slowing and occasionally bifrontal monorhythmic delta wave episodes and triphasic waves of generalised origin. Water intoxication also causes marked diffuse slowing while dehydration does not produce significant EEG change.

Changes in body temperature

Hypothermia induces slowing and attenuation of the background EEG, the changes beginning at 25°C. With hyperthermia, it is difficult to identify EEG changes that are not related to the underlying disease causing the pyrexia.

Blood sugar alterations

The first signs of hypoglycamia occur when the blood sugar falls to between 40 and 60 mg/dl, with bilateral alpha rhythm slowing and an increased delta wave response to hyperventilation. Progressive diffuse slowing continues as the blood sugar falls further. Permanent changes with generalised slowing and both focal and generalised epileptiform activity may be the outcome of severe and prolonged hypoglycaemia. Hyperglycaemia causes less EEG alteration, though diffuse slowing develops as consciousness becomes clouded.

Toxic states

Poisoning with carbon monoxide, heavy metals, organic solvents and organophosphorous compounds also cause diffuse slowing. Drug intoxication produces similar changes, prominent beta activity being an additional feature with barbiturate and benzodiazepine poisoning. In drug-induced coma, diffuse delta activity, suppression-burst activity and even electrical silence develop in temporal sequence as coma deepens. Such effects are seen with sedative/hypnotic agents, neuroleptics, antidepressants, lithium, anxiolytics, CNS stimulants, anticonvulsants, narcotics, anticholinergic drugs and steroids (Bauer 1982).

Endocrine disorders

Thyroid dysfunction has been the most carefully studied. Diffuse slowing is prominent in hypothyroidism, while lesser degrees of EEG abnormality occur in hyperthyroidism; slightly increased alpha frequency, more prominent beta rhythm and occasional irregular theta activity (Wilson 1965). Cushing's syndrome, hypopituitarism, parathyroid disorders and Addison's disease produce varying degrees of diffuse slowing, while the occurrence of epileptiform activity is more common with pseudohypoparathyroidism.

Vitamin deficiencies

Vitamin B deficiency states including pernicious anaemia are associated with generalised EEG slowing. Korsakoff's syndrome is not usually associated with EEG change, but some degree of generalised slowing is found in 50% of patients with Wernicke's encephalopathy (Victor et al 1972).

Liver and renal disease

In hepatic encephalopathy, diffuse background slowing occurs with the development of triphasic waves, bilaterally synchronous episodic runs of triphasic waves occurring in runs of tens of seconds duration (Bickford & Butt 1955). The degree of background slowing parallels the clinical state. The triphasic waves occur in only 20% of cases and are a sign of poor prognosis (Simsarian & Harner 1972). Similar changes are found in renal failure with diffuse background slowing which correlates with clouding of consciousness and blood urea levels (Bourne et al 1975, Hughes 1980). Triphasic activity has also been reported in 22% of cases, usually the more severely affected (Simsarian & Harner 1972).

Cerebral anoxia

The EEG grading of anoxic brain injury correlates well with clinical outcome; small amounts of generalised theta activity being associated with mild anoxia, more marked generalised slowing and loss of beta activity with more severe episodes and suppression-burst activity with very severe anoxia (Prior 1973).

Head injury

Minor head injuries with brief loss of consicousness, a post-traumatic amnesia of seconds, minutes or a few hours and no significant neurological sequelae (concussion) produce little change in the scalp EEG tracing examined by visual inspection. Dow et al (1944) set up an EEG laboratory in a shipyard and recorded from 213 workers within 24 hours of a mild head injury, including a number within 10 minutes of the trauma. Many showed no impairment of consciousness and a large proportion of the EEGs were within normal limits. In a minority, there were EEG changes, i.e. diffuse theta or delta activity. These correlated with clinical evidence of clouding of consciousness and tended to resolve quickly. A more recent study of accident and emergency admissions following minor head injury with concussion and transient unconsciousness used computer EEG analysis techniques and has reported significant increases in power within the theta frequency band following concussion (Montgomery et al, in preparation). Evidence of prolonged brainstem transmission times was also found in almost half the patients as well as impaired performance of a choice reaction time test (MacFlynn et al 1984).

In contusion and laceration of the brain, the EEG changes are more dramatic and depend on a number of factors including the site and extent of brain damage, the state of consciousness and the intracranial pressure. Immediately after the trauma, generalised attenuation of the EEG is probable, though, in the majority of cases this phase is over by the time EEG recordings are carried out. A contre-coup injury may cause local depression of EEG activity at a location distant from the site of injury. If this persists over days or weeks the possibility of a large accumulation of blood between the brain and the skull subdurally or extradurally must be considered. Complete and persistent generalised EEG attenuation carries a poor prognosis and is usually accompanied by deep coma giving way to death. It tends to have been a feature of those patients in whom severe hypotension or cardiorespiratory problems have accompanied or followed the head injury in the first few hours. Rarely, records obtained soon after a severe head injury may show continuous 12–15 Hz activity, again a sign of bad prognosis.

The initial attenuation is followed by the development of a higher amplitude EEG, in which disorganised slow activity of patchy distribution is dominant. A combination of generalised and local slowing is commonly seen. This slowing may increase progressively over a number of days, being presumably related to secondary effects of the injury. As the patient recovers the slow activity gradually increases in frequency and amplitude, sometimes acquiring a paroxysmal quality. Eventually the alpha rhythm returns, although at first its predominant frequency tends to be slower than the premorbid values. This gradual return towards EEG 'normality' may take months and tends to parallel clinical recovery. Paradoxically, a patient with neurological deficit who some months after a head injury shows an abnormal but 'improving' EEG is likely to exhibit further clinical recovery than one whose EEG is normal or static (Pampliglione 1975, Kiloh et al 1981, Binnie et al 1982)

EEG abnormalities over a limited area with irregular slow activity have been described in the first 24 hours after head injury due to local contusion or vascular change. These appear to be a rare finding. The occurrence of EEG epileptiform activity after a recent head injury has no predictive value for the development of late post-traumatic epilepsy (Jennett 1962).

Cerebral infections

Cerebral infections are associated with EEG changes when the brain substance is involved. Uncomplicated meningitis causes little or no EEG abnormality. In contrast, virus encephalitis is almost always accompanied by diffuse slowing. EEG normalisation within several weeks of clinical recovery is associated with a good prognosis while continued, persistent background slowing and the development of epileptiform activity are found when permanent CNS sequelae are present.Herpes simplex encephalitis affects particularly the temporal lobes and profound EEG changes occur. Asymmetrical high amplitude delta wave foci develop followed by periodic lateralised epileptiform discharges (PLEDs) recurring at 1–4 a second. These are maximal over the temporal areas predominantly affected by the disease (Illis & Taylor 1972). The PLEDs disappear over a period of days.

If the patient recovers, the slowing also gradually resolves, though this resolution is often incomplete.

CHRONIC BRAIN FAILURE

This results from progressive degeneration and death of cortical neurones and occurs as the result of specific degenerative processes such as Alzheimer's disease or patchy impairment of cerebral blood supply due to arteriosclerosis. The same diffuse EEG slowing occurs in the other dementias including that due to normal pressure hydrocephalus. The changes are often asymmetrical in multi-infarct dementia due to the patchy, multifocal nature of the ischaemic process. The EEG disturbance tends to become progressively worse as the disease process advances.

The degree of progressive slowing varies according to the nature and location of the underlying pathology, being maximal in Alzheimer's disease and less so in the other dementias, where normal EEGs and lack of progression are not uncommon. The presence of a normal EEG in the individual with dementia may result from one or more of a number of the following factors: involvement of the frontal lobes in the disease process with relative sparing of the parietal and occipital lobes and the brainstem structures as in Pick's disease, a quiescent or 'burnt-out' phase in the dementing process, or the alpha rhythm frequency slowing being still within the 'normal' 8–13 Hz range. Therefore, in patients with suspected dementia and a normal EEG serial recordings at 3–6 month intervals may well demonstrate dominant frequency slowing as the disease advances.

More specific changes are found in the following dementias — a flat EEG with little rhythmic activity in 33–83% of patients with Huntington's chorea (Scott et al 1972), transient stereotyped sharp and slow wave complexes that occur at a regular repetition rate in Creutzfeldt-Jacob disease, subacute spongiform encephalopathy and certain rare forms of progressive brain syndrome in childhood (Fenton 1986b).

THE ELECTROPHYSIOLOGY OF THE DEMENTIAS

EEG and ageing

In interpreting the EEG in the dementias, it is essential to have some knowledge of the effects of healthy ageing. The important changes due to ageing are as follows:

Alpha rhythm frequency slowing

From a young adult mean of around 10 Hz, it declines in the over-60s by about 0.05–0.75 Hz per decade; 9.0–9.5 Hz at 70 and 8.5–9.0 Hz after 80 years of age. In healthy subjects at any age, it is unusual to have a dominant (alpha) rhythm frequency of less than 8 Hz. The extent of alpha slowing is related to impaired memory function and intellectual defect in hospitalised patients with organic brain syndrome. This association does not hold true for healthy, elderly people living at home.

Low voltage fast (beta) activity

This rhythm, at 15–30 Hz, is usually less than 25 microvolts and bifrontal, rolandic or diffuse in distribution. The beta rhythm increases between 20 and 60 years especially in females. It persists into old age but diminishes greatly after 80 years.

Diffuse slowing

This consists of theta (4–7 Hz) and delta (1–3 Hz) activity of generalised distribution: rare in early senescence (7% of people under 75); over 75 the prevalence increases to 1 in 5 of community volunteers. Borderline or mild slowing does not correlate with dementia but moderate to severe slowing does. There is also a correlation with the diminished cerebral blood flow and metabolism.

Focal slow (delta) activity

Of healthy people over 60 years, 30–40% have focal anterior temporal slow waves, predominantly left-sided. These are benign. In healthy individuals, they occur in isolated runs and are strictly localised to the anterior temporal areas. Continuous focal delta slowing of more widespread distribution has a sinister significance, indicative of local pathology.

Changes in dementia

Hans Berger (1932) was the first person to report EEG abnormalities in Alzheimer's disease (AD), later confirmed histologically. There have been many EEG studies of the dementias since (Busse 1983, Pedley & Miller 1983). With important exceptions, the changes are qualitatively similar to those of healthy ageing, though much more pronounced.

Slowing of the dominant, parieto-occipital (alpha) rhythm over both hemispheres, a moderate to marked amount of diffuse theta (4–7 Hz) activity (diffuse slowing), and a bilaterally symmetrical decline in low voltage beta (fast) activity are common findings. An autopsy study reports a significant correlation between alpha frequency slowing and the number of senile plaques counted in Alzheimer's disease (Deisenhammer & Jellinger 1974). Paroxysmal runs of bifrontal delta activity, rare in healthy old people, are common in dementia patients; the main qualitative difference between the EEG manifestations of dementia and those of healthy ageing. One study has reported a relationship between such bifrontal delta episodes and degenerative brainstem changes found at autopsy (Johannesson et a 1977). The occipital responses to photic stimulation at fast flicker rates ($\geq$ 18/s) tend to disappear in a significant minority of dementia patients (1 in 5).

Studies that have compared the various types of dementing illnesses indicate that less than 5% of patients with histologically confirmed Alzheimer's disease have a normal EEG even in the early stages of the disorder (Soininen et al 1982, Gordon & Sim 1967, Johannesson et al 1979, Fenton 1986b).

Pick's disease and multi-infarct dementia (MID) differ from AD in being often associated with normal EEGs. The number of Pick's disease patients in any one study tends to be small, but a consistent finding is that 50% or more have normal EEGs. Even when diffuse alpha and delta frequencies are present in Pick's disease, the alpha activity is better preserved than in Alzheimer patients (Johannesson et al 1977, 1979, Stigsby et al 1981). This difference may relate to the fact that the histological changes in Pick's disease are confined to the frontotemporal areas of the cortex, which are relatively 'silent' electrically compared to the parieto-occipital regions, that are affected in AD. MID differs from Alzheimer's in having significantly more asymmetry between the hemispheres, localised slow-wave disturbances being particularly common, while the normal background activity, including the alpha rhythm, tends to be better preserved than in AD. For example, Constantinides et al (1969) report three times more alpha rhythm and five times more local slow-wave foci in MID. In contrast, AD patients have a significantly higher incidence of diffuse delta activity. In many cases the lateralisation of the EEG foci in MID correlates with clinical evidence of a focal ischaemic lesion.

O'Connor et al (1979) have used EEG coherence spectra to quantify asymmetries in activity between and within each hemisphere. The coherence function is essentially a frequency correlation coefficient and measures the correlation betwen pairs of EEG signals at each frequency; the range is 0 (signals quite different) to + 1.0 (signals identical). Compared with patients with functional psychiatric disorders, patients with Alzheimer type dementia had significantly higher values between the centroparietal and temporal regions within each hemisphere, while MID patients had lower values, indicating asymmetry of function between cortical areas.

Though the EEG in Creutzfeldt-Jacob disease (CJD) may only show mild generalised background slowing, which can be more marked over one hemisphere or even appear focal, distinctive periodic triphasic sharp waves of generalised origin and with a characteristic recurrence rate of 0.5–1.0 s often appear as the disease progresses. At onset the sharp waves may be unilateral, resembling periodic lateralised epileptiform discharges but they eventually become bilateral and synchronous. Their presence in a middle-aged or elderly patient with dementia due to a progressive organic brain syndrome is highly suggestive of a diagnosis of CJD.

However, it should be borne in mind that up to one-third of cases do not show this typical abnormality even with serial EEGs. Such triphasic waves with a periodicity of recurrence are seen in other conditions, notably in hepatic and other metabolic encephalopathies and subacute sclerosing leucoencephalitis. Rarely, triphasic waves may appear in advanced AD patients and in Binswanger subcortical encephalopathy but do not usually recur with such a regular periodicity nor display the characteristic evolution of CJD (Pedley & Miller 1983, Au et al 1980, Chiofalo et al 1980, Gloor 1980).

Another dementing syndrome with special EEG features is Huntington's chorea, a low voltage EEG of less than 10 microvolts being the classic finding, present in a variable number of patients (30–80%) in different series. However, such changes only become manifest when the disease is clinically well established with involuntary movements and moderate to severe dementia (Scott et al 1972, Sishta et al 1974).

EEG Cognitive and CT scan changes

Because of its insidious nature, the intellectual, emotional and behavioural deterioration caused by the degenerative process is often advanced by the time the patient presents for investigation. Hence, a substantial number of patients are already untestable because of inability to perform the standard brain damage test batteries (half to three-quarters of the series of Johannesson et al 1979). McAdam & Robinson (1956) reported a correlation of + 0.79 between ratings of EEG change and clinical severity in demented patients of mixed aetiology. This association between EEG slowing and severity of dementia has been replicated by many subsequent studies (reviewed by Busse 1983 and Fenton 1986b). However, the relationship holds for AD, but not for Pick's disease nor MID (Johannesson et al 1979).

Computerised tomography (CT) scan investigations of patients with dementia show that the best CT correlate of cognitive decline is the width of the third ventricle. Though the EEG parallels the degree of dementia, its relation to the extent of cortical atrophy is weak. Indeed the EEG and CT scan findings only correlate with each other in advanced cases.

However, combining the two improves their diagnostic power. A recent discriminant function analysis study of 56 AD patients and 84 normal elderly people found that 86% of the whole group were correctly classified using EEG variables alone. Exclusive use of the CT scan data classified 84%. The correct classification rate increased to 90% when both the EEG and CT scan findings were used (Soininen et al 1982).

There is evidence that the EEG correlates better with clinical scales sensitive to early dementia than measures of advanced dementia. The converse is true for the CT scan. These findings suggest that the EEG is more sensitive to alterations of brain function associated with early dementia while the CT scan demonstrates better the cortical atrophy of advanced dementia (Merskey et al 1980). Interestingly enough, the degree of functional brain impairment as measured by the EEG predicts prognosis for survival while the extent of cortical atrophy does not (Kaszniak et al 1978).

EEG, EPILEPSY AND BEHAVIOUR

The EEG is an invaluable aid to the investigation of the behavioural aspects of epilepsy. The clinical applications have been reviewed in detail by Fenton (1983).

Seizure-related disorders

Of the seizure related disorders, prolonged EEG/video recording has added significantly to knowledge about the clinical manifestations and electrographic features of epileptic automatism, confirming many of the previous findings based on careful clinical observation. In particular, the rarity of serious violence during ictal related automatic behaviour has been confirmed (Delgado-Escueta et al 1981).

The EEG and clinical features of complex partial seizures have been extensively studied, thus adding to the EEG/video information already accumulated about absence attacks (Delgado-Escueta et al 1982, Theodore et al 1983). Video-EEG recording technology is also being used to gather data about hysterical pseudoepileptic fits in order to improve diagnostic accuracy (Lesser 1985, Fenton 1986a). Prolonged ambulatory EEG monitoring using a portable medilog recorder is proving useful in the differential diagnosis of pseudoepilepsy.

In clouded states associated with epilepsy, the EEG helps to distinguish between automatism or confused behaviour resulting from complex partial seizures and absence status; the former being associated with focal temporal lobe spikes, sharp waves and sharp and slow wave discharges, and the latter with continuing generalised spike-wave complexes. Though a condition of children, absence status can occur in older individuals simulating a dementia or retarded depression. Postepileptic confusion, developing after one or more generalised convulsions, on the other hand, is accompanied by diffuse slowing of the EEG background activity.

These clinical observations have been confirmed by the study of a large series of short-lived psychotic episodes in epileptic patients. This work has also shown that longer psychotic episodes lasting weeks or months tend to be associated with focal temporal lobe discharges. In contrast to the brief clouded states following major seizures and during absence status, such psychoses often occurred in a setting of clear consciousness, the predominant mental state phenomena being affective, paranoid or schizophreniform symptoms. They were rarely heralded by seizures but often terminated by one. No consistent change in EEG background rhythms nor amount of focal epileptic activity during the psychoses could be demonstrated, although sometimes an apparent normalisation of the EEG occurred (Dongier 1959).

EEG and interictal psychoses

Denis Hill (1953) was the first worker to draw attention to the relation between temporal lobe epileptogenic lesions and chronic schizophrenia-like psychoses; an observation confirmed 10 years later by Slater et al (1963), who reported that 52 of the 69 patients with epilepsy and schizophrenia-like psychoses had a temporal lobe focus. Flor-Henry (1969) drew attention to the importance of the laterality of the temporal lobe dysfunction; left-sided involvement relating to schizophrenia and disorder of the right side to affective disorder. These relationships are still the subject of intense debate. Recent work suggests that left temporal lobe dysfunction may relate specifically to the syndrome of nuclear schizophrenia, while other schizophrenia-like states are associated with more diffuse brain dysfunction (Perez et al 1985). In contrast, the hypothesised link between non-dominant temporal lobe epileptogenic lesions and affective disorder is being seriously challenged (Robertson 1986, Toone 1986).

Another interesting development has been the application of intensive video-EEG monitoring methods to investigate the temporal relationship between seizures and mental state in the interictal psychoses. Ramani & Gumnit (1982) carried out a longitudinal study of 10 patients, 9 of whom had schizophreniform psychoses. Five had complex partial seizures and the rest generalised epilepsy. Only one showed a striking reduction in spiking during the psychotic phases. Further, the EEG almost 'normalised' when the patient was psychotic and a consistent inverse relation between fit frequency and the psychotic episodes was noted. EEG normalisation did not occur in the remaining patients. Therefore, the long-standing clinical observation of an inverse relation between seizures and psychosis has been confirmed by careful monitoring of individual patients but seems to be a rare event, as is the phenomenon of 'forced normalisation' (inverse relation between the degree of mental state disturbance and EEG dysfunction), first described by Landolt (1959). There is a pressing need for further such longitudinal studies of individual patients.

EEG and minor psychiatric morbidity

The relation between epilepsy, EEG epileptogenic activity and non-psychotic behaviour is also of interest to the neuropsychiatrist. When disturbed children with epilepsy are selected by EEG criteria, the site of origin of the epileptogenic process does influence the symptom profile: children with temporal lobe spikes having high aggression and low neuroticism ratings and those with generalised spike-wave complexes showing the opposite trend (Nuffield 1961). Stores (1978) has reported that children selected because of left temporal lobe epileptogenic dysfunction are specially vulnerable to a range of behavioural difficulties.

The relation in adults is less clear. The concept of a specific temporal lobe behavioural syndrome, introduced by Geschwind (1979), is theoretically attractive but is open to serious challenge (Hermann & Whitman 1984). The recent primary care study by Edeh and Toone (Edeh 1984, Toone 1986). is a significant advance in that a total general practice population of 29 822 was surveyed. Almost half of the epileptic patients had evidence of some degree of minor psychiatric morbidity. Though there were non-significant trends for more psychiatric morbidity in those with temporal lobe foci, especially on the left side, statistically significant associations were with other EEG features. The psychiatric patients had fewer normal records, slightly more lateralised or focal EEG paroxysmal abnormalities, and many more diffuse EEG background disturbances. In contrast, paroxysmal EEG abnormalities of generalised origin were more than twice as common in patients with normal mental states. Hence, in adults with epilepsy and minor psychiatric disorder, the relation between the EEG and mental state is complex. It is neither directly related to the localisation nor distribution of the EEG epileptogenic activity. The decreased number of totally normal records and greater number with diffuse EEG background activity changes amongst the patients with minor psychiatric morbidity suggest that the extent of the brain lesion causing the epilepsy and frequency of occurrence of the epileptogenic activity are important influences on mental state.

EEG in 'non-organic' psychiatric disorder

Electroencephalography is of practical value in the management of non-organic psychiatric disorders only as one of a number of special investigation techniques available for assessing the possible role of organic cerebral disease. Yet EEG abnormalities are not uncommon in these conditions in the absence of clinical or other evidence of organic pathology. In the EEG investigation of patients with these disorders it is essential to review the potential influence of the following groups of factors in a systematic fashion:

'Non-specific' abnormally of EEG background activity

A generalised excess of slower (theta/delta) background frequencies, most marked over the posterior quadrants of both hemispheres, especially in the posterior temporal regions are found in some patients in the absence of overt organic pathology. Such anomalous EEGs are common in populations of patients manifesting antisocial behaviour but are not specially found in epilepsy. Indeed their prevalence increases with the degree of maladjustment of the population studied, highest in aggressive psychopaths (50%) and lowest in people selected for stability of personality, e.g. service personnel selected for air crew duties (5%), as demonstrated by Williams (1941) and Hill (1952).

They do occur in a minority of quite healthy people (about 10%). Their significance remains unknown. The prevalence is at its peak in adolescence and early adult life and declines dramatically in the thirties (Hill 1952). The close relationship to age and the fact that such changes, anomalous in the adult EEG, are part of the normal developmental pattern in children, has led to the hypothesis that their persistence into adult life is a reflection of failure of maturation of the brain. Such a view is attractive since much of the behaviour of such individuals is 'immature'.

However, the relation between the EEG and behavioural 'immaturity' is by no means a parallel one in an individual. Further, genetic factors have been shown to be important in their genesis (Knott et al 1953). There is also some evidence linking their occurrence to perinatal brain damage (Volavka & Matousek 1969). It may be that their occurrence in psychopaths is the outcome of an interaction between genetic predisposition and the presence of mild early brain damage that interact to retard the normal processes of brain maturation.

The early environment that 'breeds' delinquency and psychopathic behaviour is often a socially disadvantaged one, where poor socioeconomic conditions prevail with disrupted family life and poor standards of health care. Such poor social circumstances and inadequate parental supervision may also increase the risk of early brain damage due either to the complications of pregnancy and childbirth, trauma or infection acquired in early childhood as a result of parental neglect or abuse. If mild, this process may delay maturation of brain activity and lead to 'immature' EEG patterns. More severe early brain damage, on the other hand, will result in organic EEG changes and/or epilepsy. This hypothesis remains to be tested. The only study in which social class was carefully controlled for, revealed no EEG differences between delinquents displaying seriously antisocial behaviour and age-matched controls (Fenton et al 1978).

In clinical practice these 'maturation' phenomena can be ignored. However, they are often prominent in the posterior temporal regions and frequently have a sharpened waveform. Such sharply formed posterior temporal slow waves can be mistaken for the EEG sharp waves of temporal lobe epilepsy (TLE). This can lead to an erroneous clinical diagnosis of TLE. Fortunately there are important differences in the location and physiological behaviour of the two waveforms. The posterior temporal slow waves are posterior in distribution, best seen in relaxed wakefulness with the eyes closed, are markedly attenuated by eye opening and disappear during sleep. Hyperventilation markedly augments them. In contrast, TLE sharp waves are located over the anterior part of the temporal lobe. They are not prominent during waking, being best seen in light sleep. They are not influenced by overbreathing.

Another association of EEG background change is abnormality in sex chromosome content. A significant generalised excess of theta activity and slow dominant rhythms are found in people with XXY and XYY karyotypes, the prevalence of EEG abnormality being higher in the XXY cases (Fenton et al 1971, 1974, Volavka et al 1977).

EEG background changes are also a feature of schizophrenia. The extent to which these changes reflect underlying subclinical organic brain damage that increases vulnerability to schizophrenia, a neurotransmitter imbalance pattern of possible genetic origin, an active brain disease process of which the psychosis is but a symptom or nonspecific changes in arousal due to the disturbed mental state remain to be determined. The observation that similar EEG changes are found in the asymptomatic children of schizophrenic parents certainly emphasises the influence of genetic factors (Itil 1977). On the other hand, observation that cases of sporadic schizophrenia have a higher incidence of EEG abnormality than patients with familial schizophrenia and the relation of EEG abnormality to a better outcome tends to support the organic vulnerability hypothesis (Kendler & Hays 1982). It is probable that all these factors are relevant to the genesis of EEG abnormality in schizophrenia, their relative contribution in each case varying from individual to individual.

More recent quantitative studies reviewed by Itil (1977) and Small (1984) confirm the visual impressions of the early workers, including Hans Berger and Denis Hill, of an excess of delta frequencies, a reduction in the amount of alpha rhythm and changes in beta (fast) activity. The beta rhythm changes are difficult to interpret because of the problem of contamination with higher frequency scalp muscle artefact. Some studies have suggested that beta activity at the high end of the frequency range (40–50 Hz) is significantly increased with a relative reduction in slower beta frequencies (14–30 Hz). There is some evidence that the frequency spectral pattern alters at different stages of the schizophrenic process, both in terms of the areas of cortex involved and the distribution of power within the frequency spectrum. One study reports that, in acute patients, alpha power alone was reduced and that this change was maximal in both temporal areas (Fenton et al 1980). In chronic patients, the changes were widespread throughout both hemispheres. Chronic day-hospital schizophrenics, well enough to live in the community, showed significantly less alpha and beta power compared to age-matched controls. Deteriorated long-stay hospital patients had a different pattern, with an excess of delta power in all areas; perhaps evidence of subclinical organic brain change with ventricular dilatation as demonstrated by CT scan studies in a significant number of schizophrenic patients (Dennert & Andreasen 1983). Visual inspection, coherence spectral analysis and brain electrical activity mapping studies have investigated lateralisation of hemisphere functioning and EEG synchrony between the hemispheres in schizophrenia. A range of findings have been reported, namely; left temporal lobe slowing, increased synchrony within the left hemisphere, decreased interhemisphere synchrony during cognitive processing and left hemisphere frequency asymmetries mainly within the beta range during brain electrical activity mapping (Abrams & Taylor 1979, Shaw et al 1979, 1983, Small 1984, Ford et al 1986, Guenther & Breitling 1985, Duffy 1986). Increased coherence values indicative of greater synchrony within the left hemisphere have recently been related to negative symptoms in chronic schizophrenia (Fenton et al 1986). These anomalies have been interpreted as either evidence of left hemisphere dysfunction or of a less lateralised brain organisation in schizophrenia. Clearly, more research is required to establish the nature of the brain processes that underlie these anomalies of lateralisation of hemisphere function.

BACKGROUND ACTIVITY CHANGES AS A CONSEQUENCE OF PSYCHIATRIC ILLNESS AND/OR ITS DRUG TREATMENT

In contrast to the 'non-specific' EEG background abnormalities, that are a constant feature of the EEG, more transient state dependent changes may occur as a consequence of the patient's mental state, changes in physical state due to illness, induced abnormal behaviour or treatment.

Mental State

Anxiety tends to attenuate the voltage and amount of alpha rhythm recorded. In some people an alpha frequency increase occurs with anxiety. Prominent low voltage beta activity is a common finding in anxious patients and low amplitude tracings dominated by diffuse beta rhythm recorded. It is likely that other abnormal mood and behavioural states such as agitation, elation, excitement and hyperactivity produce similar changes, because of the activating effect of the behavioural or emotional disturbance on the arousal system. Therefore, such changes can be expected to be a common finding in the functional psychiatric disorders and will parallel alterations in current mental state. Although not outside the range of normality, they contribute to the wide variance of EEG pattern found in psychiatric patients.

Nutritional Status

Malnutrition caused by the anorexia of severe depressive illness or alcohol abuse, self-neglect in chronic schizophrenia or severe dementia can result in folate, B_{12}, or thiamine depletion with diffuse EEG slowing. Electrolyte loss due to self-induced vomiting or purgation in patients with anorexia nervosa is associated with moderate EEG background abnormality; a diffuse excess of theta waves and sometimes dominant rhythm slowing. These changes occur in two-thirds of patients and tend to be a feature of the more chronic cases (Crisp et al 1968).

Medication

Psychotropic drugs alter the EEG background activity. Although this can complicate clinical EEG interpretation on occasions, the quantification of drug-induced EEG change has been used successfully to identify the class of psychotropic action. Itil (1974) has classified psychotropic drug action in the human into the following three main groups, according to the computer EEG (CEEG) frequency profile: 1. anxiolytics, which cause a pattern of reduced alpha and increased beta activity; 2. neuroleptics, with a profile characterised by increased delta and reduced beta frequencies; 3. antidepressants, with a pattern of increased delta, reduced alpha and slow beta and increased fast beta frequencies. This CEEG method provides a powerful tool with which to investigate the potential action of new developed psychotropic drugs.

However, the changes identified by the CEEG method during serial studies of healthy subjects in carefully controlled drug experiments are of limited value in the clinical situation. Drug-induced drowsiness alters significantly the EEG frequency pattern, reducing the alpha abundance and increasing the amounts of slower and faster frequencies. The drug effect tends to be less consistent in mentally ill patients and can be influenced by the clinical response or lack of it. There is often less change when the drug is given over a lengthy period in a psychotic patient compared to acute administration in a healthy volunteer. Further, the type of EEG effect varies according to the nature of the patient's pretreatment EEG. For example, a low voltage flat record with scanty alpha rhythm is likely to show an augmented alpha rhythm in response to a neuroleptic due to the anxiolytic effect, while a patient with a well developed alpha rhythm before treatment may respond to the same dosage of neuroleptic with a reduction in alpha abundance.

The most consistent and clearly defined drug-induced change is the beta rhythm response of the cerebral cortex to barbiturates or benzodiazepine drugs. A prominent low-voltage beta rhythm appears over both hemispheres. This is frontocentral or diffuse in distribution and is obvious to the naked eye. In addition, the benzodiazepines tend to reduce the alpha rhythm in amplitude and quantity while slightly increasing its frequency. There is often an apparent EEG 'normalisation' with reduction in slower background frequencies and suppression of focal and paroxysmal abnormalities. Similar effects can be seen whether the drugs are given in divided doses or in a single hypnotic dose at bedtime. Hence, the benzodiazepine drugs should be discontinued for 72 hours before EEG investigations are embarked upon.

On visual inspection, the neuroleptics only produce observable frequency changes when prescribed in relatively large doses (the equivalent of a daily dose of more than 600 mg of chlorpromazine). Even then, only the alpha and slower frequency changes can be detected readily by the naked eye.

Incidentally, EEG background changes induced by high-dose neuroleptic medication may take as long as 9 weeks to resolve. Antidepressants in therapeutic doses do not produce much change that is visible to the naked eye on the paper tracing. Paroxysmal abnormalities can also occur in some patients receiving neuroleptic and antidepressant medication.

At therapeutic serum levels, the EEG changes caused by lithium are slight and are likely to be missed by visual analysis (an average slowing of alpha frequency of only 0.1 Hz in one quantitative study; Reilly et al 1973). More definite frequency slowing occurs in states of lithium intoxication.

PAROXYSMAL ABNORMALITIES

Paroxysmal EEG abnormalities do occur in non-organic mental states and, indeed, in a small minority of apparently healthy people. There have been comparatively few studies of the prevalence of epileptiform activity in the latter. The most extensive study in adults is that of Robin et al (1973), who investigated more than 7000 air force personnel. 140 exhibited epileptiform EEG activity. Further enquiry revealed that half of these had in fact suffered epileptic seizures and, of the remainder, all but 15 had been excluded from flying duties on other neuropsychiatric grounds. If the data can be generalised to the population at large the prevalence of epileptiform activity in healthy people is of the order of 2–3:1000 (Binnie 1986). A number of paroxysmal abnormalities have been reported in psychiatric patients.

The 6-a-second spike-wave phenomenon

The 6-a-second spike-wave complex (6SW), also known as the fast or phantom spike-wave complex, is of special interest. The 6SW complex is of generalised origin, usually bilaterally synchronous and symmetrical over both hemispheres. In the absence of epilepsy, the 6SW discharges occur in brief paroxysmal bursts, usually lasting 0.5 to 1 second and are infrequent in recurrence in a single recording. This is in marked contrast to the slower 3-a-second spike-wave complexes associated with absence seizures. Such spike-wave bursts may be both frequent and prolonged. The 6SW phenomena also differ from classical spike-wave phenomena in being more often seen in sleep (one-third to three-quarters) and, in adults at least, having a more postcentral distribution.

Initially reports about the phantom spike-wave phenomena related its occurrence to schizophrenia. Denis Hill (1952) gave an interesting review of the clinical inter-relationships between epilepsy and schizophrenia. In a series of 80 schizophrenics, 18 had paroxysmal EEG abnormalities. He drew attention to the frequent observation in the 1940s of isolated grand mal attacks in acute catatonic states with subsequent improvement in mental state. He considered the fits and the fast spike-wave complexes as a reflection of a low convulsive threshold. He proposed that the convulsive threshold varies during the course of the psychotic illness, the process of reduction being an internal homeostatic mechanism involved in the termination of the psychosis: a sort of internal ECT. Further support for this hypothesis is the observation that insulin-induced convulsions were significantly more frequent in those schizophrenic patients who responded favourably to insulin coma therapy. These ideas gave impetus to the development of measures of convulsive threshold using combined phobic stimulation and intravenous injection of a convulsant drug, pentylenetetrazole ('metrazole'). Although changes in seizure threshold seemed to parallel the clinical course, no consistent differences were found across groups of schizophrenic patients as compared to non-schizophrenics (Smith et al 1957). Such negative findings combined with the variability and unpleasantness of the photoconvulsive threshold measurement technique led to its abandonment as a research tool.

More recently, the 6SW complex has been related to a wider range of clinical problems, though psychiatric disorder of a less specific nature than schizophrenia remains a consistent correlate. Indeed, bursts of generalised fast spike and wave activity have been reported in up to 5% of acute psychiatric admissions (Small 1968). The clinical associations are grand-mal attacks in younger patients, 'neurovegetative/dysautonomic' symptoms (headaches, gastrointestinal symptoms, syncope and dizziness), and minor affective symptoms mainly in older patients, minor head injury and drug and alcohol misuse.

The clinical significance of the 6SW phenomenon has still to be determined. In those patients with grand mal seizures, there can be little argument that the generalised, frontally predominant, relatively high-amplitude fast spike wave complexes that occur mainly in the waking state are either due to generalised epilepsy or increased cerebral excitability caused by drug or alcohol withdrawal in drug and alcohol abusers. The relation to minor head injury, neurovegetative and affective symptoms is more ambiguous. Such symptoms as well as minor head injury are not uncommon in drug and alcohol abusers and may account for the association in some cases. The relationship between the 6SW phenomenon and the symptoms may be quite coincidental in other patients since the former is rare and the latter common. The association between them may reflect referral for EEG investigation in an attempt to clarify the underlying cause of poorly defined 'neurovegetative', affective and postconcussional symptoms. Perhaps the common factor linking affective disorder and the 6SW phenomenon may be a low convulsive threshold; evidence of cell membrane instability that may make people vulnerable to depression as well as reducing the convulsive threshold.

Small Sharp Spikes

The phenomenon of small, sharp spikes (SSS) deserves consideration since a relationship with affective disorder has been reported (Small 1970). These are brief low amplitude spikes, that may be either temporal or diffuse in distribution and are best seen during drowsiness and light sleep. Some workers report a high prevalence rate (25%) in healthy people (White et al 1977). Therefore, they are best regarded as normal variants. However, an intriguing association with both bipolar and unipolar affective illness again raises questions about possible links between affective disorder and convulsive threshold.

14-and 6-a-second Positive spikes

Another paroxysmal event of ambiguous significance is the positive spindle-like bursts of 14- and 6-a-second positive spikes maximal in the posterior temporal regions and best seen during drowsiness and light sleep. Again these paroxymal events are very common in normal adolescents, reaching a peak prevalence at 13–15 years. Therefore, they have no pathological significance, though in a survey of a large survey of a large sample of healthy children and adolescents significant correlations with a range of behavioural difficulties were observed. The interested reader is referred to the detailed review by Hughes (1984).

Miscellaneous spontaneuos paroxysmal events

Other less well-defined paroxysmal events have been reported in schizophrenia: generalised sharp and slow wave episodes,bursts of bilateral fast and slow waves and focal spikes and sharp waves, mainly of temporal lobe origin (Hill 1952, Small & Small 1965).

Medication induced paroxymal abnormality

Paroxysmal abnormalities, mainly generalised bursts of theta activity, also occur in a minority of patients on antidepressant and/or neuroleptic drugs. Rarely, these phenomena may take the form of frank spike-wave complexes either during the resting record or on photic stimulation. Such paroxysmal discharges reflect the epileptogenic effects of these drugs on certain people, who are already vulnerable because of a genetically determined low convulsive threshold.

Photosensitivity

Paroxysmal discharges triggered by a flickering light stimulus (intermittent photic stimulation, IPS) are of the following two types: the photoconvulsive and photomyoclonic responses. The photoconvulsive response consists of generalised bursts of spike-wave and/or polyspike and slow wave discharges. When these outlast the stimulus by some 100 milliseconds, the probability of epilepsy is high (Binnie 1986). In contrast, the photo-myoclonic response is a non-cerebral (EMG) event; bursts of EMG potentials due to reflex and repetitive contraction of the facial and scalp muscles and eyelid flutter. This may occur in 50% of normal people when a high intensity stimulus is used (Bickford et al 1952). Its development is favoured by the presence of a high level of background scalp muscle tone, which may be a factor in determining the greater prevalence in psychiatic patients (found in 1 in 100 psychiatric patients by Small 1971). Both types of response may be found in alcohol and drug-withrawal states and in occasional patients receiving antidepressant and neuroleptic medication.

Withdrawal paroxysmal phenomena

Withdrawal states in people dependent on alcohol and drugs, including barbiturates, narcotics and benzodiazepine compounds, are often accompanied by EEG paroxysmal discharges. These may arise spontaneously or in response to photic stimulation and are usually generalised in origin. The spontaneous EEG events include brief bursts of paroxysmal theta activity and on rare occasions transient spike-wave complexes. Photoconvulsive responses may be triggered by photic stimulation.

These paroxysmal events first appear 15–20 hours after the onset of withdrawal, peak at 35–48 hours and are rare after the fifth day. Spontaneous paroxysmal abnormalities are rare during alcohol withdrawal, but common in barbiturate withdrawal. Photic-induced discharges are seen in both (Kelley & Reilly 1984). These paroxysmal discharges can be considered a manifestation of increased cerebral excitability. There is evidence that they reflect widespread excitation of subcortical nuclei, especially the limbic structures. As withdrawal proceeds, paroxysmal discharges arise in the hippocampus, amygdala, septum and thalamus and increase in intensity until they become organised into sustained paroxysmal 'seizure' discharges (Ballenger & Post 1984).

PHYSICAL TREATMENTS

The effects of ECT

Electroconvulsive therapy causes essentially similar EEG changes as those that accompany and follow a spontaneous generalised convulsion. The most commonly reported EEG change with ECT is the development of diffuse EEG slowing. This typically presents as a built-up in generalised theta and delta activity with successive treatments. The slowing affects the background activity and is often accompanied by higher voltage intermittent runs of bifrontal delta activity. Though usually symmetrical, the slowing has sometimes a left-sided predominance.

The degree of slowing varies greatly between individuals. It is more marked in patients with abnormal pretreatment EEG records and is also related to the number of treatments, seizure duration and electrode placement. More slowing occurs with bilateral ECT than with unilateral treatment. An additional finding with unilateral ECT is that, although the EEG slowing is usually symmetrical, it is occasionally greater over the stimulated hemisphere. There is some evidence that brief pulse stimuli cause less slowing than higher energy sine waves (Weiner 1984). Drugs also have an influence; anticholinergic agents, amphetamine, mescaline, LSD and diphenylhydramine causing a transient decrease while intravenous thiopentone has the opposite effect. It is reasonable to predict more slowing in the elderly, but the evidence from actual EEG studies is conflicting. Possible sex-related differences have not been extensively investigated.

The ECT-induced slowing decreases with time after completion of the course of treatment. A recent review of 21 follow-up studies shows that the slowing resolves within 1 month in most patients and is only rarely present after 3 months (Weiner 1980).

The amount of EEG slowing has no relation to the therapeutic response, but does correlate with the degree of cognitive impairment (Fink et al 1961 Stromgen & Juul-Jensen 1975), a finding that is in keeping with the current view that post-ECT slowing reflects the extent of the organic brain change caused by the ECT-induced seizures (Weiner 1984, Fink 1986).

The EEG changes immediately after stimulus application and during the actual convulsion are more or less identical with those accompanying major epileptic fits. Following stimulus onset, a brief preictal phase lasting no more than a few seconds and consisting of low amplitude beta activity is sometimes seen. Seizure onset is often accompanied by the development of 18–22 Hz rhythmic activity; evidence of recruitment of the electrical discharge within the brain. It increments in amplitude and slows in frequency and within a few seconds is replaced by the chaotic polyspike activity of the tonic phase. Both the preictal beta activity and the recruiting rhythm often cannot be identified, the irregular polyspikes of the tonic phase being the first discernable EEG change.

The tonic polyspike phase usually contains a varying amount of EMG artifact and lasts from a few seconds to tens of seconds, developing into the regular polyspike and slow wave discharges of the clonic phase of the fit, the polyspike bursts being synchronous with clonic convulsive jerks. Both these phenomena decrease in frequency from 4–6 Hz at onset to 1–2 Hz at the end of the clonic phase. This phase lasts from 10 seconds to several minutes, following which the seizure ceases.

In about two-thirds of treatments, the endpoint is clear with transient, sudden flattening of the record. This relative electrical silence lasts a few seconds only. The remaining third show a gradual resolution of the polyspike and slow wave discharges without a clear endpoint making assessment of the EEG seizure duration difficult. Diffuse slowing develops during the immediate postictal period with gradual return towards the baseline state by 10–60 minutes after cessation of the seizure.

Reduction of the EEG seizure discharge duration by a factor of more than 2 using intravenous lidocaine causes shorter clinical fits that are less potent therapeutically (Ottosson 1960). Thus it seems that EEG seizure duration is an important determinant of ECT outcome. Whether the relationship is a direct one or whether both the EEG seizure discharge and duration of the clinical fit reflect a critical level of convulsive threshold remains to be determined. It has been suggested that individual seizures require to be longer than 25 seconds to have optimum therapeutic effect (Welch et al 1982, Weiner 1984, Fink 1986).

Seizure threshold, the amount of stimulus energy needed to induce an adequate fit, varies widely between different people (by as much as a factor of 10 or more). It rises with advancing age, possibly due to increased skin resistance and lower cortical excitability (Watterson 1945). There is no sex difference. During a course of ECT, the seizure threshold rises with successive treatments. This may be a source of difficulty when constant current machines are used since the low energy stimuli delivered by such machines tend to be near threshold. Therefore, as the threshold increases with the number of treatments, the ECT stimuli may become subthreshold. Incidently, the ECT-induced rise in threshold falls after cessation of the course of treatment.

Electrodes placed too close together for the delivery of unilateral ECT tend to be associated with an apparently higher stimulus threshold, the proximity of the electrodes increasing the population of the stimulus current that is shortcircuited through scalp tissues. Other factors known to alter EEG seizure duration include the following: energetic oxygenation with concomitant hypocapnia (increase), dehydration (increase), anaesthetic agents (decrease), hypnotics, especially benzodiazepines (decrease) and anticonvulsants (decrease). It is likely that most antidepressant and neuroleptic drugs lower seizure threshold (Chadwick 1981, Luchins et al 1984).

Psychosurgery

Stereotactic subcaudate tractotomy, which involves the stereotactic placement of bilateral lesions produced by an array of radioyttrium (^{90}Y) rods in the ventromedial quadrants of the frontal lobes is used in the treatment of carefully selected patients with chronic and intractible depression, severe obsessional neurosis or incapacitating anxiety. In a recent clinical and EEG study of 35 such patients, 29% responded well, 31% were improved and 40% did not change.

High-voltage irregular bifrontal delta activity was a common immediate EEG effect. This sometimes spread widely throughout both hemispheres. In addition, about half showed a change in background activity. This usually affected the alpha rhythm, which increased in voltage and became more widespread. In the minority of patients in whom the background activity was in the theta range, it was this activity that was augmented. The presence of a marked bifrontal slow wave response to the psychosurgery predicted a good clinical outcome at one year's follow-up (Evans et al 1982). It is of interest that this bifrontal delta wave response is similar to that described following the standard prefrontal leucotomy operations in the 1940s and early 1950s.

OVERVIEW: PRESENT AND FUTURE PROSPECTS

The main clinical value of the EEG in neuropsychiatry is as a non-invasive tool for the investigation of organic mental syndromes and epilepsy. Predictions that CT scanning would render EEG redundant have not been fulfilled. Indeed, the two instruments complement each other, the EEG being a measure of function and the CT scan a reflection of brain structure. Both are proving useful in the investigation of dementia, providing different but complementary information about the extent and progress of the disease. The relation of the EEG to the other brain imaging techniques remains to be defined. Quantitative methods of EEG analysis using laboratory computer techniques are now readily available.

Significant changes in both the EEG background activity and event-related potentials have been demonstrated in the functional psychoses. These are not specific for any diagnostic condition. This implies that they reflect either long-standing 'minimal' brain dysfunction that makes the individual vulnerable to psychosis under certain conditions of stress (biological, psychological and/or social), or information processing deficits caused by the impact of the psychotic mental state on the individual's cognitive processes and level of arousal. An interaction of both sets of factors is, of course, quite plausible. The brain-imaging techniques are probably more powerful and appropriate tools to use in the exploration and identification of the brain dysfunction vulnerability factors. In contrast, the EEG and, in particular, cognitive evoked potential paradigms will facilitate the development and testing of psychophysiological models of cognitive processing, both in healthy and pathological mental states.

Though there is some evidence that the middle latency pattern reversal and visual evoked potential latencies may be useful in the early diagnosis of Alzheimer's disease, it is the late cognitive evoked potentials that are of most value in the study of cognitive processes (Wright et al 1984, Fenton 1986b, McCallum et al 1986). The new technique of brain electrical mapping permits topographic study of the EEG and facilitates the rapid visual display and analyses of maps of scalp electrical activity over short segments of time (Duffy 1986). This is a powerful new addition to the EEG study of cognitive processes.

The computerised EEG has a clearly established place in the investigation of psychotropic drug action, bypassing the blood brain barrier and providing direct access to brain activity. Clearly this approach should prove useful in the study of the effects of drug-induced change on neurotransmitter systems.

Video EEG analyses and ambulatory EEG monitoring have made major contributions to the study of the relation between electrical events and behaviour in absence and complex partial seizures. In the future it should be possible to apply similar technology to the study of states of abnormal behaviour other than seizures (Gumnit 1985).

REFERENCES

Abrams R, Taylor M A 1979 Differential EEG patterns in affective disorder and schizophrenia. Archives of General Psychiatry 36: 1355–1358

Andersen P, Andersson S A 1968 Physiological basis of the alpha rhythm. Appleton-Century-Crofts, New York

Au W J, Gabor A J, Vijayan N, Markand O N 1980 Periodic lateralized epileptiform complexes (PLEDS) in Creutzfeldt-Jacob disease. Neurology 30: 611–617

Ballenger J C, Post R M 1984 Carbamazepine in alcohol withdrawal and the schizophrenic psychoses. Psychopharmacology Bulletin 20: 572–584

Bauer G 1982 EEG, drug effects and central nervous system poisoning. In: Niedermeyer E, Lopes da Silva F (eds) Electroencephalography: basic principles, clinical applications and related fields. Urban and Schwarzenberg, Baltimore, p 479–489

Berger H 1932 Über das elektrenkephalogram des menschen. Funfte mitterlung. Archives Psychiatrik Nervenkr 98: 231–254

Bickford R G, Butt H R 1955 Hepatic coma: the elctroencephalographic pattern. Journal of Clinical Investigation 34: 790–799

Bickford R G, Sem-Kacobsen C W, White P T, Daly D 1952 Some observations on the mechanism of photic and photo-metrazol activation. Electroencephalography and Clinical Neurophysiology 4: 275–285

Binnie C D 1986 The interictal EEG. In: Trimble M R, Reynolds E H (eds) What is epilepsy? Churchill Livingstone, Edinburgh, p 116–125

Binnie C D, Rowan A J, Gutter T H 1982 A manual of electroencephalographic technology. Cambridge University Press, Cambridge, p 363

Bourne J R, Ward J W, Teschar P E, Musso M, Johnston H D Jnr., Ginn H E 1975 Quantitative assessment of the electroencephalogram in renal disease. Electroencephalography and Clinical Neurophysiology 39: 377–388

Busse E V 1983 Electroencephalography. In: Reisberg B (ed) Alzheimer's disease. Collier Macmillan, London, p 231–236

Chadwick D W 1981 Convulsions associated with drug therapy. Adverse Drug Reaction Bulletin 38: 316–319

Chiofalo N, Fuentas A, Galvez S 1980 Serial EEG findings in 27 cases of Creutzfeldt-Jacob disease. Archives of Neurology 37: 143–145

Constantinides J, Krassoievitch M, Tissot R 1969 Correlations entre les pertubations electroencephalographiques et les lesions anatour-histologiques dans les demences. Encephale 58: 19–52

Cooper R, Winter A L, Crow H J, Walter W G 1965 Comparison of subcortical, cortical and scalp activity using chronically indwelling electrodes in man. Electroencephalography and Clinical Neurophysiology 18: 217–228

Creutzfeldt O 1974 The neuronal generation of the EEG. In: Remond A (ed) Handbook of electroencephalography and clinical neurophysiology 20, vol 2, part C. Elsevier, Amsterdam p 5–157

Crisp A H, Fenton G W, Scotton L 1968 A controlled study of the EEG in anorexia nervosa. British Journal of Psychiatry 114: 1149–1160

Delgado-Escueta A V, Mattson R H, King L et al 1981 The nature of aggression during epileptic seizures, New England Journal of Medicine 305: 711–716

Delgado-Escueta A V, Bascal T E, Treiman D M 1982 Complex partial seizures on closed circuit television and EEG: a study of 691 attacks in 79 patients. Annals of Neurology 11: 292–300

Deisenhammer E, Jellinger K 1974 EEG in senile dementia. Electroencephalography and Clinical Neurophysiology 36: 91

Dennert J W, Andreasen N C 1983 CT scanning and schizophrenia: a review. Psychiatric Developments 1: 105–121

Dongier M 1959 Statistical study of clinical and electroencephalographic manifestations of 536 psychotic episodes in 516 epileptics between clinical seizures. Epilepsia 1: 117–142

Dow R S, Ulett G, Raaf J 1944 Electroencephalographic studies immediately following head injury. American Journal of Psychiatry 7: 174–183

Driver M V, McGillivray B B 1982 Electroencephalography. In: Laidlaw J, Richens A (eds) A textbook of epilepsy. Churchill Livingstone, Edinburgh, p 115–194

Duffy F H (ed) 1986 Topographic mapping of brain electrical activity. Butterworths, London

Ebersole J S, Bridgers S L 1986 Ambulatory EEG monitoring. In: Pedley T A, Meldrum B S (eds) Recent advances in epilepsy 3. Churchill Livingstone, Edinburgh, p 111–135

Edeh J 1984 Epilepsy in general practice. PhD thesis, University of London

Evans B M, Bridges P K, Bartlett J R 1982 Electroencephalographic changes as prognostic changes after psychosurgery. Journal of Neurology, Neurosurgery and Psychiatry 44: 444–447

Fenton G W 1983 Epilepsy. In: Lader M H (ed) Handbook of psychiatry 2. Mental disorders and somatic illness. Cambridge University Press, Cambridge, p 147–185

Fenton G W 1986a Epilepsy and hysteria. British Journal of Psychiatry 149: 28–37

Fenton G W 1986b The electrophysiology of Alzheimer's disease. British Medical Bulletin 42: 29–33

Fenton G W, Tennant T G, Comish K A, Rattray N 1971 The EEG in sex chromosome abnormalities. British Journal of Psychiatry 119: 185–190

Fenton G W, Tennant T G, Fenwick P B C, Rattray N 1974 The EEG in XYY and XXY karotypes. Electroencephalography and Clinical Neurophysiology 36: 551–553

Fenton G W, Fenwick P B C, Dollimore J, Foggitt R, Nicol R 1977 The EEG in antisocial behaviour: a study of borstal boys. Electroencephalography and Clinical Neurophysiology 43: 773–774

Fenton G W, Fenwick P B C, Dollimore J, Dunn L, Hirsch S 1980 EEG spectral analysis in schizophrenia. British Journal of Psychiatry 136: 445–455

Fenton G W, Fenwick P B C, Armstrong G A, Dunn L, Hirsch S 1986 Negative symptoms in schizophrenia: an electroclinical correlate. Paper presented at the Autumn Meeting of the Scottish Psychiatric Research Society

Fink M 1986 Convulsive therapy and epilepsy research. In: Trimble M R, Reynolds E H (eds) What is epilepsy? Churchill Livingstone, Edinburgh, p 217–228

Fink M, Kahn R L, Karp A E et al 1961 Inhalant-induced convulsions: significance for the theory of the convulsion therapy process. Archives of General Psychiatry 4: 259–266

Flor-Henry P 1969 Psychosis and temporal lobe epilepsy. Epilepsia 10: 363–395

Ford M R, Goethe J W, Dekker D K 1986 EEG coherence and power in the discrimination of psychiatric disorders and medical effects. Biological Psychiatry 21: 1175–1188

Geschwind N 1979 Behavioural changes in temporal lobe epilepsy, Psychological Medicine 9: 217–219

Gloor P 1980 EEG characteristics in Creutzfeldt-Jakob disease (letter), Annals of Neurology 8: 341

Goldensohn E S 1979 Neurophysiologic substrates of EEG activity. In: Klass D W, Daly D D (eds) Current practice of clinical electroencephalography. Raven Press, New York, p 421–439

Gordon E B, Sim M 1967 The EEG in presenile dementia. Journal of Neurology, Neurosurgery and Psychiatry 30: 285–291

Guenther W, Breitling D 1985 Predominant sensorimotor area left hemisphere dysfunction in schizophrenia measured by brain electrical activity mapping. Biological Psychiatry 20: 515–532

Gumnit R J 1985 Behaviour disorders related to epilepsy. In: Gotman J, Ives J R, Gloor P (eds) Long-term monitoring in epilepsy. Electroencephalography and Clinical Neurophysiology, supplement 37: 313–323

Hermann B P, Whitman S 1984 Behavioural and personality correlates of epilepsy: a review, methodological critique and conceptual model. Psychological Medicine 95: 451–497

Hill D 1952 EEG in episodic psychotic and psychopathic behaviour. Electroencephalography and Clinical Neurophysiology 4: 419–442

Hill D 1953 Psychiatric disorders of epilepsy. Medical Press 20: 473–475

Hughes J R 1980 Correlations between EEG and chemical changes in uremia. Electroencephalography and Clinical Neurophysiology 48: 583–594

Hughes J R 1984 A review of the positive spike phenomenon. In: Hughes J R, Wilson W P (eds) EEG and evoked potentials in psychiatry and behavioural neurology. Butterworths, London, p 295–324

Illis L S, Taylor F M 1972 The electroencephalogram in herpes simplex encephalitis. Lancet i: 718–721

Itil T M 1974 Quantitative pharmaco-electroencephalography. Use of computerized cerebral biopotentials in psychotropic drug research. In: Psychotropic drugs and the human EEG. Karger, Basel, p 43–75

Itil T M 1977 Qualitative and quantitative EEG findings in schizophrenia. Schizophrenia Bulletin 3: 61–78

Jennett W B 1962 Epilepsy after blunt head injuries. Heinemann, London

Johannesson G, Brun A 1977 EEG in presenile dementia related to cerebral blood flow and autopsy findings. Acta Neurologica Scandinavica 56: 89–103

Johannesson G, Hagberg B, Gustafson I, Ingvar D H 1979 EEG and cognitive impairment in presenile dementia. Acta Neurologica Scandinavica 59: 225–240

Kaszniak A W, Fox J, Gandell D L, Garron D C, Huckman M S, Ramsay R G 1978 Predictors of mortality in presenile and senile dementia. Annals of Neurology 3: 246–252

Kelley J T, Reilly E L 1984 EEG, alcohol and alcoholism. In: Hughes J R, Wilson W P (eds) EEG and evoked potentials in psychiatry and behavioural neurology. Butterworths, London, p 55–77

Kendler K S, Hays P 1982 Familial and sporadic schizophrenia: a symptomatic, prognostic and EEG comparison. American Journal of Psychiatry 139: 1557–1562

Kiloh L G, McComas A J, Osselton J W, Upton A R M 1981 Clinical electroencephalography. Butterworths, London

Knott J R, Platt E B, Ashby M C, Gottlieb J S A 1953 A familial evaluation of the electroencephalogram of patients with primary behaviour disorder and psychopathic personality. Electroencephalography and Clinical Neurophysiology 5: 363

Landolt H 1959 Serial electroencephalographic investigations during psychotic episodes in epileptic patients and during schizophrenic attacks. In: de Haas L (ed) Lectures on epilepsy. Elsevier, Amsterdam

Lesser R P 1985 Psychogenic seizures. In: Pedley T A, Meldrum B S (eds) Recent advances in epilepsy no 2. Churchill Livingstone, Edinburgh, p 273–296

Luchins D J, Oliver A P, Wyatt R J 1984 Seizures with antidepressants: an in vitro technique to assess relative risk. Epilepsia 25: 25–32

McAdam W, Robinson R A 1956 Senile deterioration and the electroencephalogram: a quantitative correlation. Journal of Mental Science 102: 819–825

McCallum W C, Zappoli R, Denoth F 1986 Cerebral psychophysiology: studies in event-related potentials. Electroencephalography and Clinical Neurophysiology, supplement 38

MacFlynn G, Montgomery E A, Fenton G W, Rutherford W 1984 Measurement of reaction time following minor head injury. Journal of Neurology, Neurosurgery and Psychiatry 47: 1326–1331

Merksey H, Ball M J, Blume W T, Fox A J, Fox H 1980 Relationships between psychological measurements and cerebral organic changes in Alzheimer's disease. Canadian Journal of Neurological Science 7: 45–49

Montgomery E A, Fenton G W, McClelland R J, MacFlynn G, Rutherford W H 1988
   Psychobiology of minor head injury. Psychological Medicine (in press)
Nuffield E J A 1961 Neurophysiology and behaviour disorders in epileptic children. Journal
   of Mental Science 107: 438–458
O'Connor K P, Shaw J C, Ongley C O 1979 The EEG and differential diagnosis in
   psychogeriatrics. British Journal of Psychiatry 135: 156–162
Ottosson J O 1960 Experimental studies on the mode of action of electroconvulsive therapy.
   Acta Psychiatrica et Neurological Scandinavica (supplement 145) 35: 1–141
Pampiglione E 1975 Early neurophysiological assessment after insult to the central nervous
   system. In: Porter R, Fitzsimmons D W Outcome of severe damage to the central
   nervous system. Elsevier, Amsterdam, p 263–273
Parsons-Smith B G, Summerskill W H J, Dawson A M, Sherlock S 1957 The
   electroencephalogram in liver disease. Lancet ii: 867–871
Pedley T A, Miller J A 1983 Clinical neurophysiology of aging and dementia. In: Mayeux
   R, Rosen W G (eds) The dementias. Raven Press, New York, p 31–48
Perez M M, Trimble M R, Murray N M F, Reider I 1985 Epileptic psychosis: an
   evaluation of PSE profiles. British Journal of Psychiatry 146: 155–163
Prior P F 1973 The EEG in acute cerebral anoxia. Excerpta Medica, Amsterdam
Pro J D, Wells C E 1977 The use of the electroencephalogram in the diagnosis of delirium.
   Diseases of the Nervous System 38: 804–808
Ramani V, Gumnit R J 1982 Intensive monitoring of interictal psychosis in epilepsy.
   Annals of Neurology 11: 613–622
Reilly E L, Halmik A, Noyes R J, 1973 Electroencephalographic responses to lithium.
   International Pharmacopsychiatry 203–213
Robertson M M 1986 Ictal and interictal depression in patients with epilepsy. In: Trimble
   M R, Bolwig T G (eds) Aspects of epilepsy and psychiatry. Wiley, Chichester, p 213–234
Robin J J, Tolan G D, Arnold J W 1973 Ten-year experience with abnormal EEGs in
   asymptomatic adult males. Aviation Space and Environmental Medicine 49: 732–736
Scott D F, Heathfield K W G, Toone B, Margerison J H 1972 The EEG in Huntington's
   chorea: a clinical and neurological study. Journal of Neurology, Neurosurgery and
   Psychiatry 35: 97–107
Shaw J C, Brooks S, Coulter N, O'Connor K P 1979 A comparison of schizophrenic and
   neurotic patients using EEG power and coherence spectra. In: Gruzelier J H, Flor-Henry
   P (eds) Hemisphere asymmetries of function in psychopathology. Elsevier, Amsterdam,
   p 257–284
Shaw J C, Colter N, Resek G 1983 EEG coherence, lateral preference and schizophrenia.
   Psychological Medicine 13: 299–306
Simsarian J P, Harner R N 1972 Diagnosis of metabolic encephalopathy: significance of
   triphasic waves in the electroencephalogram. Neurology 22: 456
Sishta S K, Troupe A, Marsalek K S, Kremer L M 1974 Huntington's chorea: an
   electroencephalographic and psychometric study. Electroencephalography and Clinical
   Neurophysiology 36: 387–393
Slater E, Beard A W, Glithero E 1963 The schizophrenia-like psychoses of epilepsy. British
   Journal of Psychiatry 109: 95–150
Small J G, Small I F 1965 A re-evaluation of clinical EEG findings in schizophrenia.
   Disease of the Nervous System 26: 345–349
Small J G, 1968 The six per second spike and wave phenomenon — a psychiatric
   population study. Electroencephalography and Clinical Neurophysiology 24: 561–568
Small J G 1970 Small sharp spikes in a psychiatric population. Archives of General
   Psychiatry 22: 277–284
Small J G 1971 Photoconvulsive and photomyclonic responses in psychiatric patients.
   Clinical Electroencephalography 2: 78–88
Small J G 1984 EEG in schizophrenia. In: Hughes J R, Wilson W P (eds) EEG and evoked
   potentials in psychiatry and behavioural neurology. Butterworths, London, p 25–40
Smith K, Ulett G A, Johnson L C 1957 The convulsive threshold in schizophrenia.
   Archives of Neurology and Psychiatry 77: 528–532
Soininen H, Partanen J V, Puranen M, Reikkinen P J 1982 EEG and computed
   tomography in the investigation of patients with senile dementia. Journal of Neurology,
   Neurosurgery and Psychiatry 45: 711–714

Stigsby B, Johannesson G, Ingvar D M 1981 Regional EEG analysis and regional cerebral blood flow in Alzheimer's and Pick's disease. Electroencephalography and Clinical Neurophysiology 51: 537–547

Stores G 1978 School children with epilepsy at risk for learning and behaviour problems. Developmental Medicine and Child Neurology 20: 502–508

Stromgen L S, Juul-Jensen P 1975 EEG in unilateral and bilateral electroconvulsive therapy. Acta Psychiatrica Scandinavica 51: 340–360

Theodore W, Porter R J, Penry J K 1983 Complex partial seizures: clinical characteristics and differential diagnosis. Neurology 33: 1115–1121

Toone B 1986 Epilepsy with mental illness: inter-relationships. In: Trimble M R, Reynolds E H (eds) What is epilepsy? Churchill Livingstone, Edinburgh, p 206–216

Victor M, Adams R D, Collins G H 1972 The Wernicke-Korsakoff syndrome. F A Davis, Philadelphia

Volavka T, Matousek M 1969 The relation of pre- and perinatal pathology to the adult EEG. Electroencephalography and Clinical Neurophysiology 27: 667

Volavka J, Medrick S A, Sergeant J, Rasmussen L 1977 Electroencephalograms of XYY and XXY men. British Journal of Psychiatry 130: 43–47

Watterson D 1945 The effects of age, head resistance, and other physical factors on the stimulus threshold of electrically-induced seizures. Journal of Neurology, Neurosurgery and Psychiatry 8: 121–125

Weiner R D 1980 Persistence of ECT-induced EEG changes. Journal of Nervous and Mental Diseases 168: 224–228

Weiner R D 1984 EEG related to electroconvulsive therapy. In: Hughes J R, Wilson W P (eds) EEG and evoked potentials in psychiatry and behavioural neurology. Butterworths, London, p 101–126

Welch C A, Weiner R D, Weir D et al 1982 Efficacy of ECT in the treatment of depression: waveform and electrode placement considerations. Psychopharmacology Bulletin 18: 31–34

White J C, Langston J W, Pedley T A 1977 Benign epileptiform transients of sleep: clarification of the small sharp spike controversy. Neurology 27: 1061–1068

Wilson W P 1965 The electroencephalogram in endocrine disorders. In: Wilson W P Applications of electroencephalography in psychiatry. Duke University Press, Durham, p 102–122

Williams D 1941 The significance of an abnormal electroencephalogram. Journal of Neurology and Psychiatry 4: 257–268

Wright C E, Harding G F, Orwin A 1984 Presenile dementia — the use of flash and pattern VEP in diagnosis. Electroencephalography and Clinical Neurophysiology 57: 405–415

Neuropsychopharmacology

In viewing the history of neurology and psychiatry, it is clear that, until recently, one of the problems practitioners have faced has been the lack of effective treatment. Although a plethora of medicaments have been prescribed over the ages for patients with neurological and psychiatric illness, it would have to be admitted that, certainly until this century, the failure to achieve any dramatic advances was remarkable.

In recent times, particularly with regard to psychiatry, there have been two important areas of therapeutic development. The first of these, which heralded a generation of 'psychological' psychiatry, was initiated by Freud, a neurologist turned psychologist whose interest in hysteria had been kindled by Charcot in Paris. One important aspect of psychoanalysis was its potential to cure the incurable, and as such it was received with alacrity by a number of psychiatrists and neurologists. Amongst the latter must be included Smith Ely Jellife and James Jackson Putnam, the latter being in part responsible for organising Freud's famous visit to Clark University, America in 1909.

The introduction of these psychological treatments which had been preceded by such movements as mesmerism and hypnotism were occurring at a time when a different, biological orientation to psychiatry was leading to the development of alternative methods. Thus, one of the great scourges of late 19th century psychiatric institutions was general paralysis of the insane (GPI), accounting for some 7–10% of hospital admissions. The recognition that this was related to syphilis, the isolation of the spirochaete within the brain and, ultimately, the development of the first effective remedy, namely malarial therapy, by Wagner-Juregg was a dramatic advance for psychiatry and its long-suffering patients. For this discovery Wagner-Juregg received a Nobel prize, the only psychiatrist so to do. Although the effective management of syphilis required the introduction of antibiotics later in the century, the therapeutic zeal of the early neuropsychiatrists with regards to this condition cannot pass without comment. For the first time in several generations, the concept that neuropsychiatric disability had an inevitable morbid outcome, being related to hereditary degeneration, was reversed, leading to a continued search for treatment for other psychopathologies. The 1920s saw the introduction of the barbiturates for the management of epilepsy, clearly a great advance over the bromides; and, in a related area, the introduction of convulsive therapy by von Meduna for psychoses. The latter ultimately led to the rapid acceptance of electroconvulsive therapy, especially in the treatment of affective disorders.

The main neuropsychopharmacological revolution however did not take place until the 1950s. Before this could proceed on a rational basis, it was important to recognise that the central nervous system was not a syncytium of joined nerve cells, but composed of neurones which communicated with each other across a synapse. The discovery of peripheral neurotransmitters in the 1930s, and the later identification of central equivalents, soon led to the acceptance of the hypothesis of central chemical neurotransmission, the cornerstone of developments in biological psychiatry since that time.

In the present era, neurologists and psychiatrists use a similar language when describing mechanisms of drug action, referring to neuroanatomical sites within the brain which seem maximally affected by the drugs they use, and words such as dopamine, noradrenaline, serotonin and endorphins, which are common to both disciplines. The mutual independence of both is demonstrated by the role that the major psychoses played in the discovery of L-dopa. Thus, chlorpromazine, although it was being developed as an antihelminthic drug, was found to have beneficial properties in psychotic patients. At this stage in its development, the underlying biochemical effects were obscure, although it was soon noted that a number of patients, as their psychosis resolved, developed an extrapyramidal motor disorder which resembled Parkinson's disease. At this time, a number of biochemists were attempting to isolate biochemical changes that were related to Parkinson's disease, and the identification of the catecholamines and indolamines was taking place. The appreciation that chlorpromazine could antagonise dopamine receptors, and that this may be responsible for the Parkinsonism, was an important piece in the jigsaw which led to the eventual development of L-dopa as a treatment for Parkinson's disease. It was also of interest that patients with that condition, when treated with L-dopa or other dopaminergic agonists, demonstrated a high incidence of psychotic behaviour.

In this chapter it is intended to review some important areas of interest to both neurologists and psychiatrists with regards to our current knowledge of psychopharmacology. It is not intended to give an exhaustive account of the various agents available for prescription, but to underline some general principles.

PSYCHOTROPIC DRUGS

A classification of psychotropic drugs is given in Table 21.1. It will immediately be obvious that a number of these compounds are

Table 21.1 Classification of psychotropic drugs

Antidepressants	Monamine oxidase inhibitors (MAOI)	hydrazines non-hydrazines
	Non-MAOI	tricyclic non-tricyclic
Major tranquillisers (neuroleptics)	Phenothiazines Butyrophenones, thioxanthines Other	
Minor tranquillisers	Barbiturates Non-barbiturates	
Psychostimulants		
Mood stabilising drugs	Lithium Carbamazepine	
Others	Beta blockers Narcotics and analgesics Anticonvulsants	

regularly prescribed by neurologists, not only in an attempt to deal with the psychiatric consequences of neurological disease, which are frequent and may be severe (Trimble 1981a), but also for neurological conditions in their own right. For example, monoamine oxidase inhibitors are now finding a place in the management of Parkinson's disease, while a number of antidepressants have been used in conditions such as migraine, which may be best described as a functional neurological disorder. The barbiturate and non-barbiturate benzodiazepine drugs are used in epilepsy, as is carbamazepine. All of these compounds have, amongst other properties, the ability to influence the activity of postsynaptic neurones, either by alteration of the amount of a neurotransmitter within a synapse, or by alteration of pre- or postsynaptic receptors and their second messengers. They thus alter CNS function maximally in highly specific areas, especially the limbic system (Trimble & Zarifian 1984), in which the neurotransmitters which regulate behaviour, such as the catecholamines and indolamines, are found in high concentration. Based on neurochemical, neurophysiological and newer neuroanatomical evidence gathered in the last 30 years, it is once again possible to recognise that the word functional has a specific and important meaning with regards to the neurosciences, namely relating to function of an underlying neurone or neuronal system. A functional disorder is one secondary to disturbed function within neuronal systems, and functional disorders may arise either secondary to structural damage or change, or as a functional disorder de novo (Trimble 1982). The border-land between neurology and psychiatry is instantly exposed to new potential for exploration when this fundamental understanding has been attained.

Antidepressants

There are two main categories, the monoamine oxidase inhibitors (MAOI) and non-MAOI drugs. The latter break down into tricyclic and non-tricyclic groups.

In many ways, the characterisation of these as antidepressant drugs is misleading. They influence synaptic neurotransmitter function and, amongst their effects, show an antidepressant or mood-elevating property. However, they find use in a number of other conditions in neurological practice, including migraine and Parkinson's disease.

The MAOI drugs act by inhibiting the activity of monoamine oxidase, an enzyme widely distributed throughout the body. It exists in two forms, MAOA and MAOB. The substrates for MAOA include noradrenaline and serotonin, while phenylethylamine is substrate a for MAOB. Tyramine and dopamine are substrates for both forms. Selective inhibitors include clorgyline, cimoxatone and moclobemide for MAOA and deprenyl for MAOB. The development of these more selective drugs has led to a renewed interest in these compounds in neuropsychiatry. In particular, an attempt is being made to develop compounds which are free from the so called 'cheese reaction', which relates to an interaction between the inhibition of peripheral monoamine oxidase activity and the ingestion of certain absorbed primary amines.

In clinical practice, the profile of patient most likely to respond to traditional MAOI drugs includes those showing hypochondriasis, somatic anxiety, irritability, agoraphobia and other social phobias, and anergia (Tyrer 1976). In particular, the presence of somatic symptoms, and of the phobic anxiety-depersonalisation syndrome, with or without the presence of panic attacks, suggest a good response. From the point of view of neuropsychiatric practice, these drugs are extremely helpful for a number of patients who present with neurological symptoms, the basis for which is psychopathology of precisely this kind. In particular, the somatic features of anxiety respond well and, for this group of patients, these drugs should be considered as first choice therapy.

Of the newer MAOI drugs, much work has recently been carried out with deprenyl, the selective inhibitor of platelet MAOB, shown to possess significant antiParkinsonian properties. Of particular interest is the potential mechanism whereby this effect occurs. It is now known that MPTP is a selective neurotoxin for cells in the substantia nigra, provoking Parkinsonism in patients, and in animal models of the disease in primates. MPTP is converted into quaternary charged amine, which is thought to be the toxic compound. Since the MPTP/MPP+ reaction is catalysed by MAOB, if endogenous neurotoxins similar to MPTP exist and play a role in the pathogenesis of Parkinson's disease, then a selective MAOB inhibitor may not only improve the efficiency of L-dopa, but have an impact on the actual course of the disease (Langston et al 1984). Deprenyl also appears to possess

Tricyclic:

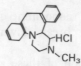

CH₂-CH₂-CH₂-N $\begin{smallmatrix} CH_3 \\ CH_3 \end{smallmatrix}$

Imipramine (Tofranil)

CH₂-CH-CH₂-N $\begin{smallmatrix} CH_3 \\ CH_3 \end{smallmatrix}$

trimipramine (Surmonil)

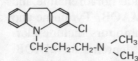

CH₂-CH₂-CH₂-N $\begin{smallmatrix} CH_3 \\ CH_3 \end{smallmatrix}$

clomipramine (Anafranil)

CH-CH₂-CH₂-N $\begin{smallmatrix} CH_3 \\ CH_3 \end{smallmatrix}$

amitriptyline (Triptyzol)

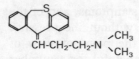

CH-CH₂-CH₂-N $\begin{smallmatrix} CH_3 \\ CH_3 \end{smallmatrix}$

dothiepin (Prothiaden)

CH-CH₂-CH₂-N $\begin{smallmatrix} CH_3 \\ CH_3 \end{smallmatrix}$

doxepin (Sinequam)

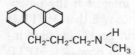

CH₂-CH₂-CH₂-N $\begin{smallmatrix} H \\ CH_3 \end{smallmatrix}$

maprotiline (Ludiomil)

Others includes:
nortriptyline (Aventyl)
protriptyline (Concordin)

NON-TRICYCLE:

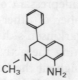

HCl

N
CH₃

mianserin (Bolvidon)

CH₃ NH₂

nomifensine (Merital)

$\overset{S}{\underset{CH-CH_2-CH_2-N}{\bigcirc}}$ CF₃
N-CH₂-CH₂-OH

flupenthixol (Fluanxol)

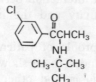

$\overset{O}{\underset{\parallel}{C}}$CHCH₃
NH
CH₃-C-CH₃
CH₃

bupropion

F₃C—⟨⟩—CH-CH₂CH₂CH₂CH₂-O-
N-OCH₂CH₂NH₂

fluvoxamine

F₃C—⟨⟩—O-C $\begin{smallmatrix} H \\ CH_2CH_2N \end{smallmatrix}$ $\begin{smallmatrix} CH_3 \\ H \end{smallmatrix}$

fluoxetine

Cl—⟨⟩—CCH₂CH₂CH₂CH₂OCH₃
N-OCH₂CH₂NH₂

clovoxamine

N-N-CH₂CH₂CH₂-N N—⟨⟩—Cl
O

trazodone

Others include:
L-tryptophan (Optimax, Pacitron)
viloxazine (Vivalan)
iprindole (Prondol)

Fig. 21.1 The structures of some non-MAOI antidepressants

antidepressant properties (Mendlewicz & Youdim 1983) and lacks the hypertensive interaction with tyramine or postural hypotension as a side effect. However, it has yet to be shown that the antidepressant effect of deprenyl is an MAOB effect, since high doses are required for the response and, at such levels, MAOA might also be inhibited.

The non-MAOI antidepressants include the tricyclic and non-tricyclic subgroups. The first be to be synthesised and used was imipramine, followed shortly by amitriptyline, both of which are probably still the most widely used. The structures of some of these are shown in Figure 21.1.

Traditionally, tricyclic drugs were thought to act by inhibition of mono-amine uptake into the presynaptic neurone, thus enhancing the availability of monoamines within the synaptic cleft. However, some of the non-tricyclic, non-MAOI drugs may have an entirely different mode of action. Precursor loading with L-tryptophan, or the use of the neuroleptic drug flupenthixol, both of which have antidepressant effects, emphasises the wide nature of chemical compounds which may have antidepressant properties. The spectrum of action of some of the antidepressants in relationship to their biochemical effects is shown in Table 21.2.

It can be seen that there are some relatively specific drugs. Selective 5-HT uptake inhibitors have recently been developed, based upon a theory of 5-HT involvement in the pathogenesis of depressive illness (see Trimble 1988). Anticholinergic effects are noted particularly with amitriptyline, clomipramine and protriptyline, and many of these compounds possess additional antihistaminic effects. Although the mode of action has tra-ditionally been related to their ability to block the reuptake of monoamines

Table 21.2 Properties for some antidepressant drugs

| | Inhibition of uptake | | | Affinities for receptor | |
	5HT	NA	DA	Muscarinic Anticholinergic	Antihistaminic
Amitriptyline	++	+++	±	+++	+++
Clomipramine	+++	+	−	++	±
Imipramine	++	+	±	+	+
Maprotiline	−	+++	±	±	+
Desipramine	+	+++	−	+	−
Nortriptyline	+	+++	±	+	+
Bupropion	−	−	++	−	−
L-tryptophan	−	−	−	−	−
Mianserin	−	+	+	−	++
Viloxazine	−	+	+	−	−
Citalopram	+++	−	−	−	−
Fluoxetine	+++	−	−	−	−
Trazadone	+	−	−	−	±
Iprindole	−	−	±	−	−
Fluvoxamine	++	−	−	−	−
Dothiepin	+	+	±	±	+++
Protriptyline	+	+++	±	+++	±

+++ = maximum
− = minimum or zero

in neurones of the CNS this effect occurs acutely, while the therapeutic effect may take several weeks to become apparent. Further, some compounds such as mianserin and iprindol minimally inhibit amine uptake in vivo. Recently, more attention has been paid to the chronic effects of these compounds and on their ability to alter the sensitivity of catecholamine receptors. In particular, they lead to down-regulation of beta receptor activity. This leads to a decrease in glycogenolysis in the postsynaptic cell, changes at the receptor being magnified by the coupler, effector and amplifier system of the postsynaptic cell membrane into larger dynamic changes. It is further known that an intact 5HT system is required for this beta receptor change. These data have led to hypotheses that relate depressive illness to a supersensitivity of these receptor sites, itself related to decreased intrasynaptic levels of neurotransmitters such as 5-HT. The mechanisms of the down-regulation and subsensitivity of noradrenergic receptors by the antidepressants is unclear, but they could be related to a change of affinity, a reduction of density or interference with cyclic AMP coupling or activity.

Attention has also been paid to the presynaptic alpha-2 adrenergic receptor, since long-term, but not short-term, antidepressant treatment reduces its sensitivity. The functional effect of this is to increase noradrenergic impulse flow and turnover with consequent behavioural activation. These hypotheses are in keeping with the suggestion that hypersensitivity of the presynaptic receptors in depression is associated with decreased release of neurotransmitters and up-regulation of the postsynaptic beta receptor. Antidepressants thus regulate the presynaptic receptor, normalising postsynaptic receptor function.

The new generation antidepressants appear to be equivalent clinically to the established tricyclic drugs, but benefit by having fewer side effects, particularly in relation to anticholinergic activity. Many of them, e.g. mianserin, are safer in overdose, although these benefits must be seen alongside the known long-term safety profile of the tricyclics. The side effects of these drugs include a number of neurological problems and are listed in Table 21.3. Nearly all the non-MAOI drugs lower the seizure threshold and may precipitate seizures, with the possible exception of viloxazine. The mechanism of this side effect is not understood, although it may be related to interference with either monoamine or GABA activity. This has significance for patients with neurological disease, many of whom have a lowered seizure threshold and therefore should be prescribed tricyclic drugs with caution. Patients with epilepsy require special consideration. Thus, many of the anticonvulsant drugs induce hepatic enzymes and, as a consequence, accelerate the metabolism of antidepressants, and the usual prescription will therefore lead to subtherapeutic doses. In general, the prescription of antidepressants should only be given after considerable thought, and although they should be introduced with an initial low-dose prescription, this will need increasing over time, often to higher oral doses than used in non-epileptic patients. This may lead to alteration and loss of seizure control, and therefore patients require careful follow up after the drugs have been given. Although viloxazine would seem a logical choice because of its minimal effect on the seizure threshold, it readily provokes carbamazepine and phenytoin intoxication, and therefore is probably best avoided (Pisani et al 1984).

Impairment of cognitive function and performance on psychological tests occurs with most non-MAOI drugs, although this has been poorly evaluated (Thompson & Trimble 1982a). Other interesting neurological complications include tremors, dyskinesia, myopathies, ataxia and peripheral neuropathy.

Major tranquillisers

These drugs group into four categories: the phenothiazines, butyrophenones, thiozanthines and others. The phenothiazines have a tricyclic nucleus, in which different configurations of the side chain lead to alteration of their properties. The butyrophenones, such as haloperidol, and related diphenyl butylpiperidines, such as pimozide, fluspiriline and penfluridol, have a different chemical structure, and some, e.g. fluspiriline and penfluridol, are long-acting oral preparations. Other major tranquillisers include molindone, reserpine, tetrabenazine, oxypertine, loxapine and the substituted benzamides such as sulpiride.

The distinguishing properties of the major tranquillisers is that they block dopamine receptors and, clinically, are antipsychotic. In addition, they evoke extrapyramidal symptoms of various types. They all inhibit apomorphine-induced stereotypy and agitation; provoke an acute increase in dopamine turnover, with raised HVA levels in brain areas such as the corpus striatum, nucleus accumbens, olfactory tubercle and frontal cortex; block the stimulation of dopamine-sensitive adenylate-cyclase; and displace receptor binding with H3-dopamine or H3-spiroperidol at postsynaptic

Table 21.3 Some side effects of non-MAOI antidepressant drugs

Sedation	Tremor
Dry mouth	Dyskynesia
Palpitations and tachycardia	Myopathy
EEG changes	Neuropathy
Visual difficulties	Convulsions
Postural difficulties	Ataxia
Postural hypotension	Delirium
Nausea, vomiting, heart burn	Agitation
Constipation	Transient hypomania
Glaucoma	Depersonalisation
Urinary retention, impotence, delayed ejaculation	Aggression
Paralytic ileus	Impairment of cognitive function
Galactorrhoea	Jaundice (cholestatic)
Sweating	Weight gain
Fever	Rashes

Table 21.4 Receptor binding properties of neuroleptics

	DA	5HT	Alpha adrenergic	Histamine	ACh
Benperidol	+++++	±	±	–	–
Droperidol	+++++	+	+	–	–
Haloperidol	+++++	–	±	–	–
Pimozide	+++++	–	–	–	–
Bromperidol	+++++	–	±	–	–
Fluspiriline	+++++	+	–	–	–
Thiothixine	++++	+	±	+	–
Trifluoperazine	++++	±	±	±	–
Perphenazine	++++	+	–	+	–
Flupenthixol	++++	+	+	±	–
Fluphenazine	+++	+	+	+	–
Penfluridol	+++	–	–	–	–
Chlorprothixine	+++	++	++	++	++
Thioridazine	++	+	++	+	++
Chlorpromazine	++	++	+++	+++	++
Sulpiride	+	–	–	–	–
Promazine	±	+	+++	+++	+++

dopamine receptor sites. Their relative potential to bind to receptors is shown in Table 21.4.

The most potent dopamine receptor antagonist used clinically is benperidol, while pimozide is the most specific. With few exceptions, their ability to block the receptor correlates with the clinical antipsychotic action, a most significant observation in attempting to understand the biochemical underpinnings of psychosis. Since the majority readily provoke extrapyramidal effects, it has been suggested that the antipsychotic potential is due to antagonism of dopamine receptors in the mesolimbic and mesocortical areas of the brain, while the motor effects relate to the nigrostriatal system.

There are some which possess minimal potential to evoke extrapyramidal disorders, in particular sulpiride, clozapine and thioridazine. One explanation for this has been the anticholinergic potential of some of these which may counteract the tendency to provoke extrapyramidal disorders. Alternatively, it has been suggested that they preferentially act on dopamine receptors on mesolimbic areas, rather than the striatum. Although studies examining dopamine metabolites do not confirm a preferential increase in levels when comparing mesolimbic to striatal structures for various neuroleptics, investigations of the disappearance or release of dopamine from selective sites do support a suggestion of a more preferential action in mesolimbic areas for these compounds (Scatton & Zivkovic 1984). Further, sulpiride does not have anticholinergic properties, supporting the suggestion that the most likely explanation for these differing clinical effects of some of the neuroleptics does indeed relate to differential antagonism of dopamine receptors in limbic, as opposed to striatal areas.

If this is the case, then it suggests an important role for dopamine within the central nervous system in its relationship to behavioural syndromes.

Thus, the main dopamine pathways originate in the region of the ventral tegmental area and substantia nigra in mid-brain, efferent neurones travelling to the caudatoputamen, limbic forebrain, including such structures as the ventral striatum and olfactory tubercle, and the orbitofrontal cortex. It is accepted that their effect at the level of the caudate-putamen relates to motor activity, influencing motor programmes and their execution. However, their link to limbic forebrain implies a role in the modulation of emotion. Clinically there can be little doubt that there is a close relationship between movements and emotion, and that abnormalities of movement are frequently associated with psychopathology and vice versa (Trimble 1981a). This not only relates to the more obvious examples of stereotypies, mannerisms, tics, choreiform movements and practical difficulties of patients with schizophrenia, but to the changes of motoric activity and posture associated with such conditions as depressive illness and mania. Neuroleptic drugs are of value in the management of psychotic conditions besides schizophrenia, especially influencing so called 'positive' symptoms, which includes hallucinations and delusions, but also excessive motor activity.

Another aspect of this link is related to the side effects of major tranquillisers, which includes a number of motor disorders. These are dystonia, akathisia, akinesia, Parkinsonism and tardive syndromes. Some of these occur acutely, e.g. dystonia, while the tardive syndromes, such as tardive dystonia or tardive dyskinesia tend to develop after several months treatment. Other neurological syndromes seen include the blepharospasm-oromandibular dystonia syndrome (Meige's or Bruegel's syndrome), catatonic reactions, the neuroleptic malignant syndrome, and tardive Gilles de la Tourette syndrome. The underlying pathogenesis of these states is thought to relate to altered dopamine activity provoked by the drugs, the acute syndromes being related to the rapid increase of dopamine turnover secondary to dopamine receptor antagonism, the chronic ones being related more to the development of supersensitivity at the postsynaptic receptor. In view of the close association between psychopathology and movement already noted, it has to be of more than passing interest that antipsychotic drugs may provoke movement disorders.

There is growing evidence that some of these disorders, e.g. tardive dyskinesia, should be accepted as part of the negative symptomatology of a progressive psychotic illness, rather than being viewed simply as a side effect of neuroleptic drug administration. There are certainly shortcomings to the concept that it is purely related to drug-induced postsynaptic dopamine receptor supersensitivity. Thus, there are discrepancies between the time of development of the clinical syndrome and the expected time of increase in dopamine receptors following the beginning of treatment, which can be shown in animal models to occur rapidly. Further, all animals given neuroleptics develop supersensitivity, whereas only some 20% of patients develop a persisting dyskinesia. In addition, in animal models where increased receptor sensitivity is shown, no equivalent of tardive dyskinesia is seen. Again, in these models, receptor changes revert to normal following withdrawal, but in patients the syndrome can persist for many years. Finally, in postmortem studies, no difference in binding is seen with respect to either dopamine 1 or dopamine 2 receptors when patients with schizophrenia, with or without movement disorders, are compared (Waddington 1985).

In a neurological setting, the same drugs are used to treat movement disorders, not only improving the clinical picture of tardive dyskinesia, but controlling the abnormal movements of, for example, Huntington's chorea, and often being used in such divergent conditions as spasmodic torticollis, the Gilles de la Tourette syndrome and the blepharospasm-oromandibular dystonia syndrome. As a general rule, drugs such as pimozide produce less in the way of cognitive dulling than haloperidol or the phenothiazines, but the incidence of unwanted extrapyramidal disorders is probably higher with the more highly selective drugs. Sulpiride, and other substituted benzamides such as tiapride, may be good alternatives, with apparently less in the way of unwanted extrapyramidal side effects. Neuroleptic use in psychoses also includes the organic brain syndromes and delirium, not an uncommon clinical problem on a neurological or neurosurgical unit. In such a setting, rapid tranquillisation is often necessary and quite large doses of medications, particularly at night, may be prescribed. It is of interest that improvement in the psychosis often does not occur until some extrapyramidal signs emerge.

Minor tranquillisers

Several generations of doctors have successfully used tranquillising drugs to aid their patients. Over the past 100 years, the bromides, barbiturates and, more recently, the benzodiazepines have been useful in many patients with minor neurotic disability. The very same drugs have been used in some neurological conditions, in particular epilepsy. The two main groups of minor tranquillisers are barbiturates and benzodiazepines, and they possess sedative, anticonvulsant and anxiolytic properties. Further, the benzodiazepines are muscle relaxant.

The barbiturate which finds most use today is phenobarbitone, introduced in the 1920s for the management of epilepsy. Although effective across a wide spectrum of seizure types, its use these days is not encouraged, in particular because of the wide range of behavioural complications it can provoke. This includes hyperactivity and conduct disorder in childhood and depressive symptomatology in adults. One effect of barbiturates is respiratory depression, leading to death in overdose. In addition, they have addictive potential and therefore benzodiazepines are preferred if possible.

The benzodiazepines have a common structure, but differ with respect

Table 21.5 Differences in potential among benzodiazepines

Drug	Anxiolytic	Anticonvulsant	Muscle Relaxing	Sedative	Amnesic
Lorazepam	++	+++	+	+	+++
Diazepam	++	+	+++	++	+
Temazepam	+	±	+	+++	±
Clonazepam	±	+++	++	+	±
Nitrazepam	+	++	+	+++	±
Clobazam	++	+++	+	±	±

to their metabolites. Many of the longer acting ones have desmethyl diazepam as their active metabolite, with a long half life of some 50 hours. However, the benzodiazepines differ with regard to their half life, and their potential for anxiolytic, anticonvulsant, muscle relaxant, sedative and amnesic effects. Some of these differences are shown in Table 21.5. On the basis of their half lives, they are divided into long, intermediate and short duration of action, as shown in Table 21.6.

In general, those with a longer duration of action tend to be prescribed as anxiolytics, while the short-acting ones are hypnotics. Several benzodiazepines are used in the management of epilepsy. While diazepam and clonazepam are well known for their potential to control status epilepticus, a number of them are useful orally (Trimble 1983). This includes nitrazepam and clonazepam in certain forms of childhood epilepsy, and the more recently introduced clobazam. The latter is a 1,5 benzodiazepine in which the nitrogen on the heterocyclic ring is moved from the 4 to the 5 position (see Fig. 21.2). This appears to confer a better therapeutic potential on the drug with regard to its anticonvulsant effect, while reducing sedative, myorelaxant and cognitive side effects. It has the advantage of having a long half life, particularly with regard to its major metabolite n-desmethylclobazam, and can therefore be given as a single night-time dose. In epilepsy, it is recommended for adjunctive treatment in intractable seizures and appears to be useful in between 10% and 20% of selected cases (Trimble 1986).

Table 21.6 Pharmacokinetic differences among benzodiazepines

Long	Intermediate	Short
Chlordiazepoxide	Alprazolam	Brotizolam
Clorazepate	Bromazepam	Midazolam
Clobazam	Flunitrazepam	Triazolam
Diazepam	Lorazepam	
Flurazepam	Lormetazepam	
Ketazolam	Nitrazepam	
Medazepam	Oxazepam	
Prazepam	Temazepam	

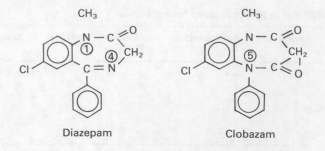

Diazepam   Clobazam

Fig. 21.2 Structures of the 1,4- (left) and 1,5-benzodiazepines (right).

The discovery of the benzodiazepine receptor has led to a clearer under-standing of their mode of action (Braestrup & Nielsen 1982). The benzo-diazepine binding site, which represents part of the GABA-receptor chloride-ionophor complex, is thought in some way to be related to the behavioural actions of these drugs, although it does not explain all of their effects. Thus, meprobamate and alcohol, both effective anxiolytics, do not appear to bind to this receptor. However, it probably does explain much of the anticonvulsant potential, which has theoretical interest. Thus, in the long history of the relationship between epilepsy and psychiatry, there is not only a link with psychotic disorders, but also with various neurotic conditions, including non-epileptic (pseudo) seizures, and anxiety symptoms (Trimble 1981b). Generally, drugs such as the benzodiazepine antagonists, which are anxiogenic, also provoke seizures, while anxiolytic drugs are anticonvulsant. These clinical observations and the identification of the benzodiazepine receptor, suggest some relationship of seizures to the neuroses, biologically hinging around the activity of the benzodiazepine-GABA-receptor complex.

Other neurological conditions in which benzodiazepines are used include spasticity, in which their muscle relaxant properties are valued, and such diverse conditions as migraine and action myoclonus. A neurological complication of treatment is seizures if the drugs are withdrawn too rapidly, particularly in a patient who has been receiving them for a long time. Side effects include oversedation, difficulty of concentration and memory and, in the elderly in particular, ataxia and confusion. A fetal benzodiazepine syndrome has been described, in which maternally derived benzodiazepines lead to hypotonus of the newborn child.

Lithium

Lithium carbonate was first introduced for the treatment of manic depress-ive illness in the late 1940s and is now the drug of choice in the prophylaxis of bipolar affective disorder. Its mode of action is unknown, but it does reduce the sodium content of the brain; increase central 5HT synthesis and noradrenaline turnover; increase platelet 5HT uptake and reduce urinary noradrenaline, MHPG, VMA, and whole body noradrenaline turnover (Coppen et al 1980, Linnoila et al 1983). It has proved useful in a number of other cyclical conditions, including recurrent aggressive disorders, particularly in those with an underlying organic brain syndrome, migraine, cluster headaches, and in organic brain syndromes with secondary affective symptoms. As such, it can be a useful drug in neurological patients with cyclical behavioural problems. Its use in association with neurological disease is not contraindicated.

Like other psychotropics, it has a number of toxic side effects (see Table 21.7), which include neurological syndromes. Severe intoxication may lead to a clear organic brain syndrome, with hyperactive reflexes, seizures and tremor. On occasions, unilateral neurological abnormalities are reported, which may be interpreted as an alternative neurological diagnosis.

Table 21.7 Toxic effects of lithium

Neuropsychiatric	Drowsiness
	Confusion
	Psychomotor retardation
	Restlessness
	Stupor
	Headache
	Weakness
	Tremor
	Ataxia
	Myasthenia gravis syndrome
	Peripheral neuropathy
	Choreoathetoid movements
	Dysarthria
	Dysgeusia
	Blurred vision
	Seizures
	Dizziness, vertigo
	Impaired short-term memory and concentration
Gastrointestinal	Anorexia, nausea, vomiting
	Diarrhoea
	Dry mouth, metallic taste
	Weight gain
Renal	Microtubular lesions
	Impairment of renal concentrating capacity
Cardiovascular	Low blood pressure
	ECG changes
Endocrine	Myxoedema
	Hyperthyroidism
	Hyperparathyroidism
Other	Polyuria and polydipsia
	Glycosuria
	Hypercalciuria
	Rashes

Anticonvulsant drugs

In the same way that the term antidepressant is a misnomer, anticonvulsant drugs possess variety of activities of which the anticonvulsant and antiepileptic potential is merely one part. Some of the anticonvulsant drugs currently in use are shown in Table 21.8. As already noted, the older, barbiturate-related compounds, but also phenytoin, are gradually being replaced by newer drugs, such as carbamazepine and sodium valproate.

The majority of anticonvulsants at one time have been used as anxiolytics, and following their introduction, most of them have been reported to have psychotropic properties. This has always been the subject of considerable controversy, not the least problem being that patients are usually given newer drugs as older ones are removed. The psychotropic effect may therefore relate to the removal of some impairment provoked by the compound removed, as opposed to a new biological property of the anticonvulsant introduced.

It is of considerable interest to both psychiatry and neurology that carbamazepine has recently been demonstrated to have psychotropic properties in a variety of different settings. This particular drug, structurally related to the tricyclic antidepressants, has therefore not only a structure but also a mode of action different from phenytoin and the barbiturates. Its biochemical actions include partial agonism of adenosine receptors. It acutely increases the firing of the locus coeruleus, and decreases CSF somatostatin and HVA accumulation after probenocid loading (Post et al 1985). Further, in animal models, carbamazepine is shown to be relatively more effective than other anticonvulsants in inhibiting seizures developed

Table 21.8 Some anticonvulsant drugs in current use

Name	Half-life, h	Recommended serum level μmol/l	Indications
Carbamazepine (Tegretol)	8–45	16–40	generalized seizures; simple or complex partial seizures; secondary generalised seizures
Clobazam (Frisium)			
Clonazepam (Rivotril)	20–40	—	myoclonic epilepsy
Ethosuximide (Zarontin)	30–100	300–700	'petit mal' epilepsy
Phenobarbitone (Epanutin)	36 (children)	60–180	generalized or simple partial seizures
Phenytoin (Epanutin)	—	40–100	generalized seizures: simple or complex partial seizures
Primidone (Mysoline)	3–12	—	generalized seizures: simple or complex partial seizures
Sodium Valproate (Epilim)	10–15	—	'petit mal': generalised seizures: myoclonic epilepsy; simple or complex partial seizures

from amygdala kindling, suggesting some limbic system selectivity (Albright & Burnham 1980).

Ever since its introduction for the management of epilepsy, it has been reported to have psychotropic properties, and this has been constantly sought in epileptic patients. There are few systematic studies, but, interestingly, in the literature there are four investigations which imply a psychotropic effect of the drug, based upon pharmacokinetic-pharmaco-dynamic relationships. Trimble & Corbett (1980) examined behaviour disorders in a large population of epileptic children and identified those where conduct disturbance was a problem. In examining the relationship between anticonvulsant drugs and conduct disorder, the latter rated on a standardised scale, a significant negative correlation was noted between conduct disorder scores and the serum carbamazepine level. In this study some 50% of the children receiving phenobarbitone were rated as having a conduct disorder.

In adults, Robertson & Trimble (1987) investigated patients with affective disorder and epilepsy in combination, and rated the phenomenology of the depression with standardised rating scales. A significant negative correlation was noted between the scores of an anxiety rating scale and the serum levels and dose of carbamazepine. Reynolds and his colleagues (Andrewes et al 1986) noted a similar relationship between rating scales for both anxiety and depression and the serum carbamazepine levels in a population of patients being placed on anticonvulsant drugs for the first time following diagnosis of their epilepsy. Once again, a higher level of carbamazepine was associated with lower scoring on the affective disorder rating scales. Finally, Rodin & Schmaltz (1983) have reported a significant negative correlation between serum levels of carbamazepine and the scores of a number of items of the Bear-Fedio rating scale, a rating scale of psychopathology in epilepsy. Taken together with the large number of anecdotal suggestions that carbamazepine has psychotropic effects, these studies all imply some influence of carbamazepine on mood, and hint at relationships between this and serum levels, similar to the relationship between serum levels and control of seizures.

These data, the interpretation of which is complicated by such problems as controlling for seizure variables, are complimented by the extensive studies of the use of carbamazepine as a mood stabiliser in psychiatric illness (Post & Uhde 1986). Thus, it has been shown to be as effective as conventional neuroleptics in the management of acute mania and to be better than placebo and similar to lithium in the long-term prophylaxis of bipolar affective disorder. Although some trials have been carried out on patients who are lithium resistant, neither this, nor the presence of EEG abnormalities are related to a beneficial clinical response. Some patients do well on a combination of carbamazepine and lithium, while not responding to either individual drug alone. Other psychiatric indications for carbamazepine include schizoaffective disorders, aggression and episodic dyscontrol, and some schizophrenic patients, particularly for the more difficult to control aggressive episodes.

Sodium valproate, thought to be a GABA agonist, may also possess some mood stabilising properties (Emrich et al 1984), although to date further investigations of this are required. In epilepsy it has been shown to be useful in the management of generalised tonic-clonic, and generalised absence seizures, and possesses less in the way of cognitive impairment as a side effect, compared with the older drugs.

The hazards of long-term anticonvulsant therapy have been well reviewed elsewhere (Reynolds 1975), but include a number of neuropsychiatric side effects. These are an encephalopathy, particularly with phenytoin, deterioration of intellectual function, apathy, depression, dysphoria, irritability, and hyperactivity. These occur particularly in patients on polytherapy with barbiturates. The profile of epileptic dysphoria, not uncommonly seen in outpatient clinics, may well be related to the prescription of polytherapy. It has been shown in controlled trials that rationalisation of polytherapy with an attempt to achieve monotherapy, particularly with carbamazepine, leads to significant improvements in rating scale scores of depression and anxiety (Thompson & Trimble 1982b), and it is customary these days to avoid polytherapy where possible, particularly in patients complaining of possible neuropsychiatric consequences.

Chronic dyskinesias are occasionally seen, and an acute dystonic reaction has been noted following carbamazepine.

Some other neuropharmacological treatments

The majority of the drugs so far described, with the exception of the anticonvulsants, find major use in the treatment of psychiatric illness, but, as emphasised, are used in some neurological conditions and quite frequently by neurologists as psychotropic agents. Within the range of drugs which alter neurotransmission some, such as the dopamine agonists, are used primarily by neurologists, but influence and may provoke psychopathology. Thus, L-dopa, originally introduced for the treatment of Parkinson's disease, was soon shown to provoke psychosis. The phenomenology of the psychosis has never been well described, and neither have the patients who are most susceptible to the development of the psychosis been identified. Generally, this may emerge as the effect of the L-dopa on the motor symptoms is declining, although this is not inevitably the case. The psychosis usually resembles an organic brain syndrome in the sense of provoking visual rather than auditory hallucinations, often of a complex nature. The psychosis may be associated with an accompanying paranoid disorder, and fluctuation of the mental state with nocturnal arousal may provide a clue to the diagnosis. In this setting, it is germane to try to control the psychosis, if it is troublesome, with a dopamine antagonist, although the danger of exacerbating the Parkinson's disease then emerges. Generally, drugs such as thioridazine with minimal Parkinsonian properties should be tried initially.

Other dopamine agonists that have been introduced, including bromocryptine, also provoke psychoses, the receptor agonists probably doing so with a greater frequency than L-dopa. The more recently introduced lisuride pumps may be particularly powerful with regard to their psychotogenic properties.

CONCLUSIONS

In this review, some overlapping areas of neuropsychopharmacology of interest to both psychiatrists and neurologists have been presented. The emphasis has been to demonstrate how drugs which influence neurotransmitter function within the brain are of value in the management of functional disorders, the use of functional here referring to its original physiological meaning. Many of the same drugs also find use in functional neurological conditions, and are readily and frequently prescribed by both psychiatrists and neurologists. The introduction of these medications has given us tools for the investigation of the relationship of the central nervous system to behaviour, but has also allowed the generation of hypotheses about, and further understanding of, the underlying neurochemical bases for psychopathology. Biological psychiatry is now firmly based in neurophysiology and neurochemistry, and its links with neurology are obvious. The fact that many of the neurotransmitters influenced by the drugs described are to be found in limbic system structures emphasises the latter's importance for psychiatry. The understanding of much psychopathology is firmly based on an understanding of the neurology, neurophysiology and neurochemistry of the limbic system.

REFERENCES

Albright P S, Burnham W I 1980 Development of a new pharmacological seizure model: effects of anticonvulsants on cortical and amygdala kindled seizures in the rat. Epilepsia 21: 681–689

Andrewes D G, Bullen J G, Tomlinson L, Elwes R D C, Reynolds E H 1986 A comparative study of the cognitive effects of phenytoin and carbamazepine in new referrals with epilepsy. Epilepsia 27: 128–134

Braestrup C, Nielson M 1982 Anxiety. Lancet ii: 1030–1034

Coppen A, Swade S, Wood K 1980. Lithium restores abnormal platelet 5-HT transport in patients with affective disorders. British Journal of Psychiatry 136: 235–238

Emrich H M, Dose M, von Zerssen D 1984 Action of sodium valproate and of oxcarbazepine in patients with affective disorders. In: Emrich H M et al (eds) Anticonvulsants in affective disorders. Excerpta Medica, Oxford, p 44–45

Langston J W, Irwin I, Langston E B, Foono L S 1984 Pargyline prevents MPTP induced Parkinsonism in primates. Science 225: 1480–1482

Linnoila M, Karoum F, Rosenthal N, Potter W Z 1983 ECT and lithium carbonate. Archives of General Psychiatry 40: 677–680

Mendlewitz J, Youdim M B H 1983 L-deprensil — a selective MAOB inhibitor in the treatment of depression: a double-blind evaluation. British Journal of Psychiatry 142: 508–511

Pisani F, Narbone M C, Fazio A et al 1984 Increased serum carbamazepine levels by Viloxazine in epileptic patients. Epilepsia 25: 482–485

Post R M, Uhde T W, Joffe R T, Roy-Byrne P P, Kellner C 1985 Anticonvulsant drugs in psychiatric illness: New treatment alternatives and theoretical implications. In: Trimble M R (ed) The psychopharmacology of epilepsy. John Wiley, Chichester

Post R M, Uhde T W 1986 Anticonvulsants in non-epileptic psychosis. In: Trimble M R, Bolwig T G (eds) Aspects of epilepsy and psychiatry. John Wiley, Chichester, p 177–212

Reynolds E H 1975 Chronic antiepileptic toxicity. A review. Epilepsia 16: 319–352

Robertson M M, Trimble M R 1987 Phenomenology of depression in epilepsy. Epilepsia 28: 364–372

Rodine E, Schmaltz S 1983 Folate levels in epileptic patients. In: Parsonage M et al (eds) Advances in epileptology: the 4th epilepsy international symposium. Raven Press, New York, p 143–153

Scatton B, Zivkovic B 1984 Neuroleptics and the limbic system. In: Trimble M R, Zarifian E (eds) Psychopharmacology of the limbic system. Oxford University Press, Oxford, p 174–197

Thompson P J, Trimble M R 1982a Non-MAOI antidepressant drugs and cognitive function: a review. Psychological Medicine 12: 539–548

Thompson P J, Trimble M R 1982b Anticonvulsant drugs and cognitive functions. Epilepsia 23: 531–544

Trimble M R 1981a Neuropsychiatry. John Wiley, Chichester

Trimble M R 1981b Hysteria and other non-epileptic convulsions. In: Reynolds E H, Trimble M R (eds) Epilepsy and psychiatry. Churchill Livingstone, Edinburgh, p 92–112

Trimble M R 1982 Functional disorders. British Medical Journal 285: 1768–1170

Trimble M R 1983 Benzodiazepines in epilepsy. In: Benzodiazepines divided. John Wiley, Chichester, p 277–289

Trimble M R 1986 Recent contributions of benzodiazepines to the management of epilepsy. Epilepsia 27: Suppl 1

Trimble M R 1988 Biological psychiatry. John Wiley, Chichester

Trimble M R, Corbett J 1980 Anticonvulsant drugs and cognitive abilities. In: Canger R, Angeleri F, Penry J K (eds) Advances in Epileptology: 11th International Epilepsy Symposium. Raven Press, New York, p 199–204

Trimble M R, Zarifian E 1984 The psychopharmacology of epilepsy. John Wiley, Chichester

Tyrer P 1976 Towards rational therapy with MAOI. British Journal of Psychiatry 128: 354–360

Waddington J L 1985 Further anomalies in the dopamine receptor supersensitivity hypothesis of tardive dyskinesia. Trends in Neurosciences 8: 200

22   *S. A. Whatley   M. J. Owen   R. M. Murray*

Neuropsychiatric disorders and the new genetics

There has been a revolution in molecular genetics during the last decade, and, as a result, medical genetics now occupies a central position in the 'new medicine' that is beginning to take shape. Knowledge about the genetic make-up of individuals is becoming important not only in the diagnosis of those already exhibiting disease, but also in the detection of those who may be liable to it. We can now sometimes tell by direct examination of DNA whether an abnormal gene is present or not. In other conditions the genetic status of a patient can be determined indirectly from the presence or absence of genetic markers known to be near the crucial gene. These techniques have, for example, greatly enhanced our understanding of the molecular pathology in disorders such as cystic fibrosis, the haemoglobinopathies and polycystic kidney disease (Weatherall 1985). Neurological disorders have been a major area of endeavour and these efforts have been amply rewarded for single gene disorders such as Duchenne muscular dystrophy and Huntington's chorea. Although psychiatric disorders are more complex in their aetiology than most neurological conditions, the expectation that molecular biology would contribute significantly to our understanding of psychiatric illness has already been rewarded for Alzheimer's disease and manic-depression. There are high hopes that these techniques will advance our knowledge of the genetic basis of other neuropsychiatric disorders as well as those associated with mental handicap in the near future. In this chapter we shall present some of the basic principles of molecular genetics, review some of the advances that have been made and describe some of the directions that future research into neuropsychiatric disorders may take.

THE GENOTYPE, THE ENVIRONMENT AND THE PHENOTYPE

In disorders where heredity is involved we must consider both the genotype and the phenotype as well as the relationship between them.

The human genome consists of some 100 000 genes strung along 23 pairs of chromosomes. The term genotype refers to the collection of genes inherited by an organism whose genetic individuality is due to differences in the form of the genes (termed alleles) occupying each site or locus. Genes consist of DNA which is made up of two chains of nucleotide bases wrapped around each other in the form of a double-helix. There are four bases in DNA; adenine (A), guanine (G), cytosine (C) and thymine (T), which can lie in any order along the sugar-phosphate backbone. The two chains are held together by hydrogen bonds between the bases. Because of their particular steric properties A always pairs with T and C with G. Genetic information is encoded by the sequence of bases: different base triplets code for different amino acids, the order of which determines the structure of protein molecules.

Genetic information is transported from the cell nucleus to the cytoplasm by a type of RNA known as *messenger RNA (mRNA)*. This is copied directly from one strand of the DNA. Each molecule of mRNA therefore contains bases in a sequence complementary to that found on the portion of the DNA molecule (gene) from which it was copied. The transfer of genetic information from the gene to mRNA is known as *transcription*. Once in the cytoplasm mRNA then acts as a template from which protein

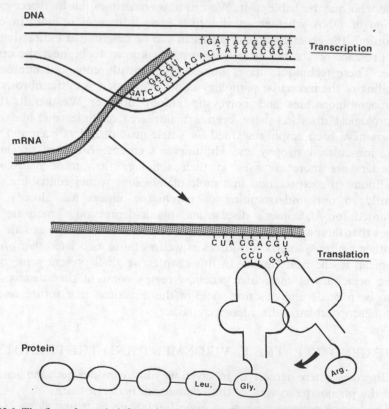

Fig. 22.1 The flow of genetic information in the cell. The linear information contained in the base sequence of DNA is converted to structural information by the process of transcription of DNA to mRNA followed by translation of mRNA into protein.

molecules are assembled. Genetic information is thus converted into either a structural protein or an enzyme. This is known as *translation* (see Fig. 22.1).

From the foregoing it is clear that understanding the molecular basis of the genetic contribution to a disease will lead to considerable insight into the biological mechanisms involved. In time this may result in biological therapies and ultimately perhaps even treatment aimed at reversing the genetic abnormality; manipulation of DNA has already been tried, although unsuccessfully, in an attempt to cure two patients terminally ill with thalassaemia.

The term phenotype refers to the recognisable characteristics of an individual. Originally the term was used to describe features such as height and hair colour. With the development of biological techniques we can now recognise characteristics that are more fundamental, such as blood group and products of metabolism. These are known as *endophenotypes* as opposed to *exophenotypes*.

Clearly there are many steps, and many endophenotypes, between the genotype and a complex exophenotype, such as the signs and symptoms of schizophrenia. Indeed, most phenotypes are not determined solely by the genotype but reflect an interaction between the genotype, or endophenotypes deriving from it, and the environment. The importance and the nature of environmental influence varies greatly between phenotypes. Nowhere is this more apparent than in psychiatry where the exophenotypes of interest (i.e. clinical disorders) can be influenced to different extents by environmental events ranging through all the different organisational levels from the molecular to the social.

Further complexity is added by the fact that different aetiologies, either genetic or environmental, may be present in individuals of identical diagnosis. In other words, apparently identical phenotypes may have heterogeneous bases. This has been shown particularly clearly in the case of the thalassaemias where 40 different structural changes in DNA cause the same clinical disorder of β-thalassaemia. Moreover, a clinical syndrome which, in some individuals, has a genetic basis may, in others, reflect only environmental factors. These latter cases are said to be *phenocopies*. Other individuals may possess a defective gene which is not expressed exophenotypically, in which case the gene is said to have a *penetrance* of less than 100%. Where penetrance is low environmental influences may be crucial in producing illness. Finally, it is theoretically possible for the environment to interact with the genotype in ways other than the additive fashion described above. For example, genes may determine sensitivity to specific environmental factors or even influence the degree of exposure to them (Kendler & Eaves 1986).

The identification of endophenotypes is important because this is likely to throw light upon pathological processes which, in turn, may have therapeutic implications. Indeed, in disorders with a complex genetic component, or those where the environmental determinants are more distinctive than the genetic, characterisation of endophenotypes is arguably more likely to be of therapeutic relevance than an understanding of the genotype. Moreover, in psychiatry, where precise definitions of categories of exophenotype is difficult and consequently there are interminable arguments about diagnostic concepts, the need for endophenotypic characterisation is especially pressing.

Both endo- and exophenotypes can be trait- or state-specific. Trait-specific phenotypes are present in those who are liable to develop the illness, whether or not signs or symptoms are present at the time of investigation. In contrast, state-specific phenotypes are the signs and symptoms themselves or phenomena present only in association with them. Trait-specific markers may be genotypic as well as phenotypic. Genotypic markers may consist of probes for the crucial allele itself or may label a gene which is close enough on the chromosome so as to be 'linked' to it. That is to say the linked gene is extremely unlikely to be separated from the disease gene during meiosis and therefore serves as a marker for it in studies of multiply affected families. Trait markers may therefore allow the pre- and postnatal identification of those at risk as well as the detection of carriers in recessive conditions.

Genetic diseases range from those due to single gene defects or gross chromosomal disorders to those which result from multiple (polygenic) factors. Thus Huntington's disease is due to a single dominantly inherited gene and Down's syndrome results from a gross chromosomal aneuploidy. However, the majority of pyschiatric illnesses are due to an as yet ill-defined balance between genetic and environmental factors. We therefore have to consider both complex as well as simple genetic models.

THE 'NEW GENETICS'

Whereas classical genetics derives inferences from an examination of the phenotype, recent advances in molecular biology have provided techniques to enable the progressive characterisation of genetic disorders more directly in terms of both genotypic and endophenotypic abnormality. The former, of course, refers to studies of DNA itself whereas the latter consists in the definition of alterations in its expression. We provide here a simple guide to the techniques of molecular biology. More technical discussions are found in Steel (1984a, 1984b) and Weatherall (1985).

The study of DNA

Since all the cells of an individual person have essentially the same genotype, DNA can be obtained and prepared quite easily from peripheral blood leucocytes. However, one of the daunting aspects of the study of this genetic material is its sheer size in molecular terms (about 10^8 base pairs of DNA per chromosome). A key development in modern molecular genetics has been the discovery of restriction enzymes (or restriction endonucleases), which act as chemical scissors to cut DNA, not at random, but where specific base sequences occur in the molecule. This results in fragments of easily manageable size (10^3–10^4 base pairs) and therefore enables genes to be handled more or less in isolation rather than as part of a single very long molecule.

The second major development has been the ability to purify specific pieces of DNA and then to use them to recognise corresponding sequences in the genome, i.e. use them as gene 'probes'. There are two main types of gene probe; those made from genomic DNA extracted and digested with restriction enzymes, and those made from complementary DNA (cDNA). cDNA is synthesised from mRNA by the action of an enzyme called reverse transcriptase. These genomic or cDNA pieces can be inserted into the genome of a bacterial plasmid or bacteriophage (again using restriction enzymes), which has ability to replicate freely within bacteria such as *Escherichia coli* and from which they can be recovered. The preparation is treated in such a way that only one DNA fragment is inserted into each bacterium.

If the collection of bacteria is then diluted and plated out, individual bacteria will give rise to bacterial colonies each containing many copies of the DNA fragment which was inserted into the founder. This process is known as 'molecular cloning' and can be considered as a process of biological purification and amplification of specific DNA fragments (see Fig. 22.2). The collection of bacterial colonies is termed a 'library', in which there is a certain probability that any given sequence from the starting DNA mixture will be represented. (It has been pointed out that while British molecular geneticists refer to 'libraries', their Californian and Swiss equivalents talk of 'pools' and 'banks' respectively.)

These technological advances are combined in one of the most fundamental techniques of molecular genetics which is called Southern mapping after its inventor Dr E. M. Southern. Firstly, genomic DNA is cut with a restriction enzyme. This produces a large number of different sized DNA fragments which can be separated according to their size by electrophoresis on an agarose gel. Because of the specificity of the enzyme, only a few particular fragment sizes will contain the gene of interest. In order to detect these fragments, the DNA has to be treated with alkali to denature it to single stranded DNA, i.e. the molecular equivalent of unzipping a zip fastener. The DNA is then transferred to a sheet of nitrocellulose by a blotting procedure. This results in a copy of the gel which retains the original arrangement of DNA fragments. The blot is then exposed to a gene 'probe' radioactively labelled for easy detection. *Gene probes* consist of many small identical pieces of single-stranded DNA. It is an essential property of single stranded DNA that it will 'hybridise', in other words combine to form a double strand, with another single strand composed of a complementary

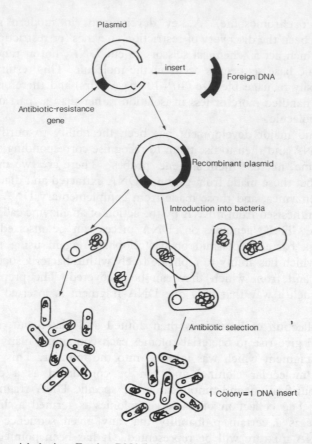

Fig. 22.2 Bacterial cloning. Foreign DNA is inserted into a bacterial plasmid which contains an antibiotic resistance gene. On infection, bacteria which contain plasmid are able to grow in the presence of antibiotics whereas those without plasmids cannot. Plating bacteria on antibiotic selection medium therefore produces bacterial colonies each of which is derived from a single bacterium and which contains a pure population of recombinant plasmid.

base sequence: A opposite T and G opposite C. Surplus DNA probe will not bind elsewhere and can be washed away. The position on the nitro-cellulose filter of the fragments containing the gene to be analysed can then be determined by autoradiography (see Fig. 22.3).

Any cloned piece of DNA from a DNA library can be labelled with a radioactive marker and used as a probe in a Southern blot. However, if these are unknown sequences probing genes of unknown function, how can they be useful?

We have seen that restriction enzymes cleave DNA at specific base sequences. However, the positions of these 'restriction sites' vary from one individual to another (except in identical twins). This variability is due to random base substitutions in the DNA sequences which may have no

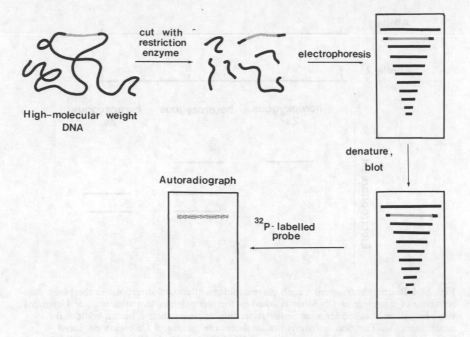

High–molecular weight DNA

cut with restriction enzyme

electrophoresis

denature, blot

Autoradiograph

^{32}P- labelled probe

Fig. 22.3 'Southern blot' analysis. Genomic DNA is cut with restriction enzyme and subjected to agarose gel electrophoresis. The gel is then blotted into nitrocellulose producing a replica which can be hybridised to a suitable radiolabelled probe. If the probe is complimentary to the shaded piece of DNA, the position of this particular fragment will show up on subsequent autoradiography.

phenotypic effect and which are inherited in a simple Mendelian fashion. Thus the fragments produced by digestion of one individual's DNA by a restriction enzyme will not be the same as those produced by digestion of DNA from someone else. Appropriate probes may be used to detect changes in length of specific restriction fragments and the resulting *restriction fragment length polymorphisms (RFLPs)* therefore provide a potentially large number of genetic markers since, using these, one can distinguish different alleles and follow their inheritance through families (Fig. 22.4). It is from this fortuitous phenomenon that much of the diagnostic usefulness of modern molecular genetics derives. DNA samples are obtained from members of a family in which several people are affected by a condition which is suspected to result from a single gene defect. The samples are then digested with a restriction enzyme and converted to a Southern blot. A selection of probes from a DNA library is then applied to the blots in the hope of finding a polymorphism in the family. A polymorphism is only discovered when the probe is homologous to DNA close to the restriction site in question.

The next step is to determine whether the polymorphism is 'linked' with the putative abnormal gene. This occurs when one variant of the poly-

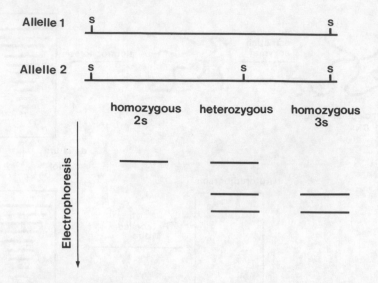

Fig. 22.4 Restriction fragment length polymorphisms. Random alterations in the base sequence of this piece of DNA has resulted in the formation of two alleles: allele 1 contains two recognition sites (S) for a particular restriction enzyme; allele 2 has an additional recognition site. The electrophoresis profile shows the pattern of fragments produced following digestion by restriction enzyme of DNA from individuals representing the three possible combinations of genotype. This fragment pattern can therefore be used to analyse the genotype of a particular individual at this locus.

morphism is reliably present in individuals suffering from the disease but not in those who are disease-free within the same family (Fig. 22.5). This implies that the gene which has been labelled by the probe is close to the pathological gene on the chromosome (and may be the same), and that recombination between the abnormal gene and the marker DNA sequence is therefore very rare. How close the two are linked is expressed as the recombinant fraction — the proportion of individuals in whom the abnormal gene and the marker are not inherited as a unit. Once a linked marker has been discovered it can be used to aid diagnosis, to discover carriers and for prenatal diagnosis.

Finding a suitable probe and determining which restriction enzymes to use is almost always a matter of trial and error. In spite of this, the technique has already given spectacular results in diseases such as Duchenne muscular dystrophy and Huntington's chorea. Moreover, once a linked marker has been found it is possible to find markers even more closely linked by using a series of overlapping fragments of DNA obtained from DNA libraries as probes. In this way it is possible to 'walk the genome' towards the abnormal gene itself.

Unknown gene probes selected randomly are not the only probes in use. A number of specific, known sequences are available which can be employed to probe genes of known function. These can be produced in

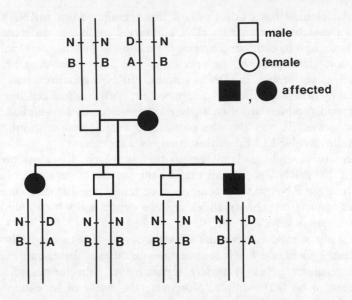

Fig. 22.5 Linkage analysis. The diagram represents a family in which there is an autosomal dominant genetic disease. The gene involved therefore can exist as disease (D) and normal (N) alleles. A polymorphic marker locus which has two alleles (A and B) is closely linked to the disease allele on the same chromosome. The chromosome carrying the defective gene also carries allele A of the marker gene. Consequently, allele A is co-inherited with the disease (unless genetic recombination occurs). If the position of the marker locus is known, this helps to define the position of the disease locus.

several ways (see Steel 1984a for a review), and their number is increasing rapidly. Every time a gene which may be important in a particular disorder is cloned, it is used to see whether an abnormality is present exclusively in those suffering from the illness in question by looking for RFLPs. For example, one might suspect that genes coding for various enzymes involved in the monoamine neurotransmitter systems might be of relevance to psychiatric disorders. This is known as the 'candidate gene strategy'. It has the advantage over linkage analysis that large pedigrees are not required. However, it is clearly something of a shot in the dark. Another approach is to use probes for genes whose position in the genome is roughly known when one suspects that the abnormal gene in question might be close to it. This is the 'favoured locus' strategy.

The study of mRNA

mRNA exist in the cell as a mixture of many different sequences, each destined to be translated into separate proteins. It can be extracted easily from brain tissue either postmortem or from neurosurgical specimens. As in the case DNA, the complexity of this mixture used to be a severe handicap to its analysis, but the ability to purify individual species using molecular cloning has made the task much easier. Thus mRNA's can be used as templates to construct cDNA libraries specific to different regions of the brain and to compare libraries from control and diseased individuals. Any clones that appear to be specific to the illness can then be used as candidate-gene probes in DNA studies. mRNA mixtures may also be analysed by first using them to direct protein synthesis in a cell-free system. The protein products are then analysed themselves by two-dimensional gel electrophoresis. It may thus be possible to characterise a specific protein or proteins involved in the pathogenesis of a disease.

There are several disadvantages to this approach, the most obvious of which is that mRNA populations reflect the pattern of gene expression only at the time the RNA was extracted. It is certainly possible that some mental illnesses result from abnormalities of gene expression which only occur at certain stages in development.

The study of mRNA has some advantages too. It is theoretically possible for a disease to have a fairly complex genomic basis, for example involving several regulator genes at widely separate loci, but for the disorder in expression to be fairly simple. Moreover, the study of an endophenotype allows the identification of state- as well as trait-markers which might well afford insight into the biological basis of a relapsing and remitting condition.

DISORDERS WITH A KNOWN PATTERN OF INHERITANCE

Not surprisingly, molecular genetics has made most progress in those single gene disorders where the mode of transmission was already known. These disorders, which act as Mendelian inherited recessive or dominant traits, may be divided into a) those where both inheritance pattern and locus are defined and b) those where the gene locus remains undefined.

Lesions where the locus is defined

Where the locus of a disease is well defined it is now a fairly simple task to characterise the molecular basis of the lesion. Gross chromosome deletions or point mutations may be characterised by Southern mapping and DNA sequencing respectively. Southern mapping techniques also enable us to detect carriers and to carry out prenatal diagnosis. Moreover, these techniques allow an estimation of the heterogeneity in the population of disease alleles. Both the disorders that we shall use to illustrate this type of condition are associated with mental deficiency.

Phenylketonuria

Phenylketonuria (PKU) is an autosomal recessive disorder resulting in a deficiency of the liver enzyme phenylalanine hydroxylase, which converts phenylalanine to tyrosine. This leads to a build-up of serum phenylalanine which causes severe mental retardation unless dietary restriction of this amino acid is implemented early in life. Subtle neuropsychological deficits, such as in conceptual and visuospatial skills, have also been described in some cases even after early treatment (Pennington et al 1985). (Apart from the classical infantile form, other hyperphenylalaninaemias have been described with higher residual phenylalanine hydroxylase levels. These may be due to biopterin and dihidropteridine reductase deficiencies as well as phenylalanine hydroxylase with altered kinetic properties.)

The availability of cloned DNA probes homologous to the gene for phenyl-alanine hydroxylase has now enabled not only prenatal diagnosis but also the identification of carriers in families with at least one affected child (Woo et al 1983, Daiger et al 1986). For their child to have PKU both parents must be heterozygous, i.e. each must carry one defective and one normal copy of the phenylalanine hydroxlase gene. It is therefore possible, by examining DNA from the affected child and both parents, to establish which restriction fragment is associated with the mutant gene, and then to go on to see whether it is present also in an unaffected child; if so the child is a carrier for PKU.

Although classical PKU appears to involve a single locus, it seems to be heterogeneous both at the genomic level and when analysed phenotypically in terms of mRNA levels for phenylalanine hydroxylase (DiLella et al 1985). However, recent work indicates that this heterogeneity is restricted. Analysis of the DNA base sequence of the phenylalanine gene of affected individuals showed that just two specific mutations account for as much as half of the cases of PKU in a North European sample of 33 families (DiLella et al 1987). This is surprising for such a common disease (1 per 10 000 live births), which would normally be expected to arise from a high rate of mutation in the gene involved. This raises the possibility that possession of one copy of the PKU allele actually confers a selective advan-tage to carriers. Such a 'balanced polymorphism' is seen in sickle cell disease where heterozygous carriers are protected against malaria. In addition, there are important implications for genetic screening, since we may expect to identify half of the carriers of PKU in this population by simple tests to identify these mutations, without the necessity for any family history.

Lesch-Nyhan syndrome

Lesch-Nyhan syndrome is an X-linked recessive disorder of purine meta-bolism caused by a deficiency of hypoxanthine-guanine phosphoribosyl-transferase (HPRT). This results in severe mental retardation, hyperactivity, aggression and bizarre self mutilation. The enzyme deficiency also results in hyperuricaemia, but this does not appear to be associated with the neuro-logical manifestations of the disease. One hypothesis is that neurones which employ purines as transmitters may be affected. In addition a recent report has linked self mutilation with supersensitivity to dopamine (Goldstein et al 1985).

DNA clones for human HPRT are available and have been used to study the molecular basis of the mutations in Lesch-Nyhan patients (Yang et al 1984). Interestingly, 7 out of 28 patients studied showed major alterations (deletions or insertions) of the HPRT locus. According to Haldane's principle, because there is strong selection pressure against the disease, new mutations must be arising frequently in order to maintain the syndrome in the population. In agreement with this, all 7 detectable changes were different, and 1 appeared to be a new mutation as assessed by DNA analysis of the family. Other patients appear to have more subtle gene alterations, such as point mutations, causing amino acid substitutions, several of which have been characterised (Wilson et al 1983).

Lesch-Nyhan syndrome can now be diagnosed prenatally from samples of chorionic villi (Gibbs et al 1984). Chorionic villus biopsy allows diagnosis to be made in the first trimester of pregnancy; much earlier than is possible when amniocentesis is used, and enough tissue can be obtained for DNA analysis. It therefore offers, together with recombinant DNA technology, a real hope for the early diagnosis of genetic conditions. However, in the case of Lesch-Nyhan syndrome, diagnosis can also be made upon the basis of low levels of HPRT, which is expressed in the foetus, and this is quicker and cheaper than using a DNA probe (Gibbs et al 1984). In many other conditions, however, this approach will not be possible and methods based upon recombinant DNA technology will have to be employed.

Complete delineation of the particular molecular defects in Lesch-Nyhan syndrome will require characterisation of the appropriate genomic sequences. This type of analysis has been applied most successfully to the study of the haemaglobinopathies (Weatherall & Clegg, 1982). Although these consist of alterations at a single locus (the globin gene cluster) they too exhibit a wide range of clinical severity and, even in cases of identical clinical presentation, there are a wide range of molecular lesions. Almost all the possible types of defects that could be imagined to disrupt the function of the globin genes (deletions, insertions, point mutations, frameshift mutations, abberant mRNA processing, abberant translation) have been described. It seems likely that Lesch-Nyhan syndrome will involve molecular pathologies that are just as varied.

Lesions where the locus is incompletely defined

For the genetic diagnosis of conditions in which the primary biochemical lesion is unknown and in which the affected gene cannot be identified, we must fall back upon the technique of linkage. This has long been employed in classical genetics to map chromosomes, but the discovery of RFLPs and their use as linkage markers has dramatically increased its potential applicability. Indeed, the availability of RFLPs should result in a comprehensive human gene map in the foreseeable future. One of the most spectacular successes so far using this approach has been the identification of a linked marker in Huntington's chorea.

Huntington's chorea

Huntington's chorea is an autosomal dominant disorder of complete penetrance. The children of an affected person therefore have a 50% chance of inheriting the defective gene, and individuals who do so will develop choreiform movement and progressive dementia usually between 35 and 45 years of age. There are about 6000 people with Huntington's chorea in Britain, and another 50 000 who are at risk of developing it. The disease has been described as 'genetically programmed cell death' for, while neurological development is normal, selective neuronal loss subsequently takes place, most notably in the basal ganglia. A wide range of psychiatric manifestations occur and may precede both chorea and dementia.

Although subjected to intensive research, the primary biochemical abnormality of the disease is not yet known. Gusella and his colleagues (1983) began a systematic search for linkage with the disease locus in two large affected American and Venezualan families. Unexpectedly, one of the first DNA probes tested (termed G8) revealed a DNA polymorphism which was linked to the disease locus at a distance of about 2 centimorgans (cm) (Gusella et al 1984). This distance represents a mere 2% chance of recombination occurring between the two loci at meiosis, but in physical terms represents 2 million base pairs (bp) of DNA.

Since the G8 marker is known to come from chromosome 4, the Huntington's gene must be there also. The progressive characterisation of the genome in the region of this locus should eventually lead to the precise identification of the genetic lesion. One approach is to try and find flanking markers, located on the opposite side of the Huntington's gene to the G8 marker. There is, however, a gap between the resolution obtainable by linkage analysis (down to about 0.5 cm), and the size of DNA which can be easily characterised by DNA technology (up to about 100 000 bp or 0.1 cm). A number of strategies have been proposed to try and bridge the gap between marker and disease loci, and it now remains to be seen which of these will succeed. It is possible that the occurrence of Huntington's patients with deletions in the chromosome may provide a way of reducing the DNA segment of interest to manageable size, as has occurred in the study of Duchenne muscular dystrophy (Monaco et al 1985, 1986).

While the determination of the basic defect in Huntington's disease is the ultimate goal of this research, it should be possible in the immediate future to use these findings as a presymptomatic test. The linked marker makes it possible to decide, long before the first manifestation of symptoms, if a person at risk carries the Huntington's gene. In various surveys at least half of all such individuals have indicated that, should a definitive test be available, they would wish to be tested. Unfortunately, the marker test is not applicable to everyone at risk. At least one living grandparent must be available, in order to tell whether the person at risk has inherited from the affected parent the gene that has come from the affected grandparent or the healthy grandparent. In one study this criterion was fulfilled for only 15% of individuals at risk (Harper 1986).

The marker test is likely to be more useful for prenatal diagnosis where the fetus now represents the third generation, although here the situation is more complex. The majority of fetuses at risk will be the offspring of potential carriers who may, or may not, subsequently develop the illness. Essentially the test will determine whether the fetus received a marker gene from its at-risk parent that came down from the healthy grandparent, in which case it should be unaffected, or whether the marker from the affected grandparent has been transmitted, in which case the conceptus has the same 50% risk as the parent. It should be emphasised that such knowledge provides no further information concerning risk in the parent. This may well be an advantage because many parents will not wish to know whether or not they will become affected.

It seems likely that, given the low rate of spontaneous mutation in Huntington's (Harper 1986), a combination of prenatal diagnosis and genetic counselling should ensure that the prevalence of this disorder will fall to a fraction of its present level. Nevertheless, the ability to test asymptomatic at-risk individuals for the presence of a lethal late onset gene is unique, and will undoubtedly lead to new ethical dilemmas. Not the least of these is the advisability of abortion for a fetus which, even if affected, could be expected to live quite healthily for 30–40 years before the onset of a dreadful illness. The most famous modern victim of Huntington's chorea was the folk singer Woodie Guthrie; America's musical heritage would have been considerably poorer without him!

CHROMOSOMAL DISORDERS

Down's syndrome

Both autosomal and sex-chromosome aneuploidy are known to cause neuropsychiatric disorders, and the techniques of molecular biology are being deployed in an effort to delineate the manner in which these defects are expressed. The most important of these is Down's syndrome which has an incidence of about 1 per 1000 live births. It results in mental retardation, as well as a wide variety of physiological defects (Crome & Sterne 1972). Monoclonal trisomy for the whole of chromosome 21 accounts for 95% of all cases. This is caused by non-disjunctive meiosis either in the mother or the father, the extra chromosome being twice as likely to be of maternal origin (Wagenbichler et al 1976). However, the phenotype arises from

trisomy for just a small part of the long arm of chromosome 21, and trans-
locations of this portion to a D or G group chromosome are known also to
cause the syndrome. In addition, abnormal mitosis in the zygote may result
in genetic mosaicism with a 21-trisomic cell clone.

Down's syndrome is known to cluster in certain families and it appears
that, in these cases, there may be a genetic tendency for non-disjunction.
The basis for this is not yet understood. It is not clear whether chromosome
21 is particularly affected or whether there is a general increase in non-
disjunctions with relatively few of those affecting chromosomes other than
21 being viable. Some evidence in support of the former explanation comes
from the finding of Anotonarakis et al (1985) that a particular DNA
haplotype on chromosome 21 is found more commonly in parents and their
children with Down's syndrome than in a control population. This raises
the possibility that chromosome 21 may contain a site which predisposes
to its non-disjunction. This observation is potentially of considerable
importance and need replication.

Whilst the chromosomal basis for the syndrome is known (LeJeune et
al 1959) the molecular mechanisms governing expression of the phenotype
are poorly understood. In contrast to defects like PKU, it is generally
accepted that Down's syndrome results from dosage-dependent transcription of qualitatively normal genetic material (Kurnit 1979). Evidence for
this explanation comes from the demonstration that both the activity and
synthesis of specific enzymes with structural loci in chromosome 21 are
dependent upon the number of gene copies present (Feaster et al 1977). In
addition, dosage-dependent transcription of chromosome 21 sequences has
been shown to occur in human fibroblast strains (Kurnit 1979). However,
the demonstration of changes in the activities of enzymes which do not map
to chromosome 21 (Hsai et al 1971) indicates that a combination of primary
and secondary effects is responsible for phenotypic expression of the
trisomy. Such interactions may have the effect of amplifying the original
effect of abnormal gene dosage, particularly when the primary change either
represents, or interacts directly with, regulatory elements within the cell.

The multigenetic nature of the defect in Down's syndrome makes linkage
mapping an inappropriate strategy to study its molecular pathology.
However, one approach to disorders involving the interaction of several
genetic systems is to study the proteins produced by translation of mRNA
in vitro. The complex mixtures which result can then be separated by two-
dimensional electrophoresis and those species that are differentially
expressed identified by their co-ordinates on the gel. Using these techniques, gene expression has been studied in fetal Down's syndrome brains.
It appears that, in the developing brain, the Down's syndrome phenotype
is associated with alterations in the levels of a limited number of mRNA
species. Moreover, these alterations are specific to the brain (Whatley et al
1984, Whatley, unpublished observations). One of these affected species of
mRNA codes for a protein which is associated specifically with synaptic

membranes and synaptic vesicles. The further characterisation of this and other altered products of gene expression may lead to a greater understanding of the phenotypic effects of trisomy 21 in the brain.

Fragile X syndrome

Fragile sites have been detected on various human chromosomes and are expressed as poorly-staining chromosomal 'stalks' when cells are cultured in a medium deficient in folate and thymidine. Unlike aneuploidies, they are inherited in a Mendelian fashion. Although autosomal fragile sites do not appear to be associated with any specific pathology, a fragile site on the X chromosome (Xq 27) results in a form of mental retardation (Sutherland 1979). In the past decade it has become apparent that this syndrome, which affects nearly one in 1000 males, is the second commonest form of mental retardation after Down's syndrome. Whilst males are primarily affected, a proportion of heterozygous females also appear to be below average in intelligence (Chudley et al 1983). The existence of a number of other X-linked conditions leading to moderate retardation (Fishburn et al 1983) indicates the importance of genes on the X chromosome in the development of normal cognitive function.

Although the cause of the fragile site is unknown, it appears that it does correspond to a genetic lesion, since the phenotypic expression of the disorder has been shown to be linked to coagulation factor IX in the Xq 26–27 region (Camerino et al 1983). This has again provided a means of prenatal diagnosis, which is fortunate since fragile sites can be difficult to detect, especially in carriers. However, the transmission of the syndrome through cytogenetically normal males and the existence of phenotypically normal males with fragile X sites makes interpretation of linkage data for carrier detection and prenatal diagnosis difficult in certain families. It is obvious that more information on the inheritance of fragile X syndrome and the role of secondary factors in its expression is needed before linkage analysis can be used in clinical practice. In addition, the molecular mechanisms responsible for the appearance of the fragile site are obscure. It is possible that an investigation of the mechanisms of DNA condensation at mitosis may provide clues to the processes involved.

DISORDERS WITH ILL-DEFINED PATTERNS OF INHERITANCE

In order to illustrate the possible application of the 'new genetics' to neuropsychiatric disorders with ill-defined patterns of inheritance we shall discuss five conditions: narcolepsy and Gilles de la Tourette's syndrome, which straddle the borders between neurology and psychiatry; Alzheimer's disease, where the pathology is partially characterised; schizophrenia and affective disorder, where the biochemical and neurological bases are obscure. Molecular biology is currently being employed to investigate several other conditions, for example autism and panic disorder. The interested reader is referred to a recent review by Gurling (1986).

In their separate ways, two uncommon disorders; Gilles de al Tourette's syndrome and narcolepsy have long intrigued behavioural neurologists and neuropsychiatrists, the latter including Sir Denis Hill. In recent years they have begun to attract the attention of geneticists, not only for themselves, but also because they show how genes may influence very specific behaviours and offer interesting models for the more common, and more complex, psychiatric disorders. Although the mode of inheritance remains unknown, there has been remarkable progress, particularly in narcolepsy.

Narcolepsy

Narcolepsy is characterised by attacks of unwanted sleep and periods of drowsiness during the day. Cataplexy, in which muscle tone is abruptly lost, also occurs in many cases. Other features are sleep paralysis and hypnagogic hallucinations, but cases showing all components of the tetrad are the exception rather than the rule. There are about 20 000 suffers in the UK. Because some of these symptoms simulate psychiatric illness, a psychogenic aetiology (e.g. due to guilt or anxiety) was at one time proposed, but this now seems unlikely although emotional factors are clearly involved, particularly in the precipitation of cataplectic episodes. The condition also appears to be associated with a range of psychiatric and psychosocial difficulties, such as depression, alcoholism and personality disorders (Krishnan et al 1984).

Various studies have estimated that between 10% and 50% of sufferers have an affected relative. The exact pattern of inheritance is not clear, but a single dominant mode is found in some families (Kessler et al 1974). Recent studies have indicated an astonishing association between HLA antigens and narcolepsy: almost all the affected individuals studied so far have been found to be positive for the HLA antigen DR2 (Langdon et al 1984, Juji et al 1984). Only 1–2% of patients with typical narcolepsy do not have the DR2 haplotype; this is the closest known association between a disease and an HLA type and gives strong support for a genetic and organic basis to the disease. Although DR2 is associated with narcolepsy, it does not itself cause the disease; indeed, it occurs in one in five of the British population. However, the strength of the association indicates that the disease susceptibility locus must be very close to, if not within, the DR2 locus for such tight linkage disequilibrium to exist in different ethnic groups. The disease allele could well be a subtle variant of the DR2 complex. One hypothesis is that possession of DR2 antigens renders an individual more susceptible to some environmental agent which precipitates an immunological reaction with resultant disorder (Parkes et al 1986).

The clinical diagnosis of narcolepsy can be difficult, and sleep-onset REM activity is not always found. The association between narcolepsy and DR2 may therefore be valuable in diagnosis and also in identifying at-risk family members. Moreover, further study of the DR2 locus in affected individuals using molecular genetic techniques should lead to considerable advances in understanding both the pathophysiology of the condition and the brain mechanisms involved in sleep.

Gilles de la Tourette's syndrome

Tourette's syndrome is a lifelong disorder characterised by multiple motor and vocal tics (Corbett et al 1969, Corbett & Turpin 1985). A familial aggregation has long been suspected and has now been confirmed (Pauls et al 1981). Price et al (1985) have further shown concordance rates of 53% and 8% in MZ and DZ pairs of twins respectively; when other milder tics are included, the MZ concordance rate rises to 77%. This is in line with other reports that there is a common aetiology between Tourette's syndrome and milder tics. Various models of transmission have been proposed. Currently the most favoured is that of Comings et al (1984), which postulates a major semidominant gene with 94% of homozygotes and 47% of heterozygotes manifesting multiple tics. The fact that multiply affected families are relatively common makes this disorder a well-suited candidate for molecular genetic analysis. The discovery of a patient and family with abnormalities on the long arm of chromosome 18 makes this a favoured locus for molecular genetic study (Donnai 1987). The gene for human myelin basic protein is located in this region and will be an obvious candidate for linkage studies.

Alzheimer's disease (AD)

AD is characterised by progressive failure in the performance of every day activities, memory defects and decline in general intellectual abilities, such as reasoning and conceptual thought. Finally, disorganisation of personality occurs, with deterioration in self care, blunting of affect and markedly impaired social adjustment. The major neuropathological findings are senile plaques and neurofibrillary tangles in the brain.

There is a significantly increased risk of primary dementing illness among the relatives of patients with AD (Heston 1981). The evidence for a genetic basis to the condition also includes a number of pedigrees in which the disease appears to be segregating as a Mendelian dominant with full penetrance (e.g. Nee et al 1983), suggesting that an abnormality at a single locus might be important in at least a proportion of cases. This makes AD a particularly appealing candidate for study of molecular genetic analysis. The degree of aetiological heterogeneity is difficult to determine because, in a disease that usually occurs late in life, unrelated illness may cause death in many predisposed relatives. Folstein and colleagues (Breitner & Folstein 1984) have argued that, if this is taken into account, in nearly 80% of cases the risk to first-degree relatives of developing AD appears close to 50%; that which would be expected on the basis of autosomal dominant transmission with full penetrance. Unfortunately, the late age of onset and short life-span of affected individuals mean that pedigrees with living affected members in more than one generation are rare. The collection of DNA from enough family members for linkage analysis therefore requires some investment of time, effort and resources. It appeared, however, that this effort would be likely to be worthwhile, since there were both genetic and biochemical clues to the aetiology of AD.

Associations between Down's syndrome and AD led to speculation that the genetic abnormality might be located on chromosome 21. People with Down's syndrome commonly develop the neuropathological stigmata of AD between the ages of 35 and 45, and the prevalence of Down's syndrome is reported to be increased among relatives of probands with AD (reviewed by Oliver & Holland 1986). In addition, both AD families and Down's syndrome are associated with an increased risk of leukaemias (Heston 1981). These shared phenomena suggested common pathophysiological mechanisms and hence a possible shared genetic susceptibility locus. Over the last few years, therefore, a considerable effort has been made to determine whether there is linkage between AD and gene markers for loci on chromosome 21. This has recently culminated in the demonstration of linkage by a large international group centred on Boston (St George-Hyslop et al 1987). These investigators used several polymorphic DNA markers spanning the long arm of chromosome 21 to study the inheritance of the disease in four large pedigrees. Linkage analysis revealed that two of these probes (designated D21 S/6 and D21 S1/D21 S11) are linked to the expression of AD with a highly significant probability.

AD, unlike many psychiatric illnesses, is associated with characteristic neuropathological findings. The molecular composition of neuritic plaques, neurofibrillary tangles and amyloid angiopathy has been the focus of much recent investigation. This work has converged strikingly upon the genetic studies. The first breakthrough was the isolation of the amyloid protein found in the core of senile plaques and in the blood vessels of those with AD. This protein, which is also abnormally deposited in Down's syndrome, has been termed A4 protein or B-Amyloid. Needless to say, a good deal of excitement was generated when the gene coding for A4 protein was located on chromosome 21 close to the linked probes of the Boston group (Tanzi et al 1987a). Furthermore, it has been claimed that a small portion of chromosome 21 containing the A4 gene is duplicated in AD so that, as in Down's syndrome, three copies are present (Delabar et al 1987).

Taken together, these data appeared to represent strong circumstantial evidence that the A4 gene is the locus of the defect causing AD. However, evidence that this is not the case has come from two studies in which the A4 locus was only weakly linked to the disease. Moreover, in several families, there was recombination between the A4 gene and AD (Van Broeckhoven et al 1987, Tanzi et al 1987b). These findings suggest that in these families the disease locus is on the neighbouring portion of chromosome 21.

Attempts are currently being made in a number of centres to locate the pathological gene more precisely and it should only be a matter of time before it is identified.

There is also interest in the question of genetic heterogeneity. All the families in which linkage to chromosome 21 has been demonstrated have suffered from illness of early onset. We do not yet know if familial cases with an older age of onset are carried by a defect at the same locus. Work is also underway to resolve this issue.

Schizophrenia

The genetic contribution to schizophrenia is the only clearly established aetiological factor and evidence comes from each of the three classic models of psychiatric genetic research; family, twin and adoption studies (Murray et al 1986). Although these data strongly indicate the existence of a gene, or genes, which predispose to schizophrenia, the disorder does not generally appear to segregate in an obvious Mendelian fashion within families. In addition, the shortfall below 100% concordance in monozygotic twins indicates that the genotype is not sufficient in all cases to explain the expression of the illness. This indicates that environmental mechanisms of aetiology exist. Three main models can be postulated which could either separately or in combination produce these data.

1. A single major gene of variable and incomplete penetrance requiring environmental factors for phenotypic expression in some, if not all, cases.

2. Heterogeneity: multiple aetiologies both genetic and environmental with sporadic as well as familial cases. This could produce the same pattern of results as 1. despite fully penetrant genes being present in some families.

3. The existence of polygenic/multifactorial causation. According to this hypothesis, disease in an individual reflects the presence of a number of genetic factors and the influence of environmental events.

The single gene model probably has the least support though a major gene against a polygenic background remains a distinct possibility (Murray et al 1986). The heterogeneity approach holds that there are sporadic as well as familial schizophrenias. While this is certainly the case, for example in temporal lobe epilepsy, proponents of the polygenic/multifactorial view hold that such *phenocopies* are rare.

It will be apparent to the reader that, within general medicine, the most impressive results have come from the application of molecular techniques to single gene disorders. However, a start has been made in dissecting out the genetic component of disorders such as diabetes and coronary artery disease which, like schizophrenia, are both more common and more complex in their aetiology. For example, while the genetic basis of coronary artery disease remains obscure, it appears that particular polymorphisms are associated with premature vascular disease and with abnormalities of lipid metabolism in certain families; thus, one can identify individuals at particular risk of coronary artery disease. In schizophrenia, as in coronary artery disease, several approaches should be made.

Specific genetic linkage markers will only be found if schizophrenia is caused to a large extent by a single gene or by a small number of genes having a major effect. According to the polygenic model, the schizophrenic genotype consists of a particular combination of a number of genes, each of which would be common in the general population. If schizophrenia has a heterogeneous aetiology, then we might expect to find a particular genetic marker or abnormality in only a subgroup of schizophrenics.

Up until now studies of genetic markers have been disappointing with initially optimistic reports not confirmed (McGuffin et al 1983). A great deal of effort was spent on seeking linkage with the HLA system, but the only consistent finding has been a weak association (not linkage) between paranoid schizophrenia and A9. The significance of this is quite uncertain (McGuffin & Sturt 1986). However, the advent of RFLP analysis has dramatically increased the chances of finding a linkage marker, or markers, in schizophrenia should single loci be important in its aetiology. As candidate genes are being cloned, so they are being tested (Gurling 1986). So far results have been negative, but these are very early days. In addition, the development of 'minisatellite' gene probes have further increased the power of the linkage method. These are small pieces of DNA homologous to a 10–15 bp 'core' sequence which is repeated a variable number of times at various points in the genome. The number of repeats is very highly variable between individuals, which means that the restriction fragments after endonuclease digestion are also extremely variable. However, large multiply affected families are required for the investigation of linkage with minisatellite markers and pedigrees of this sort are rare with schizophrenia though not with manic depressive psychosis.

Another approach is to look for abnormalities of gene expression in schizophrenia by the analysis of mRNA. Various lines of research can be envisaged. First, mRNA could be obtained postmortem from different regions of normal and schizophrenic brains. The most common gene products could then be compared by translating mRNA in vitro and then subjecting the resultant protein populations to two-dimensional gel electrophoresis. Changes in less common species could be determined by the differential screening of cDNA libraries from patients and controls. Of course, if changes were observed then one could not necessarily tell whether they were related causally to the illness or whether they were secondary to some other factor, for example, treatment with drugs. However, cDNA probes could be constructed from differentially expressed mRNA and employed as candidate genes in studies of multiply affected families.

A third strategy, complementary to the second, would be to study the effects of antipsychotic drugs upon gene expression either in the brains of experimental animals or in peripheral human lymphocytes. The reasoning behind this approach is that genes whose expression is altered by drug action may, a priori, be envisaged to play a part in the biological processes of the illness itself. In support of this line of enquiry, clinical studies suggest that the antipsychotic effects of neuroleptics in schizophrenia are delayed by between two and three weeks (Johnstone et al 1978, Garver et al 1984). Given that neurotransmitter receptor blockade takes place almost immediately, this suggests the mechanism of action may be mediated by other, longer-term, processes occurring secondarily to the action of the drug on receptors. It seems highly likely that such processes will involve changes in protein synthesis, in turn reflecting changes in mRNA production. If these changes could be identified then they would certainly increase present understanding of how antipsychotic drugs work, and also possibly throw some light upon the biological basis of the psychoses.

Affective disorder

Until a short time ago our understanding of affective disorder in genetic terms closely resembled that of schizophrenia, with the prospects of genetic analysis being just as uncertain, although large multiply affected families were known to be more common in bipolar disorder. Evidence for a single major locus was stronger in bipolar illness than for schizophrenia (O'Rourke & McGuffin 1983) but the question of whether its effect was dominantly or recessively inherited remained unclear. Family and twin studies suggested, however, that bipolar and unipolar disorders were genetically related (Smeraldi et al 1977).

Preliminary evidence with protein markers suggested that inheritance in a small proportion of families was consistent with X-linked transmission (Risch & Baron 1982), although this is excluded in most families by the observation of father-to-son transmission. Attempts to identify a major locus on the autosomes using protein markers, however, had not been successful.

Despite the lack of clues which have benefitted research into the molecular genetics of Alzheimer's Disease, much insight has been gained from the study of the old order Amish community of Pennsylvania. This population is highly suitable for genetic research as families are large, emigration rare and paternity relatively certain. Moreover, religious convictions proscribe the use of alcohol or drugs and thereby facilitate unambiguous diagnosis of affective disorder. Segregation analysis of data from the families of probands with bipolar disease provided evidence for a single genetic locus with autosomal dominant transmission. Initial studies of

RFLPs in a large Amish pedigree using a number of probes suggested that the disease might be linked to two markers on the short arm of chromosome 11, the insulin gene (INS) and the cellular oncogene Ha-ras-1 (HRAS 1). These two markers have recently been employed in a more extensive study of the same pedigree which has produced quite convincing evidence for linkage (Egeland et al 1987). This suggests that, in this pedigree at least, a dominant gene which confers a strong predisposition to bipolar affective disorder lies on the tip of the short arm of chromosome 11. It is of considerable interest that the structural gene for tyrosine hydroxylase is located upon the same segment of the chromosome. This enzyme catalyses an important step in the synthesis of the neurotransmitters dopamine and noradrenaline, which have both been implicated in the pathogenesis of mental illness.

However, the generality of findings in the Amish has already been called into question by two studies, one of American and the other of Icelandic pedigrees (Detera-Wadleigh et al 1987, Hodgkinson et al 1987), which managed to rule out linkage of INS and HRAS1 to bipolar affective disorder. This discrepancy is probably not due to methodological differences, but rather suggests that there is more than one gene responsible for the condition. Further support for genetic heterogeneity comes from recent studies showing linkage of bipolar illness to various X chromosome markers in Israeli and Belgian pedigrees (Baron et al 1987, Mendlewicz et al 1987). It seems likely, therefore, that there are at least three genes predisposing to bipolar disorder.

Several interesting issues arise from the demonstration of genetic heterogeneity. First, we must ask whether this is associated with clinical heterogeneity. There do not appear to have been gross clinical differences between the patients in the above studies. However, it may be possible to detect more subtle differences in symptoms or variations in course or outcome associated with different genetic defects. The second question, which may well turn out to be related to the first, concerns the degree of similarity between the various disturbances of brain function that result from the different genetic lesions. For example, each gene might code for a subunit of the same complex molecule, such as a receptor. Conversely, they might have quite different effects whose consequences eventually converge upon the final common pathway to affective disorder.

CONCLUSIONS

We have tried to give a brief introduction to some of the techniques of molecular genetics and to show their application in several conditions of relevance to psychiatrists and their potential in others. There have been many false dawns in biological psychiatry and still distressingly little is understood of the aetiology of major mental illness. In the past, psychiatric genetics has been accused of providing little more than a counsel of despair by pointing out the hereditary basis of many psychiatric conditions. In the light of the 'new genetics', the message is rather more hopeful.

As we have seen, it is now possible to analyse the structure of human genes directly and to determine the underlying molecular pathology of single gene disorders. This has been achieved in part for several conditions associated with mental handicap, such as phenylketonuria and Lesch-Nyhan syndrome. Molecular genetics has also provided us with a series of DNA markers scattered throughout the human genome to which we can link genes for disorders of completely unknown aetiology; thus, the gene for Huntington's chorea has been located to chromosome 4, and genes of major effect have been located on chromosome 21 for Alzheimer's disease and chromosome 11 for affective disorder.

One of the great advantages of the new techniques described in this chapter is that they will allow the investigation of many psychiatric and neurological illnesses at the level of the gene in the absence of detailed knowledge about brain mechanisms. The insights gained will then provide new starting points for the study of disturbed brain function. This, in turn, will lead to advances in understanding of neurological mechanisms. A firm bridge between neurology and psychiatry can be built only when students of the two disciplines share a common language; that of neurobiology.

REFERENCES

Antonarakis S E, Kittur S D, Metaxotou C, Watkins P C, Patel A S 1985 Analysis of DNA haplotypes suggests a genetic predisposition to trisomy 21 associated with DNA sequences on chromosome 21. Proceedings, National Academy of Sciences 82: 3360–3364

Baron M, Risch N, Hamburger R et al 1987 Genetic linkage between X-chromosome markers and bipolar affective illness. Nature 326: 289–292

Breitner J C S, Folstein M F 1984 Familial Alzheimer dementia: A prevalent disorder with specific clinical features. Psychological Medicine 14: 63–80

Camerino G, Mattei M G, Mattei J F, Jaye M, Mandel J L 1983 Close linkage of fragile X — mental retardation syndrome to haemophilia B and transmission through a normal male. Nature 306: 701–704

Chudley A E, Knoll J, Gerrard J W, Shepel L, McGahey E, Anderson J 1983 Fragile (X) X linked mental retardation 1: Relationship between age and intelligence and the frequency of expression of fragile (X) (q28). American Journal of Medical Genetics 14: 699–712

Comings D E, Comings B G, Devor E J, Cloninger C R 1984 Detection of major gene for Gilles de la Tourette's syndrome. American Journal of Human Genetics 36: 586–600

Corbett J A, Matthews A M, Connell P H, Shapiro D A 1969 Tics and Gilles de la Tourette's syndrome: A follow up study and critical review. British Journal of Psychiatry 115: 1229–1241

Corbett J A, Turpin G 1985 Tics and Tourette syndrome. In: Rutter M, Hersov L (eds) Child and adolescent psychiatry — modern approaches, 2nd edn. Blackwell Scientific Publications, Oxford, p 516–525

Crome L, Sterne J 1972 Pathology of mental retardation. Churchill Livingstone, Edinburgh

Daiger S P, Lidsky A S, Chakraborty R, Koch R, Guttler F, Woo S L C 1986
Polymorphic DNA haplotypes at the phenylalanine hydroxylase locus in prenatal
diagnosis of phenylketonuria. Lancet i: 229–231

Delabar J-M, Goldgaver D, Lamour Y et al 1987 B amyloid gene duplication in
Alzheimer's disease and karyotypically normal Down syndrome. Science 235: 1390–1392

Detera-Wadleigh S D, Berrettini W H, Goldin L R et al 1987 Close linkage of C-Harvey-
ras-1 and the insulin gene to affective disorder is ruled out in three North American
pedigrees. Nature 325: 806–808

DiLella A G, Hedley F D, Ray F, Murnick A, Woo S L C 1985 Detection of
phenylalanine hydroxylase messenger RNA in liver biopsy samples from patients with
phenylketonuria. Lancet i: 160–161

DiLella A G, Morvit J, Brayton K, Woo S L C 1987 An amino acid substitution involved
in phenylketonuria is in linkage disequilibrium with DNA haplotype 2. Nature
327: 333–336

Donnai D 1987 Gene location in Tourette syndrome. Lancet i: 627

Egeland J, Gerhard D S, Pauls D L et al 1987 Bipolar affective disorders linked to DNA
markers on chromosome 11. Nature 325: 783–787

Feaster J, Kwok L W, Epstein C J 1977 Dosage effects for superoxide dismutase 1 in
nucleated cells aneuploid for chromosome 21. American Journal of Human Genetics
29: 563–570

Fishburn J, Turner G, Daniel A, Brookwell R 1983 The diagnosis and frequency of X-
linked conditions in a cohort of moderately retarded males with affected brothers.
American Journal of Medical Genetics 14: 713–724

Garver D L, Zemlam F, Hirshowitz J, Hitzemann R, Mavoidis M L 1984 Dopamine and
non-dopamine psychosis. Psychopharmacology 84: 138–140

Gibbs D A, McFadyen I R, Crawfurd M et al 1984 First trimester diagnosis of Lesch-
Nyhan syndrome. Lancet ii: 1180–1183

Goldstein M, Anderson L T, Reuben R, Dancis J 1985 Self-mutilation in diagnosis of
Lesch-Nyhan disease is caused by dopaminergic denervation. Lancet i: 338–339

Gurling H M D 1986 Candidate genes and favoured loci: Strategies for molecular genetic
research into schizophrenia, manic depression, autism, alcoholism and Alzheimer's
disease. Psychiatric Developments 4: 289–309

Gusella J F, Wexler N S, Conneally P M et al 1983 A polymorphic DNA marker
genetically linked to Huntington's disease. Nature 306: 234–238

Gusella J F, Tanzi R E, Anderson M A et al 1984 DNA markers for nervous system
diseases. Science 225: 1320–1326

Harper P S 1986 Genetic studies of dementia with emphasis on Parkinson's disease and
Alzheimer's neuropathology. In: Mortimer J A, Shuman L M (eds) The epidemiology of
dementia. Oxford University Press, Oxford p 101–116

Heston L L 1981 Genetic studies of dementia with emphasis on Parkinson's disease and
Alzheimer's neuropathology. In: Mortimer J A, Shuman L M (eds) The epidemiology of
dementia. Oxford University Press, Oxford p 101–116

Hodgkinson S, Sherrington R, Gurling H M D et al 1987 Molecular genetic evidence for
heterogeneity in manic depression. Nature 325: 805–806

Hsai D Y, Justice P, Smith G F, Dowbon R M 1971 Down's syndrome: a critical review of
the biochemical and immunological data. Journal of Diseases of Children 12: 153–162

Johnstone E C, Crow T J, Frith C D, Carney M W P, Price J S 1978 Mechanism of the
antipsychotic effect in the treatment of acute schizphrenia. Lancet i: 848–851

Juji T, Satake M, Honda Y, Doi Y 1984 HLA antigens in Japanese patients with
narcolepsy. All the patients were DR2 positive. Tissue Antigens 24: 316–319

Kang J, Lamaire H-G, Unterbeck A et al 1987 The precursor of Alzheimer's disease
amyloid A4 protein resembles a cell surface receptor. Nature 325: 733–736

Kendler K S, Eaves L J 1986 Models for the joint effect of genotype and environment on
liability to psychiatric illness. American Journal of Psychiatry 143: 279–289

Kessler S, Guilleminault C, Dement W 1974 A family study of 50 REM narcoleptics. Acta
Neurologica Scandinavica 50: 503–512

Krishnan R R, Valow M R, Miller R P, Carwile S T 1984 Narcolepsy: Preliminary
retrospective study of psychiatric and psychosocial aspects. American Journal of
Psychiatry 141: 428–431

Kurnit D M 1979 Down's syndrome: Gene dosage at the transcriptional level in skin fibroblasts. Proceedings of the National Academy of Sciences USA 76: 2372–2375

Langdon N, Welsh K I, VanDam M, Vaughan R W, Parkes D 1984 Genetic markers in narcolepsy. Lancet ii: 1178–1180

LeJeune M, Gauttier M, Turpin R 1959 Etude des chromosomes somatiques de neuf enfants mongoliens. Comptes rendus hebdomadaires des seances de l'Academie des Sciences 248: 13260–1321

McGuffin P, Festenstein H, Murray R M 1983 A family study of HLA antigens and other genetic markers in schizophrenia. Psychological Medicine 13: 31–43

McGuffin P, Sturt E 1986 Genetic markers in schizophrenia. Human Heredity 36: 65–88

Mendlewicz J, Simon P, Sevy S et al 1987 Polymorphic DNA marker on X chromosome and manic depression. Lancet i: 1230–1232

Monaco A P, Bertelson C J, Middlesworth W et al 1985 Detection of deletions spanning the Duchenne muscular dystrophy locus using a tightly linked DNA segment. Nature 316: 842–845

Monaco A P, Neve R L, Colletti-Feeno C, Bertelson C J, Kurnitt D M, Kunkel L M 1986 Isolation of candidate cDNAs for portions of the Duchenne muscular dystrophy gene. Nature 323: 646–650

Murray R M, Reveley A M, McGuffin P 1986 Genetic vulnerability to schizophrenia. Psychiatric Clinics of North America 9: 3–16

Nee L E, Polinsky R J, Eldridge R, Weingartner H, Smallbert S, Ebert M 1983 A family with histologically confirmed Alzheimer's disease. Archives of Neurology 40: 203–208

O'Rourke D H, McGuffin P 1983 Genetic analysis of manic depressive illness. American Journal of Physical Anthropology 62: 51–59

Oliver C, Holland A J 1986 Down's syndrome and Alzheimer's disease: A review. Psychological Medicine 16: 307–322

Parkes J D, Langdon N, Lock C 1986 Narcolepsy and immunity. British Medical Journal 292: 359–360

Pauls D L, Cohen D J, Heimbuch R C, Detlor J, Kidd K K 1981 The familial pattern and transmission of Tourette syndrome and multiple tics. Archives of General Psychiatry 38: 1091–1093

Pennington B F, Van Doorninck W J, McCabe L L, McCabe E R B 1985 Neuropsychological defects in early treated phenylketonuric children. American Journal of Mental Deficiency 89: 467–474

Price R A, Kidd K K, Cohen D J, Pauls D L, Leckman J F 1985 A twin study of Tourette syndrome. Archives of General Psychiatry 42: 815–820

Risch N, Baron M 1982 X-linkage and genetic heterogeneity in bipolar-related major affective illness: Reanalysis of linkage data. American Journal of Human Genetics 46: 153–166

Smeraldi E, Negri F, Melica A M 1977 A genetic study of affective disorders. Acta Psychiatrica Scandinavica 56: 382–398

St George-Hyslop P H, Tanzi R E, Polinsky R J et al 1987 The genetic defect causing familial Alzheimer's disease maps on chromosome 21. Science 235: 885–890

Steel C M 1984a DNA in medicine: The tools. Part I. Lancet ii: 908–911

Steel C M 1984b DNA in medicine: The tools. Part II. Lancet ii: 966–968

Sutherland G R 1979 Hereditable fragile sites on human chromosomes II. Distribution, phenotypic effects and cytogenetics. Human Genetics 53: 136–148

Tanzi R E, Gusela J F, Watkins P C et al 1987a Amyloid B protein gene: cDNA, mRNA distribution and genetic linkage near the Alzheimer locus. Science 235: 880–884

Tanzi R E, St George-Hyslop P H, Haines J L et al 1987b The genetic defect in familial Alzheimer's disease is not tightly linked to the amyloid B protein gene. Nature 329: 156–157

Van Broeckhoven C, Gentle A M, Vanderberghe A et al 1987 Failure of familial Alzheimer's disease to segregate with the A4 amyloid gene in several European families. Nature 329: 153–156

Wagenbichler P, Killian W, Ritt A 1976 Origin of the extra chromosome no. 21 in Down's syndrome. Human Genetics 32: 13–16

Weatherall D J 1985 The new genetics and clinical practice, 2nd edn. Oxford, Oxford University Press

Weatherall D J, Clegg J B 1982 Thalassaemia revisited. Cell 29: 7–9

Whatley S A, Hall C, Davison A N, Lim L 1984 Alterations in the relative amounts of specific mRNA species in the developing human brain in Down's syndrome. Biochemical Journal 220: 179–187

Wilson J M, Young A B, Kelly W N 1983 Hypoxanthine–guanine phosphoribo-syltransferase deficiency: the molecular basis of the clinical syndromes. New England Journal of Medicine 309: 900–910

Woo S L C, Lidsky A S, Guttler F, Chandra T, Robson K J H 1983 Cloned human phenylalanine hydroxylase gene allows prenatal diagnosis and carrier detection of classical phenylketonuria. Nature 306: 151–155

Yang T P, Patel P I, Chinault A C et al 1984 Molecular evidence for new mutations at the hprt locus in Lesch-Nyhan patients. Nature 310: 412–414

Neurotransmitters in neuropsychiatry

INTRODUCTION

Since the early researches of Franz Gall, cortical localisation has proven to be a powerful strategy in the understanding of higher cerebral functions and their disturbance. This approach, which has utilised the correlation of clinical features with discrete areas of cortical damage found at autopsy, has been refined by the development of in vivo imaging techniques such as computerised cranial tomography and magnetic resonance imaging. This conceptual approach however has had its critics (for review see Meyer 1974). It might be argued that the discrete anatomical localisation of disordered function and the associated concept of disconnection syndromes (Geschwind 1965) have been particularly valuable in analysing the cortical dysfunction that arises from the discrete pathologies seen with tumours and cerebral infarcts. It may be less successful in understanding neuropsychiatric diseases, in which discrete neuropathological lesions are not readily discernible, such as schizophrenia and the affective disorders, or in degenerative conditions in which changes may be diffuse, such as Alzheimer's disease. An alternative approach to the interpretation of disturbances of higher cortical function in neuropsychiatric disease derives from the dramatic advances made in the pharmacology and biochemistry of brain transmitter systems. The discovery that drugs known to be effective in certain diseases, e.g. neuroleptics in schizophrenia, have precise and powerful effects at neurotransmitter specific synapses, and the changes in neurotransmitter markers in certain degenerative diseases, offer the possibility of correlation of cortical dysfunction with changes in defined neurotransmitter systems. This strategy presupposes that changes may occur in a diffuse neuronal network which can be uniquely defined by virtue of the neurotransmitter utilised (Drachman 1978). Although changes in such a network may subsume important structural loci, the changes cannot be readily defined in anatomical terms and it remains to be seen to what extent such an approach offers an advance on the classical localisation concept. A neurochemical approach has been successful in relation to the dopamine disturbances in schizophrenia and Parkinson's disease and has also been valuable in the investigation of Alzheimer's disease. The various techniques used in the study of neurotransmitters in neuropsychiatric disease will be discussed and then illustrated by reference to Parkinson's disease, Huntington's disease, Alzheimer's disease and schizophrenia.

METHODOLOGY

Important advances have followed from the discovery of drugs found to be effective in the treatment of neuropsychiatric disorders. Both neuroleptics and antidepressant drugs were found to be clinically valuable before their precise mechanism of action had been elucidated. For example, the development of radioligand binding techniques to quantitate receptor sites within brain tissue established the pharmacological action of neuroleptics long after their clinical application. They were found to be potent dopamine antagonists and the efficacy of drug action defined in terms of the average clinical dose bore a relationship to the K_d or affinity for the dopamine receptor (Snyder et al 1974). This established that the antipsychotic action of neuroleptics was related to dopamine antagonism and from this arose the 'dopamine hypothesis' of schizophrenia. This concept, i.e. that excess dopaminergic activity is the cause of the schizophrenic syndrome, has been more difficult to establish (see below) and may be inadequate to explain the heterogeneity of disease, but nevertheless it has been an important and fertile area of investigation (for review see Crow 1980). Animal studies have developed using drugs to increase dopaminergic transmission and the clinical syndrome of amphetamine psychosis has been interpreted in terms of excessive dopamine activity.

Alternatively, the clinical efficacy of drugs may confirm and extend studies obtained at postmortem. The classical example is the use of levodopa and dopamine agonists in the treatment of Parkinson's disease; these were developed directly from the observed neurochemical changes in Parkinson's disease (Ehringer & Hornykiewicz 1960) and confirmed the central role of the dopamine deficit in the pathophysiology of the disease. However, such clinical pharmacological studies can only provide indirect evidence of neurotransmitter disturbances; direct measurements require postmortem determinations of neurotransmitter markers or in vivo imaging.

Postmortem studies

The techniques of direct analysis of neurotransmitter systems in postmortem brain tissue have been a major source of data on neurotransmitter changes in neuropsychiatric disease. A stable chemical marker is necessary, which can be measured in the disease group and compared directly with a normal control population; an important assumption is that postmortem stability does not differ between the disease and control group. In general, this assumption appears to be valid although some exceptions have been reported, e.g. choline acetyltransferase (ChAT) activity (Davies & Terry

1981) and cholecystokinin (Perry et al 1981) in Alzheimer's disease (for review see Rossor 1986). The choice of chemical marker is dictated by adequate postmortem stability and the analysis of certain neurotransmitters is precluded in routine autopsy material, acetylcholine, for example, is relatively unstable in contrast to its biosynthetic marker enzyme ChAT. Neurotransmitter receptors are generally stable, as are neuropeptides. The unexpected stability of peptides within postmortem brain tissue has permitted detailed immunohistochemical studies in addition to classical regional dissection followed by radioimmunoassay. This does not provide such detailed quantitation but can provide anatomical precision of changes in defined peptidergic pathways. It has been possible to carry out such studies on some peptides such as substance P and enkephalin from routine autopsy material that has been formalin fixed (for review see Shiosaka & Tohyama 1986).

More recently, the collection of autopsy tissue within hours of death has demonstrated that the analysis of less stable systems is feasible. For example, functional polyribosomes can be extracted from tissue up to six hours postmortem, and can then be 'read' in cell-free protein synthesis systems (Marotta et al 1981, Gilbert et al 1981). Viable synaptosomes can also be isolated from rapid autopsy samples and this has proved useful in the measurement of amino acid uptake sites to determine the integrity of glutamate and GABA in Alzheimer's disease (Hardy et al 1987a, 1987b) Although many chemical markers are stable, there are many factors that need to be considered before differences between the groups can be attributed to the disease itself (for review see Rossor 1986). Two important factors which may be difficult to control for in studies of neuropsychiatric disease are the agonal state and antemortem drug treatment. It is common for patients with degenerative disease of the central nervous system to die from bronchopneumonia following a period of inanition. Prolonged terminal illness, particularly if associated with hypoxia, may profoundly affect the postmortem neurochemical profile. The best studied example is glutamic acid decarboxylase (GAD), in which a non-specific reduction in activity occurs following a prolonged terminal illness, although this does not appear to affect GABA concentration (Bowen et al 1976, Spokes et al 1979). Drug treatment is a major source of error in interpretation as it uncommon for patients with neuropsychiatric disease to remain entirely unmedicated. This is best illustrated by the postmortem studies in schizophrenia, since increased numbers of dopamine receptors can be seen following neuroleptic treatment and this may account for a major proportion of the increased D_2 receptor binding observed in the disease (Mackay et al 1982).

However, although one may allow for these non-specific influences, there remains a major problem of interpretation arising from the analysis of end-stage disease if there is a delay between clinical assessment and death. This is of particular importance in the analysis of conditions such as the affective disorders, in which the clinical syndrome may fluctuate considerably during life. The relationship of any observed change at death to a clinical symptom months or years earlier may be obscure, although this problem has been partially circumvented by the analysis of suicide victims. However, even with degenerative disease in which there may be a relatively stable neurological deficit, further problems of interpretation arise. It is always tempting to interpret the reduced concentration of a chemical marker as being due to neuronal loss or neuropil attrition, but this need not necessarily be so. Reductions in a chemical marker may arise from changes in the functional state of the neurone, such as an increased firing rate (Ekstrom 1978). Neurochemical changes may, therefore, reflect compensatory activity in surviving neurones, rather than direct involvement in the disease process. When the problem of interpreting concentrations of a chemical marker in the presence of tissue shrinkage is also considered, it is clear that postmortem data should be interpreted with considerable caution. However, these problems may, to some extent, be overcome by a combination of classical quantitative radioimmunoassay, immunohistochemistry and the recent techniques of specific messenger RNA determinations which may distinguish functional changes in turnover from neuronal loss (Shiosaka & Tohyama 1986). Since autopsy studies may provide very detailed information on a large variety of neurotransmitter systems, it is likely that it will remain a central technique to transmitter studies of neuropsychiatric disease. A variety of systems in many different brain areas can be studied and specific changes determined which can then direct in vivo imaging studies.

Cerebrospinal fluid

The analysis of neurotransmitters and associated chemical markers in cerebrospinal fluid (CSF) offers the opportunity of monitoring specific neurotransmitter systems during life. This has led to a plethora of reports of metabolic abnormalities in neuropsychiatric disease (for review see Wood 1980). However, many of these reports are conflicting and show considerable overlap with a control population; for example, inconsistent findings have been reported of changes in acetylcholinesterase, in Alzheimer's disease and monoamine levels in patients with depression (Davies 1979, Soininen et al 1984).

Similar problems to those encountered in autopsy studies occur with the interpretation of neurochemical changes in CSF. In addition, however, are problems specific to CSF. A major drawback is that the anatomical origin of the chemical marker cannot be known with certainty; there may, for example, be a major contribution from lumbar spinal cord when discrete nuclei within the forebrain are the structures of interest. In those circumstances where the marker is derived predominantly from brain, there is usually a rostrocaudal gradient in the CSF which needs to be taken into account by removing the same aliquots of lumbar CSF for biochemical determination. An additional problem with degenerative disease is that an increase in the volume of the ventricular system may produce low concentrations of a chemical marker due to a dilutional effect. Despite the disadvantages, the examination of CSF still provides one of the few means of access to the CNS in vivo. The reports of specific protein abnormalities in Alzheimer's disease (Wolozin et al 1986) await confirmation on a larger population, but may herald renewal of interest in CSF examination in neuropsychiatric disease.

In vivo imaging techniques

Positron emission tomography (PET) and single photon emission tomography (SPECT) have allowed detailed regional analysis of blood flow and metabolism in a variety of neuropsychiatric diseases. The development of specific labelled ligands has greatly enhanced the value of these techniques for transmitter studies and have already made a major impact on research. The development of pre- and postsynaptic markers of dopamine systems have focussed studies on Parkinson's disease and schizophrenia. The use of ^{11}F-fluorodopa (Garnett et al 1983) has demonstrated a unilateral deficit in hemi-Parkinson's disease but also differences between patients with and without on/off phenomena, suggesting that these patients develop a presynaptic storage abnormality (Leenders et al 1986). The recent development of the highly specific D_2 antagonist ^{14}C-raclopride is likely to prove valuable in PET studies of the dopamine system (Farde et al 1986).

Most studies of Alzheimer's disease have examined regional metabolism using oxygen-15 or (^{18}F) fluorodeoxyglucose. These demonstrate a predominantly parietotemporal hypometabolism (Frackowiak et al 1981). SPECT cannot provide the same quantitative analysis, but is more readily available and is reported to be of value in the diagnosis of Alzheimer's disease on the basis of regional metabolism. A SPECT study with iodine-123-labelled 3-quinuclidinyl-4-iodobenzilate (^{123}I-QNB) found a reduction in muscarinic acetylcholine receptor binding throughout the cortex (Holman et al 1985). The lack of reliable cholinergic markers for PET studies has proved a disappointment. Magnetic resonance imaging has made a dramatic impact on neuroradiology, providing high resolution of posterior fossa structures and changes in white matter. However, it is likely that the in vivo resonance spectra of the amino acid GABA and glutamate may be resolved, which would confer considerable benefit for the analysis of transmitter systems in neuropsychiatric disease.

MOVEMENT DISORDERS: PARKINSON'S DISEASE, PROGRESSIVE SUPRANUCLEAR PALSY AND HUNTINGTON'S DISEASE

Parkinson's disease remains the best example of a disorder of the central nervous system which can be described in terms of damage to a specific neurotransmitter system. The demonstration of reduced dopamine concentrations in the striatum at postmortem (Ehringer & Hornykiewicz 1960), and the subsequent development of levodopa and dopamine agonists in the treatment of Parkinson's disease, attest to the value of neurotransmitter analysis. The reduced concentrations of striatal dopamine reflects damage to the ascending nigrostriatal projection and it appears that substantial dopamine loss needs to occur before the clinical syndrome is apparent (for review see Marsden 1982). Since the original description of the dopamine deficit, many other neurotransmitters have been measured in the basal ganglia of patients dying with Parkinson's disease and a variety of deficits have been observed (for review see Marsden 1982, Hornykiewicz & Kish 1986). In addition to the ascending nigrostriatal projection, other ascending systems from the basal forebrain and brain stem are involved.

Adjacent to the substantia nigra, dopaminergic neurones in the ventral tegmental area project to the cerebral cortex and limbic areas and cortical concentrations of dopamine are reduced (Hornykiewicz & Kish 1986, Agid et al 1987). The noradrenergic locus coeruleus neurones, which project throughout the cerebral cortex from the pons, are also reduced in number with a concomitant reduction in cortical noradrenaline. Recently the loss of neurones from the nucleus basalis, an area originally shown to contain Lewy bodies, has been confirmed and shown to be associated with a reduction in ChAT activity in cerebral cortex (Ruberg et al 1982, Perry et al 1985). These changes in ascending systems are of particular interest in relation to the cognitive and affective disorders reported in Parkinson's disease. A small proportion of patients with Parkinson's disease develop dementia (Brown & Marsden 1984). In some this may be due to the coexistence of Alzheimer pathology (Quinn et al 1986), but even in patients with early untreated Parkinson's disease, subtle cognitive deficits in tests which are believed to be sensitive to frontal lobe function can be demonstrated (Lees & Smith 1983).

The neurotransmitter correlates of the frontal cognitive abnormalities have not been established with certainty, but both the cholinergic and cortical dopamine deficit have been implicated. The cognitive deficit arising from cholinergic blockade (Drachman 1977) and the comparison to Alzheimer's disease suggest that the nucleus basalis lesion is relevant and a correlation has been demonstrated between the severity of the cholinergic deficit and dementia in some patients (Ruberg et al 1982). However, it is probable that damage to the dopamine projection from the ventral tegmental area to frontal cortex is also important. Gotham et al (1986) have recently shown differences in performance on frontal lobe tasks in patients on and off treatment. Performance on some frontal lobe tasks improved on levodopa, while others deteriorated, suggesting that treatment itself may impair some cognitive functions while improving motor function. A number of reports have suggested that patients with Parkinson's disease are more likely to develop a depressive illness (Mindham 1970). The abnormalities of catecholamines and serotonin in frontal cortex and limbic structures may relate to the depressive symptomatology and patients rarely respond to levodopa (Mayeux et al 1986).

Of particular note is the large variety of peptides which have been found in lowered concentration (Agid et al 1986a). The significance of the peptide changes is unknown and it is possible that they represent secondary changes. The fact that Parkinsonian symptoms can be relieved by increasing dopaminergic transmission supports the central role of dopamine in the pathophysiology of the disease, although it is possible that some of the peptide changes, e.g. cholecystokinin which coexists with dopamine in the mesolimbic projection, may contribute to some of the clinical features. The description of many peptide changes which may be secondary functional changes illustrate the difficulties of interpretation with postmortem studies.

Progressive supranuclear palsy shares many of the clinical and biochemical features of Parkinson's disease. Cognitive impairment may be prominent and it was the early studies of Albert et al (1974) on the dementia in progressive supranuclear palsy that gave rise to the concept of subcortical dementia. They drew attention to the impaired memory, apathy, difficulty with handling learned skills and slowness of response, together with an absence of dyspraxia, agnosia and dysphasia, which contrasted with the abnormalities in Alzheimer's disease. The term subcortical dementia was proposed to reflect the prominent neuropathological abnormalities in subcortical structures with sparing of the cerebral cortex. At the same time, McHugh & Folstein (1975) reported on the 'subcortical' dementia of Huntington's disease, but the concept has remained controversial. The nomenclature has attracted criticism because subcortical structures are also affected in Alzheimer's disease and cortical changes can be observed in progressive supranuclear palsy and other subcortical dementias (D'Antona et al 1985, Agid et al 1986b). It has also been argued that a consistent clinical difference between cortical and subcortical dementia cannot be demonstrated (Mayeux et al 1983), although in this study the cortical and subcortical groups were poorly matched for severity. The term subcortical dementia is useful clinically to describe patients who are slow cognitively and who show a cluster of predominantly frontal lobe deficits and it has been recommended that the term frontosubcortical dementia replaces subcortical dementia (Freedman & Albert 1985). In keeping with the predominant frontal abnormalities in subcortical dementia is the frontal hypometabolism in progressive supranuclear palsy demonstrated on PET scan (D'Antona et al 1985). Some of the brain stem and basal forebrain nuclei which are damaged in progressive supranuclear palsy project to the frontal lobes and it is tempting to attribute the subcortical dementia to damage to these ascending systems. However, recent work by Agid et al (1986b) fails to confirm this and the neurotransmitter correlates remain to be determined.

HUNTINGTON'S DISEASE

In Huntington's disease there is a variable relationship between chorea, cognitive impairment and behavioural abnormalities. In some patients cognitive impairment and behavioural abnormalities, such as schizophreniform psychoses, may present early, whereas in others involuntary movement may be prominent with relative preservation of intellect until later on in the disease. The loss of striatal type II spiny projection neurones, which leads to a loss of GABA markers in striatum, has been known for more than a decade (Perry et al 1973, Bird & Iversen 1974). More recently a variety of peptide abnormalities have been reported (Emsom 1986) and using immunohistochemical techniques the loss of immunoreactivity can be attributed to coexistence of peptide and GABA within spiny projection neurones. Some of these cells contribute to a striatonigral projection and hence reductions in substance P and metenkephalin can also be observed in the substantia nigra (Emsom 1986). In contrast to most of the peptides studied is a marked increase in concentration of somatostatin and neuropeptide Y immunoreactivity. Aspiny somatostatin immunoreactive cells can be shown to be spared immunohistochemically and undoubtedly some of the increase is due to shrinkage of tissue compartments although additional alterations in turnover may be observed (Aronin et al 1983, Ferrante et al 1985). Intrastriatal quinolinic acid can cause damage to striatal neurones with sparing of the somatostatin neurones and reproduces many of the amino acid changes seen in the disease (Ellison et al 1987). By contrast to the intrinsic striatal cell damage, the substantia nigra pars compacta is preserved and, presumably due to shrinkage, the concentration of dopamine in striatum is increased (Spokes 1980). By comparison to the dyskinesia induced by levodopa it has been suggested that this imbalance between dopamine and GABA in the striatum is the cause of the involuntary movements. A similar argument has been proposed for the psychosis that may occur, since the nucleus accumbens is relatively preserved in Huntington's disease with an increased dopamine concentration (Spokes 1980) a pattern which shows similarities to that seen in schizophrenia (Mackay et al 1982).

ALZHEIMER'S DISEASE

The early autopsy studies of Alzheimer's disease demonstrated reduced ChAT activity in cerebral cortex and generated a great deal of optimism that a specific deficit in the cholinergic system might underlie the pathophysiology. However, it was already known that undercutting the cortex markedly reduced the ChAT activity and further animal studies elucidated the detailed anatomy of the cholinergic pathway to cerebral cortex. It was demonstrated that the majority of enzyme activity could be located to the nerve terminals of cell bodies in the basal forebrain (Mesulam et al 1983a, 1983b, 1984). This discrepancy between a cholinergic deficit related to damage to an ascending input and the observed intrinsic cortical neuro-pathology of Alzheimer's disease has weakened a central role for the cholinergic system. Nevertheless, the pharmacological evidence that the cholinergic system may be important in cognitive functioning has continued to attract attention and this will be considered first. The original obser-vation that the cholinergic biosynthetic marker enzyme ChAT is reduced in cerebral cortex has been confirmed in many subsequent studies (for review see Perry 1986a). The reduction is greatest in younger patients and in the temporal and parietal cortex, hippocampus and amygdala (Rossor et al 1982). Substantial reductions are also seen in the caudate, septal nuclei and the nucleus basalis but not all cholinergic neurones are involved and some areas, such as the putamen and red nucleus, are spared. The reduced ChAT activity in the basal forebrain is assumed to reflect damage to the cholinergic cell bodies (Whitehouse et al 1982) and immunohistochemical staining with ChAT antisera have confirmed the cholinergic cell loss (McGeer et al 1984). The muscarinic cholinergic receptors assayed using ^{3}H-QNB were initially found in normal concentrations, but later studies reported small reductions. This may have been resolved by the work of Mash et al (1985) who defined two subclasses of muscarinic receptor using agonist displacement. On the basis of animal studies the M_I receptor is believed to be postsynaptic and the M_2 receptor presynaptic and located on the cholinergic terminals. In Alzheimer's disease the M_I receptor number is normal but the M_2 binding is reduced by about 25%. This would be compatible with loss of the ascending cholinergic projection, but preser-vation of the postsynaptic site. The reduced QNB binding is similar to that reported in a preliminary in vivo SPECT study (Holman et al 1985).

Early studies of the nicotinic receptor using alpha bungarotoxin binding were inconsistent and may have been due to postmortem degradation. However, a reduction in receptor concentration has been reported (White-house et al 1986, Perry et al 1986). Some of the nicotinic receptors may be presynaptic and so may reflect the cholinergic cell loss. The muscarinic receptor data have implications for therapy since an intact postsynaptic receptor population would be necessary for successful cholinergic replace-ment. The role of the cholinergic projection in memory and learning and its potential significance in Alzheimer's disease has been recently reviewed by Collerton (1986). Both pharmacological antagonism of cholinergic recep-tors and lesion of either the septohippocampal or nucleus basalis-neocortex projections do cause impairment in a number of animal learning paradigms. The administration of scopolamine in man may also induce amnesia, although the disruption of attentional processes may be important (Drachman 1977). The functional abnormalities in lesioned animals and in man following pharmacological cholinergic blockade can be reversed with anticholinesterases, such as physostigmine. However, despite the reversi-bility of the functional deficit consequent upon cholinergic damage in the experimental situation cholinergic strategies in Alzheimer's disease have been unsuccessful when compared to the efficacy of levodopa in Parkinson's disease. Small, clinically insignificant improvement may be seen with physostigmine, but the benefit is often limited by side effects (Mohs et al 1985). A recent study reporting major improvement with the anticholinesterase tetrahydroaminoacridine (THA) is of considerable interest but remains to be confirmed (Summers et al 1986). One of the reasons for the failure of cholinergic replacement therapy may be the lack of specificity of the cholinergic deficit, since many other neurotransmitter abnormalities have now been reported.

Non-cholinergic ascending systems

The dopamine, noradrenaline and serotonin projections to the cerebral cortex share many of the characteristics of the cholinergic projection in that they all arise from the brain stem and project in a diffuse manner. Of these systems the dopamine appears to be relatively spared, in that dopamine concentrations within cerebral cortex are normal (Arai et al 1984). The nigrostriatal dopamine system may be affected in some patients with reduced striatal concentrations of dopamine and HVA (Arai et al 1984, Palmer & Bowen 1985). Some of these patients may have coincidental Lewy body disease (Quinn et al 1986). By contrast, concentrations of noradrenaline and serotonin are reduced in cerebral cortex together with changes in specific uptake systems in synaptosome preparations (Adolfsson et al 1979, Benton et al 1982, Arai et al 1984). Cell counts in the locus coeruleus, the origin of the noradrenergic projection and to a lesser extent in the raphe nucleus, the origin of the serotonin projection, are reduced (Bondaroff et al 1982, Curcio & Kemper 1984) and neurofibrillary tangle formation is also prominent within the raphe nucleus (Ishii 1966). The cognitive and behavioural effects of abnormalities in the noradrenergic and serotonin projection systems are less well established than for the cholinergic system. However, abnormalities of learning in animals are reported following lesions of the dorsal noradrenergic projection and it has been suggested that the serotonergic abnormality may contribute to aggressive behaviour.

Intrinsic cortical systems

Although consistent changes are found in the ascending projections to cerebral cortex, the associated biochemical changes provide no information about the abnormality of cortical neurones. The cell loss and formation of intraneuronal neurofibrillary tangles occur predominantly within the pyramidal neurones of layer three of the association cortices (Perry 1986a). The neurotransmitter associated with these neurones has not been established with certainty, but is likely to be the excitatory amino acid glutamate. Both glutamate concentration and receptor numbers are reduced in postmortem brain (Greenamyre et al 1985). However, a major problem with the determination of glutamate in postmortem brain is the inability to distinguish reliably between the metabolic and neurotransmitter pools. A more specific technique is to measure the high affinity glutamate uptake in synaptosomes obtained from rapid autopsy samples. Hardy et al (1987a) used D-aspartate as a stable analogue and demonstrated reduced uptake throughout the cerebral cortex in Alzheimer's disease. The other major cortical neurotransmitter is the inhibitory amino acid gamma aminobutyric acid (GABA) and a similar approach demonstrates reduced uptake (Hardy et al 1987b). The metabolic pool of GABA is smaller than for glutamate and so the reported reductions in GABA concentrations may be an adequate reflection of damage to GABA neurones (Rossor et al 1982, Ellison et al 1986).

One of the first abnormalities in an intrinsic cortical transmitter reported in Alzheimer's disease was a reduction in the concentration of somatostatin immunoreactivity (Davies et al 1980, Rossor et al 1980). Somatostatin is one of a number of neuropeptides which include cholecystokinin, vasoactive intestinal polypeptide (VIP) and neuropeptide Y, all of which are found in relatively high concentration in cerebral cortex and which serve as intrinsic cortical neurotransmitters (for review see Emson 1983). The other peptides of this group have been examined and cholecystokinin and vasoactive intestinal polypeptide are found in normal concentration (Rossor & Iversen 1986). The data on neuropeptide Y are conflicting with reports of both normal (Allen et al 1984, Dawbarn et al 1986) and reduced concentration (Beal et al 1986). Immunohistochemical studies in primates have demonstrated that these peptides coexist with GABA in cortical neurones (Hendry et al 1984) and so the observed reduction in somatostatin may be a further reflection of the involvement of GABA neurones. The reported normal concentrations of neuropeptide Y is notable. There is immunohistochemical evidence to suggest that, in human brain, peptide Y coexists with somatostatin in GABA neurones (Vincent et al 1982) and that one would expect there to be a commensurate loss of neuropeptide Y. The reported normal concentrations may therefore reflect differences in turnover between somatostatin and neuropeptide Y or that only a subset of the somatostatin neurones, i.e. those not containing neuropeptide Y, are involved. This serves to illustrate the considerable difficulties in the interpretation of postmortem data. Recently corticotropin releasing factor (CRF) has been reported to be reduced in the cerebral cortex in Alzheimer's disease (Bissette et al 1985, DeSouza et al 1986). Less is known about the contribution and possible coexistence of this peptide, although it may relate to cholinergic neurones. CRF receptors are increased in number suggesting an up regulation in response to the CRF deficit (DeSouza et al 1986). This provides important evidence of selective vulnerability since the ability to up regulate in response to a presynaptic deficit implies intact, fully functional, postsynaptic neurones.

Immunohistochemistry has made an important contribution towards correlating the biochemical changes observed at postmortem and the histological abnormalities. Most of the peptides can now be visualised in postmortem human brain and recently monoclonal antibodies against choline acetyltransferase have also become available for use on human material. Loss of choline acetyltransferase positive neurones from the nucleus basalis and of dopamine hyroxylase neurones from the locus coeruleus confirm damage to the ascending cholinergic and noradrenergic projections. Immunostaining within the cerebral cortex has been less consistent. Somatostatin immunoreactivity has been observed within neurones containing neurofibrillary tangles, but staining for the other neuropeptides VIP, cholecystokinin and neuropeptide Y was not seen (Roberts et al 1985). Immunostaining for both somatostatin and neuropeptide Y also visualise cells with profiles suggestive of degenerating neurones indicative of selective damage (Chan Palay et al 1985). In general, immunostaining of nerve terminals is more prominent in postmortem material than perikaryal staining. Thus the identification of the nerve terminals which contribute to senile plaques has been an easier task. It is apparent that there is no neurotransmitter selectivity but rather that nerve terminals adjacent to a nascent plaque are involved non-specifically. All neurotransmitter markers examined to date have been found within the dystrophic neurites of senile plaques (for review see Price et al 1986).

The effects on cognition of specific lesions of cortical neurotransmitter systems has only recently been investigated due to the lack of selective toxins or antagonists. However, abnormalities in learning paradigms have been reported both with glutamate antagonists (Morris et al 1986) and with cysteamine, which reduces brain somatostatin (Bakhit & Swerdlow 1986).

SCHIZOPHRENIA

The absence of prominent neuropathological abnormalities together with the induction of a schizophreniform psychosis by drugs such as amphetamine, has focussed attention on schizophrenia as a neuropsychiatric disease which would be explicable in terms of a chemical imbalance. The pendulum has swung from the initial view of Kraepelin that schizophrenia was due to structural brain pathology, to a psychoanalytic interpretation and back to a neuropathological basis (Brown et al 1986).

Much attention has focussed on the dopamine system. The induction of a schizophreniform illness by amphetamine, the similarity between stereotypy induced in animals by dopaminergic drugs and the behavioural abnormalities in schizophrenia, plus the demonstration that the efficacy of neuroleptics is proportional to their affinity for the dopamine receptor (Snyder et al 1974), all supported a central role of the dopamine system. However, although there is good evidence that neuroleptic drugs owe their efficacy to dopamine antagonism, this need not necessarily imply a primary dopaminergic excess in the disease. A parallel can be drawn to Parkinson's disease, in which anticholinergics are effective, but the disease is not due to a primary overactivity of the cholinergic system. Postmortem studies have demonstrated increase both in dopamine concentrations and an increase in the number of dopamine receptors (Bird et al, 1977, Owen et al 1978, Mackay et al 1982). One of the major problems, as discussed above, is that antemortem drug treatment may profoundly alter the post-mortem findings. However, Reynolds (1983) reported a neurochemical asymmetry with abnormally high concentrations of dopamine in the left amygdala in brains of schizophrenic patients. This observation suggests that the dopamine abnormality cannot be explained by drug effects alone, which would be expected to be symmetrical. It also accords with earlier clinical and electrophysiological observations of a left temporal abnormality in schizophrenia (Flor Henry & Koles 1980). Postmortem peptide measure-ments by Crow and colleagues also confirm abnormalities in temporal lobe studies with changes in VIP, cholecystokinin and somatostatin in the amyg-dala, hippocampus and temporal neocortex particularly in type 2 cases (Roberts et al 1983, Ferrier et al 1983). Recently abnormalities in meten-kephalin and substance P have also been reported and the abnormally high VIP concentrations in the amygdala confirmed (Bissette et al 1986, Tyrer & Mackay 1986).

There is general agreement that abnormalities in the dopamine system can be demonstrated postmortem and it is likely that some of the peptide changes are secondary and arise from known dopamine/peptidergic inter-action. However, the difficulty of relating the postmortem changes to clinical features and of excluding drug effects remains a major problem (Mackay et al 1982). The most promising area of research at present is the use of PET scanning to obtain quantitative measures of dopamine systems in vivo and an increase in dopamine receptors has been recently demon-strated in drug-naive patients (Wong et al 1986), but not confirmed (Farde et al 1987). It is likely that further studies of the pre- and postsynaptic dopamine systems will resolve the controversy.

CONCLUSION

The strategy of identifying biochemical changes in neuropsychiatric disease has been valuable. The rationale is identical to that of relating localised pathology to clinical features and has the same potential for errors of interpretation. The value of such an approach will ultimately depend upon whether disease processes affect the central nervous system by virtue of selective vulnerability based on neurotransmitter systems. In diseases such as Parkinson's disease and myasthenia gravis and probably schizophrenia this has proved to be a valuable approach. For Alzheimer's disease the evidence of selective vulnerability is far less. Nevertheless, it is possible that characteristic clinical features can be related to damage to defined neuro-transmitter systems within a wider spectrum of abnormalities. The ultimate advantage of such an approach is the efficacy with which drugs can manipu-late synaptic activity and offer strategies for therapeutic intervention.

REFERENCES

Adolfsson R, Gottfries C G, Roos B E, Winblad B 1979 Changes in the brain catecholamines in patients with dementia of Alzheimer type. British Journal of Psychiatry 135: 216–223

Agid Y, Taquet H, Cesselin F, Epelbaum J, Javoy-Agid F 1986a Neuropeptides and Parkinson's disease. In: Emsom, P C, Rossor M, Tohyama M (eds) Peptides and neurological disease. Progress in Brain Research 66: 107–116

Agid Y, Javoy-Agid F, Ruberb M et al 1986g Progressive supranuclear palsy: anatomoclinical and biochemical considerations in Parkinson's disease. In: Yahr M D, Bergmann K J (eds) Advances in Neurology 45: 191–206

Agid Y, Javoy-Agid F, Ruberb M 1987 Biochemistry of neurotransmitters in Parkinson's disease. In: Marsden C D, Fahn S (eds) Movement disorders 2. Butterworths, London, p 166–230

Albert M L, Feldman R G, Willis A L 1974 The 'subcortical dementia' of progressive supranuclear palsy. Journal of Neurology, Neurosurgery and Psychiatry 37: 121–130

Allen J M, Ferrier L N, Roberts G W, Cross A J, Adrian T E, Crow T J, Bloom S R 1984 Elevation of neuropeptide Y (NPY) in substantia innominata in Alzheimer's type dementia. Journal of the Neurological Sciences 64: 325–331

Arai H, Kosaka R, Iizuka T 1984 Changes of biogenic amines and their metabolites in postmortem brains from patients with Alzheimer-type dementia. Journal of Neurochemistry 43: 366–393

Aronin N, Cooper P E, Lorenz L J et al 1983 Somatostatin is increased in the basal ganglia in Huntington's disease Annals of Neurology 13: 519–526

Bakhit C, Swerdlow N 1986 Behavioural changes following cerebral injection of cysteamine in rats. Brain Research 365: 159–163

Beal M F, Mazureck M F, Chattha G et al 1986 Neuropeptide Y is reduced in cerebral cortex in Alzheimer's disease. Annals of Neurology 20: 282–288

Benton J S, Bowen D M, Allen S J et al 1982 Alzheimer's disease as a disorder of isodendritic core. Lancet i: 456

Bird E D, Iversen L L 1974 Huntington's chorea — post mortem measurement of glutamic acid decarboxylase, choline acetyltransferase and dopamine in basal ganglia. Brain 97: 457–472

Bird E D, Spokes E G, Barnes J, Mackay A V P, Iversen L L, Shepherd M 1977 Increased brain dopamine and reduced glutamic acid decarboxylase and choline acetyltransferase in schizophrenia and related psychoses. Lancet ii: 1157–1159

Bissette G, Reynolds G P, Kilts C D 1985 Corticotrophin-releasing factor-like immunoreactivity in senile dementia of the Alzheimer type. Journal of the American Medical Association 254: 3067–3069

Bissette G, Nemeroff C B, Mackay A V P 1986 Neuropeptides and schizophrenia. In: Emson P C, Rossor M N, Tohyama M (eds) Peptides and Neurological disease. Progress in Brain Research 66: 161–174

Bondareff W, Mountjoy C Q, Roth M 1982 Loss of neurons of origin of the adrenergic projection to cerebral cortex (nucleus locus coeruleus) in senile dementia. Neurology 32: 164–168

Bowen D M, Smith C B, White P & Davison A N 1976 Neurotransmitter-related enzymes and indices of hypoxia in senile dementia and other abiotrophies Brain 99: 459–496

Brown A G, Marsden C D 1984 How common is dementia in Parkinson's disease? Lancet ii: 1262–1265

Brown R, Coltes N, Corsellis J A N et al 1986 Postmortem evidence of structural brain changes in schizophrenia. Archives of General Psychiatry 43: 35–42

Chan Palay V, Long W, Allen Y S, Haesler V, Polak Y M 1985 Cortical neurones immunoreactive with antisera against neuropeptide Y are altered in Alzheimer-type dementia. Journal of Comparative Neurology 238: 340–400

Colleston D 1986 Cholinergic function and intellectual decline in Alzheimer's disease. Neuroscience 19: 1–28

Crow T J 1980 Molecular pathology of schizophrenia: more than one disease process? British Medical Journal 280: 66–68

Curcio C A, Kemper T 1984 Nucleus raphe dorsalis in dementia of the Alzheimer type: neurofibrillary changes and neuronal packing density. Journal of Neuropathology and Experimental Neurology 43: 359–368

D'Antona R, Baron J C, Samson Y et al 1985 Subcortical dementia: frontal cortex hypometabolism detected by positron tomography in patients with progressive supranuclear palsy. Brain 108: 785–799

Davies P 1979 Neurotransmitter related enzymes in senile dementia of the Alzheimer type. Brain Research 171: 319–327

Davies P, Terry R D 1981 Cortical somatostatin-like immunoreactivity in cases of Alzheimer's disease and senile dementia of the Alzheimer type. Neurobiology of Aging 2: 9–14

Davies P, Katzman R & Terry R D 1980 Reduced somatostatin-like immunoreactivity in cerebral cortex from cases of Alzheimer's disease and Alzheimer senile dementia. Nature 288: 279–280

Dawbarn D, Rossor M N, Mountjoy C Q, Roth M, Emsom P C 1986 Decreased somatostatin immunoreactivity but not neuropeptide Y immunoreactivity in cerebral cortex in senile demetia of Alzheimer type. Neuroscience Letters 70: 154–159

De Souza E B, Whitehouse P J, Kuhar M J, Price D L, Vale W W 1986 Reciprocal changes in corticotropin-releasing factor (CRF)-like immunoreactivity and CRF receptors in cerebral cortex of Alzheimer's disease.

Drachman D A 1977 Memory and cognitive function in man. Does the cholinergic system have a specified role? Neurology 27: 783–790

Drachman D A 1978 Central cholinergic systems and memory. In: M A Lipton, A Dimascio, K F Killan (eds) Psychopharmacology: a generation of progress. Raven Press, New York p 651–652

Ehringer R, Hornykiewicz O 1960 Verteilung von Noradrenalin und Dopamin (3-Hydroxytyramin) im Gehirn des Menschen und ihr Verhalten bei Erkrangungen des extrapyramidalen Systems. Klinische Wochenschrift 38: 1236–1239

Ekstrom J 1978 Acetylcholine synthesis and its dependency on nervous activity. Experientia 34: 1247–1251

Ellison D W, Beal M F, Mazurek M F Bird E D, Martin J B 1986 A study of aminoacid neurotransmitters in Alzheimer's disease. Annals of Neurology 20: 616–621

Ellison D W, Beal M F, Mazurek M F, Malloy J R, Bird E D, Martin J B 1987 Aminoacid neurotransmitter abnormalities in Huntington's disease and the quinolinic acid animal model of Huntington's disease. Brain 110: 1657–1673

Emson P C 1983 Chemical neuroanatomy. Raven Press, New York

Emson P C 1986 Neuropeptides and the pathology of Huntington's disease In: Emson P C, Rossor M N, Tohyama M (eds) Peptides and neurological disease. Progress in Brain Research 66: 91–105

Farde L, Hall H, Ehrine et al 1986 Quantitative analysis of D_2 dopamine receptor binding in the living human brain by PET. Science 231: 258–261

Farde L, Wiesel F-A, Hall H et al 1987 No D_2 receptor increase in PET study of schizophrenia. Archives of General Psychiatry 44: 671–672

Ferrante R J, Kowall N W, Beal M F, Richardson E P, Bird E D, Martin J B 1985 Selective sparing of a class of striatal neurons in Huntington's disease. Science 230: 561–563

Ferrier I N, Roberts G W, Crow T J et al 1983 Reduced cholecystokinin-like and somatostatin-like immunoreactivity in limbic lobe is associated with negative symptoms in schizophrenia. Life Sciences 33: 475–482

Flor Henry P, Koles Z J 1980 EEG studies in depression, mania and normals; evidence for partial shift of laterality in the affective psychoses. Advances in Biochemical Psychopharmacology 4: 21–43

Frackowiak R J S, Pozzilli C, Legg N J et al 1981 Regional cerebral oxygen supply and utilisation in dementia. Brain 104: 753–778

Freedman M, Albert M L 1985 Subcortical dementia. In: Freideriks J A M (ed) Handbook of clinical neurology: Neurobehavioural disorders. Elsevier, Amsterdam

Garnett E S, Firnau G, Nehmias C 1983 Dopamine visualised in the basal ganglia of living man. Nature 305:137–138

Geschwind N 1965 Disconnexion syndromes in animals and man. Brain 88: 237–294, 585–644

Gilbert J M, Brown B A, Strocchi P, Bird E D, Marotta C A 1981 The preparation of biologically active messenger RNA from human postmortem brain tissue. Journal of Neurochemistry 36: 976–984

Index

399